EXECUTIVE FUNCTIONING

AMERICAN ACADEMY OF CLINICAL NEUROPSYCHOLOGY

Series Editors

Susan McPherson, *Editor-in-Chief*
Ida Sue Baron
Richard Kaplan
Sandra Koffler
Greg Lamberty
Jerry Sweet

Volumes in the Series

Mild Cognitive Impairment and Dementia
Glenn E. Smith and Mark W. Bondi

Neuropsychology of Epilepsy and Epilepsy Surgery
Gregory P. Lee

The Business of Neuropsychology
Mark T. Barisa

Adult Learning Disabilities and ADHD
Robert L. Mapou

Board Certification in Clinical Neuropsychology
Kira E. Armstrong, Dean W. Beebe, Robin C. Hilsabeck,
Michael W. Kirkwood

Understanding Somatization in the Practice of Clinical Neuropsychology
Greg J. Lamberty

Mild Traumatic Brain Injury and Postconcussion Syndrome
Michael A. McCrea

Ethical Decision Making in Clinical Neuropsychology
Shane S. Bush

Intellectual Disability: Civil and Criminal Forensic Issues
Michael Chafetz

Executive Functioning: A Comprehensive Guide for Clinical Practice
Yana Suchy

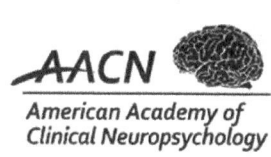

American Academy of
Clinical Neuropsychology

EXECUTIVE FUNCTIONING
A Comprehensive Guide for Clinical Practice

Yana Suchy

OXFORD WORKSHOP SERIES

OXFORD
UNIVERSITY PRESS

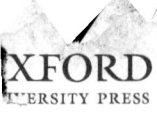

Oxford University Press is a department of the University of
Oxford. It furthers the University's objective of excellence in research,
scholarship, and education by publishing worldwide.

Oxford   New York
Auckland   Cape Town   Dar es Salaam   Hong Kong   Karachi
Kuala Lumpur   Madrid   Melbourne   Mexico City   Nairobi
New Delhi   Shanghai   Taipei   Toronto

With offices in
Argentina   Austria   Brazil   Chile   Czech Republic   France   Greece
Guatemala   Hungary   Italy   Japan   Poland   Portugal   Singapore
South Korea   Switzerland   Thailand   Turkey   Ukraine   Vietnam

Oxford is a registered trademark of Oxford University Press
in the UK and certain other countries.

Published in the United States of America by
Oxford University Press
198 Madison Avenue, New York, NY 10016

© Oxford University Press 2016

All rights reserved. No part of this publication may be reproduced, stored in
a retrieval system, or transmitted, in any form or by any means, without the prior
permission in writing of Oxford University Press, or as expressly permitted by law,
by license, or under terms agreed with the appropriate reproduction rights organization.
Inquiries concerning reproduction outside the scope of the above should be sent to the
Rights Department, Oxford University Press, at the address above.

You must not circulate this work in any other form
and you must impose this same condition on any acquirer.

Library of Congress Cataloging-in-Publication Data
Suchy, Yana, author.
Executive functioning : a comprehensive guide for clinical practice / Yana Suchy.
    pages cm. — (Oxford workshop series)
Includes bibliographical references and index.
ISBN 978–0–19–989032–3 (alk. paper)
1. Executive functions (Neuropsychology)   2. Neuropsychology.
3. Clinical neuropsychology.   I. Title.
QP405.S86 2016
612.8—dc23
2015026011

9 8 7 6 5 4 3 2 1
Printed in the United States of America
on acid-free paper

To my husband:
With gratitude for your patience, support, and love.

Contents

PART ONE **BEYOND THE FRONTAL LOBES** *1*

Chapter 1 Executive Functions as a Neurocognitive Construct *3*

PART TWO **EXECUTIVE SUBDOMAINS AND THE ASSOCIATED SYNDROMES** *13*

Chapter 2 Executive Cognitive Functions and the Dysexecutive Syndrome *15*

Chapter 3 Meta-tasking and the Disorganized Syndrome *37*

Chapter 4 Response Selection and the Disinhibited Syndrome *51*

Chapter 5 Initiation/Maintenance and the Apathetic Syndrome *69*

Chapter 6 Social Cognition and the Socially Inappropriate Syndrome *83*

PART THREE	CLINICAL ASSESSMENT OF EXECUTIVE FUNCTIONS *101*
Chapter 7	Gathering Background Information *103*
Chapter 8	Challenges in the Use of Standardized Tests of Executive Functions *121*
Chapter 9	Interpretive Considerations *145*
PART FOUR	EXECUTIVE DYSFUNCTION IN CLINICAL POPULATIONS *163*
Chapter 10	Neurodevelopmental Disorders *165*
Chapter 11	Neurodegenerative Disorders *177*
Chapter 12	Neuropsychiatric Disorders *191*
Chapter 13	Acquired Brain Insults and Medical Conditions *203*
	Appendix *215*
	References *221*
	Index *321*

EXECUTIVE FUNCTIONING

PART ONE

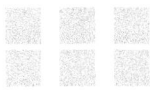

BEYOND THE FRONTAL LOBES

Just as one is unaware of the effortlessness of breathing until deprived of air, one is unaware of the covert neurocognitive underpinnings of self-control until deprived of them. Historically, many components of cognition did not come to the attention of researchers until their *absence* became evident among patients with brain injury. The first well-known description of the absence of executive control dates back to the mid-19th century: On September 13, 1848, Phineas Gage, a railroad foreman, sustained an injury in which a tamping iron penetrated his skull and severely damaged his frontal lobes. Although Gage survived the accident, his behavior and personality evidenced a profound change, from previously thoughtful and even-tempered to subsequently childish, socially inappropriate, and emotionally dysregulated (Macmillan, 2000). Despite the prominence of this case study, it would be nearly another 100 years before systematic linkages between the damage to the frontal lobes and changes in volition and personality would begin to be made; the emergence of these linkages then also precipitated the emergence of the terms *frontal lobe syndrome* and *frontal lobe functions* (Alford, 1943; Halstead, 1947, 1950; Ruffin, 1939; Russell, 1948; Wittenborn & Mettler, 1951).

The term *executive functions* initially emerged in parallel to the literature on frontal lobe functioning. The focus of these early writings was on "will and temperament" (Downey, 1923), "synthetic ability" (Dyrud & Donnelly, 1969), and "intention, initiation, and organization of motor output" (Guilford, 1972). The link between frontal lobe functions and executive functions did not begin to appear in the literature until the 1980s (Goldberg, Bilder, Hughes, & Antin, 1989; Grafman, 1988; Morice, 1986; Sandson & Albert, 1984; Stuss & Benson, 1987; Welsh & Pennington, 1988), undoubtedly in response to Muriel Lezak's second edition of *Neuropsychological Assessment* (1983), which in turn likely drew upon Alexander Luria's (1973) and Karl Pribram's (1973) conceptualizations. Interestingly, the early 1980s also brought the first explicit treatment of executive functions as an entity that is fundamentally different from other cognitive processes in that *it is not readily measurable*: It was described as less related to concrete performance scores (such as IQ) and more to "*how* a person goes about doing something or *whether* he does it at all" (Lezak, 1982, p. 282).

Since the 1980s, the terms frontal lobe functioning and executive functioning have been used virtually interchangeably, despite evidence that executive deficits sometimes do not appear in patients with frontal lobe injuries, and that injuries elsewhere in the brain sometimes lead to executive problems. This continued reliance on frontal lobes as a synonym for a functional domain perhaps stems from the fact that our understanding of what executive functioning actually means continues to be a source of debate and controversy. For this reason, Chapter 1 reviews some of the sources of this ongoing controversy and offers explanations for the conceptual and theoretical choices taken in writing this book.

I

Executive Functions as a Neurocognitive Construct

Evolutionary Purpose of Executive Functions

In order to facilitate the conceptual understanding of executive functioning (EF), let us consider EF's *overarching evolutionary purpose*. Specifically, EF confers an evolutionary advantage on an organism by providing the option to override prepotent responses, whether they be hardwired reflexes or overlearned habits. Put another way, EF frees an organism from the mandatory laws of stimulus-response. Unlike a moth that is necessarily drawn to a light source (even if it means burning its wings), and unlike newly hatched turtles that are always drawn to the sea (even if it means a virtual certainty of relentless predators), higher-order species can adapt their behavioral responses to newly emerging contingencies in their environment.

What is more, with increasing sophistication of the EF system (such as the EF capabilities found in humans), any response to a given stimulus can simultaneously consider not only immediately available contingencies or feedback from the environment, but also knowledge acquired in the past as well as long-term goals envisioned for the future. Long-term goals, in turn, can be achieved *only* if a person pursuing these goals is capable of consistently overriding responses that are *not* consistent with such goals. Thus, EF necessarily involves both moment-to-moment control over discrete cognitive, behavioral, and affective processes and more overarching control responsible for generation of future plans and organization of complex actions. In layperson's terms then, EF essentially is what allows us to make it from Point A to Point B, both on a daily basis and in the long run.

In determining how to more precisely define not only what EF does but also what it *is*, many issues need to be considered. These include (a) whether the construct should be defined based on function versus structure, (b) whether the construct is unitary versus multifaceted, (c) what type of research should serve as the basis for the definition (e.g., relying on healthy versus compromised populations, behavioral versus imaging research), (d) at what level of analysis one should consider relevant processes, and (e) whether only effortful versus both effortful and automatic processes should be included. Readers may vary in their assumptions about the "correct" answers to these questions. To avoid confusion or perhaps even frustration on the part of the readers, each of these issues is addressed in some detail later.

Issues to Consider

(1) Function Versus Structure. In clinical neuropsychology, it is customary to define neurocognitive domains in terms of their practical, or evolutionary, function. For example, we refer to vision, rather than occipital functions; to memory, rather than mesial temporal functions; and to language, rather than Broca's and Wernicke's functions. However, EF does not appear to follow this tradition. The reason for this divergence perhaps lies in the fact that visual abilities, memory abilities, or language abilities represent rather obvious and discrete cognitive processes; in other words, people are clearly aware of the nature of their difficulty if they cannot see, remember, or speak. Hence, labels for these cognitive processes are readily available in all languages.

In contrast, the ability to control one's behavior has *not* been traditionally associated with some obvious and discrete cognitive processes, nor has it been historically viewed as a product of the brain. Instead, behaviors that are thoughtful, planful, or otherwise carefully executed have typically been viewed as products of one's personality, temperament, or even moral fiber, with no clear notion of their reliance on the brain. Consequently, a "cognitive" label for behavioral control did not traditionally exist. By extension then, when the association between brain damage and the capacity to control one's behavior became evident, no single term that could describe the deficit existed. In fact, the description of Phineas Gage's "mental manifestations" by his physicians clearly reflects the lack of available labels: He was described as having lost "the balance between his intellectual faculties and animal propensities" (Harlow, 1868, p. 14).

Subsequent research on the association between brain damage and behavioral control continued to be plagued by a lack of appropriate labels, necessitating the reliance on the term *frontal lobe functions* (Alford, 1943; Halstead, 1947, 1950; Ruffin, 1939; Russell, 1948; Wittenborn & Mettler, 1951). This problem was not sufficiently remedied by the emergence of the term *executive functions*; this is perhaps because EF, unlike vision, memory, or speech, seems more like a man-made construct and less like a concrete, readily observable cognitive capacity. And constructs, unlike concrete entities, need to be defined lest they be misunderstood. Unfortunately, no universally accepted definition of EF exists. To make matters worse, available definitions span the gamut, ranging from laundry lists of terms that themselves need further defining, to definitions of convenience that are based on some salient characteristic of a single test (Suchy, 2009). For this reason, some theoreticians have begun to argue that the study of EF represents a futile exercise; the term itself, they argue, should be avoided, and neuropsychological research should focus on identifying cognitive processes that are subserved by the frontal lobes rather than attempting to understand a construct that is as elusive as it is ill-defined (Stuss & Alexander, 2000).

Although the frustration expressed by these authors is understandable (and understood), this text nevertheless holds the position that the difficulty with defining EF is not a sufficient reason to avoid the construct altogether. In fact, with continued advances in neuroimaging, clinical practice increasingly focuses less on lesion localization and more on characterization of patients' *functioning*. From that standpoint, the term frontal lobe functions not only is inconsistent with neuropsychological tradition but also is clinically and practically highly unsatisfying. As is evident from the title of this book, the term executive functioning is held in high regard here, and *it*, rather than frontal lobe functions, is consistently used throughout. By extension, then, *EF will not be defined here by the presumed neuroanatomical underpinnings but instead by its functional or evolutionary purpose.*

(2) Unitary Versus Multifaceted Conceptualization. To some researchers and clinicians, viewing EF as an umbrella for an entire suite of cognitive processes is a virtual truism, and the notion of unitary EF seems obsolete or perhaps even foolish (Parkin, 1998; Stuss & Alexander, 2000, 2008). Nevertheless, it needs to be acknowledged that the discussion about the possibility of unitary EF continues. Perhaps the most cited construct that is purported to undergird all of EF is the so-called central executive, which is presumed to coordinate lower-order processes that make up working memory (Baddeley & Della Sala, 1998; Baddeley, Chincotta, & Adlam, 2001; Baddeley, Della Sala, Roberts, Robbins, & Weiskrantz, 1998). Other unifying constructs that have been proposed include inhibitory control (Aron, Robbins, & Poldrack, 2014) and cognitive control (E. K. Miller & Cohen, 2001), and some factor analytic research does in fact offer support for such unitary explanations (Baddeley & Jarrold, 2007; Brydges, Fox, Reid, & Anderson, 2014; Brydges, Reid, Fox, & Anderson, 2012; Garon, Bryson, & Smith, 2008; Gligorović & Đurović, 2014; Wiebe et al., 2011).

By the same token, most studies that directly test the unitary versus multifaceted structure of EF find multiple components (Cona, Arcara, Amodio, Schiff, & Bisiacchi, 2013; Friedman et al., 2006; Lehto, 1996; Lerner & Lonigan, 2014; M. R. Miller, Giesbrecht, Müller, McInerney, & Kerns, 2012; Tsuchida & Fellows, 2013; Whitney, Arnett, Driver, & Budd, 2001). Unfortunately, there is imperfect agreement among researchers about what the different components mean, or even how many there are. For example, although a model of EF that has recently gained some prominence (Miyake, Friedman, Emerson, Witzki, & Howerter, 2000) proposes three main components (updating information in working memory, inhibiting prepotent responses, and switching between tasks), other researchers have identified as few as two (Adrover-Roig, Sesé, Barceló, & Palmer, 2012) and as many as six (Testa, Bennett, & Ponsford, 2012) factors.

Of note, as reviewed earlier, much of the research on determining the unitary versus multifaceted nature of EF relies on factor analysis, an approach that has been criticized. First, as discussed in more detail in Chapter 8, available measures of EF have many limitations, and many EF constructs are potentially not tapped by tests that are included in most factor analytic studies. Of course the results of any factor analysis are only as good as are the measures that are included in the study. Second, it is well recognized that factor analyses conducted with different populations will yield different factor structures (Delis, Jacobson, Bondi, Hamilton, & Salmon, 2003). For example, although immediate and delayed memory recall load on a single factor in healthy individuals, they become dissociated in patients characterized by rapid forgetting. Similarly, then, many EF tests may load on a single factor in a healthy population, but a different factor solution may emerge when patients with different types of EF dysfunction are examined.

Given the limitations of factor analysis, perhaps a more appropriate approach is to conceptually and theoretically consider various components of behavioral and cognitive control, as well as the different syndromes that are associated with EF dysfunction. Using such an approach, Norman and Shallice's (1986) model proposes two components, including the supervisory attentional system and contention scheduling, and Lezak, Howieson, and Loring's (2004) model proposes four components, including volition, planning, purposive action, and effective performance. Finally, although Stuss's (2011) work, by self-description, focuses on localization of function within the frontal lobes rather than EF modeling, he nevertheless describes five processes that could be viewed as components of EF; these are energization, monitoring, task setting, behavioral and emotional self-regulation, and meta-monitoring.

In sum, although there is not much agreement regarding the exact components of EF, there is considerable support for the construct of EF being multifaceted. For that reason, *the conceptualization of EF used in this book assumes that the construct is multifaceted. Given the problems with factor analytic approaches to modeling cognition, the model used in this book relies on conceptual and theoretical understanding of the construct based on the presentations of different clinical syndromes.*

(3) Healthy Versus Compromised Brain. In building a model of EF, one can either attempt to identify cognitive processes that contribute to healthy cognitive and behavioral control, or, conversely, examine which aspects of cognitive and behavioral control are lacking in different patient populations. These two approaches typically rely on different methodologies, and as such they tend to lead to somewhat different results. Specifically, much research with healthy populations tends to examine discrete control processes, such as inhibitory control (e.g., go/no-go tasks), working memory (e.g., span tasks), or the ability to switch (e.g., switching tasks). Such studies do in fact find individual differences in highly fine-grained aspects of cognition, enhancing our understanding of the constructs at hand. However, among patients who present with considerable EF dysfunction, such subtle distinctions may become obscured by larger problems with cognitive and behavioral regulation. For example, a patient may have difficulty even just attending to a given task, let alone present with differential strengths in inhibition versus switching; another patient may perseveratively respond by pressing the same button regardless of the task, precluding a meaningful interpretation of results. Still another patient may perform perfectly well on such tasks, yet exhibit difficulties staying organized in daily life, or may behave inappropriately with the examiner. Clearly, then, although certain discrete processes may evidence individual differences among healthy study participants and may offer valuable insights into the elemental components of larger EF constructs, such discrete processes may not always adequately capture *the gamut* of executive dysfunction present among patients.

Relatedly, in identifying neuroanatomical networks that subserve EF, one can rely on functional imaging research conducted with healthy participants, or one can examine which types of lesions lead to deficits in EF. On the one hand, functional imaging research enhances our understanding of complex neuroanatomical networks. On the other hand, such research often does not fully answer the question of which brain regions are truly *necessary* for certain functions. In fact, it is commonly found that although complex networks become activated by a given task in functional imaging paradigms, lesions in only some subset of such networks lead to disruption of function (Shamay-Tsoory, Tomer, Berger, & Aharon-Peretz, 2003; Shamay-Tsoory, Tomer, Goldsher, Berger, & Aharon-Peretz, 2004); such findings once again show that there is dissociation in conclusions based on research conducted with healthy versus impaired populations.

In sum, some questions can be answered with healthy populations, whereas others require that patient populations be examined; vice versa, some questions cannot be adequately addressed in patient populations, and examination of the healthy brain is necessary. For these reasons, *this text comprehensively integrates research from both healthy participants and patient populations, as well as behavioral research and research employing functional neuroimaging.*

(4) Levels of Analysis. Although, as discussed earlier, the study of healthy populations can facilitate a highly fine-grained understanding of discrete elemental processes that contribute to cognition, our understanding of such elemental processes is useful to us (as clinicians) only if it can be translated into a level of analysis that is clinically meaningful. Admittedly, some discrete details are sometimes unavoidably lost in such a translation. For example, even though certain disorders differentially target specific subregions of the hippocampus, clinical assessments of memory fail to differentiate among them; similarly, clinical assessments of EF generally fail to differentiate among, for example, the exact information-processing time points at which inhibition of a response breaks down. Such apparent clinical failures may frustrate behavioral and cognitive neuroscientists who devote their careers to careful and

painstaking mapping of subregions of the hippocampus or to manipulation of stimulus onset asynchronies in inhibition paradigms. However, until proved otherwise, the only information that is generally of clinical relevance in both examples is the fact that the patient cannot learn new information or inhibit responses.

That is not to say that no fractionation into subdomains and elemental processes should be attempted. In fact, clinically relevant subcomponents of memory are routinely examined (e.g., immediate vs. delayed recall, delayed recall vs. delayed recognition) because they offer better insight into a patient's daily functioning while also affording some degree of diagnostic specificity. Similarly, differentiating between perseverative responding due to a failure to inhibit versus a failure to register corrective feedback can, and should, be accomplished in a clinical assessment of EF. Importantly, it is the fine-grained insights into cognitive processing that allow clinical neuropsychologist to identify those processes that warrant more fine-grained assessment, as well as to have a better conceptual grasp of component processes that contribute to test performance.

Consistent with the preceding examples, *this text conceptualizes EF at a level of analysis that integrates what is known about brain-behavior relationships with what is understood about neurobehavioral manifestations of neurological disorders, while also considering what is practical and realistic from functional and diagnostic standpoints.* To that end, EF is divided into *subdomains* that correspond to major clinical syndromes, with each subdomain further divided into *elemental processes* that facilitate conceptualization of patients' difficulties and generation of rehabilitation or compensation strategies.

(5) *Effortful Versus Automatic Processes.* Executive functioning has traditionally been described as effortful by definition (Shallice, 1990; Suchy, 2009). It has been said that EF is employed only in situations that are novel, as opposed to situations in which automatic or overlearned responses suffice (Lezak, Howieson, Bigler, & Tranel, 2013; Shallice, 1990). In the same vein, tests presumed to assess EF are typically effortful and novel by design, and require a great deal of cognitive focus.

Although this conceptualization offers a nice way of delineating EF boundaries and differentiating EF from other cognitive processes, it is unfortunately fraught with paradoxical assumptions that may have contributed to the general dissatisfaction with the construct itself, as well as the frustration with EF assessment instruments. Specifically, by insisting that EF is purely effortful, we implicitly reject any possibility that it may possess a mechanism that is responsible for turning the effortful processing on. In other words, according to the prevailing conceptualization, while a person is engaged in automatic behaviors, EF is presumably turned off; the logical consequence of this is that some other (non-EF) process must be responsible for turning EF on. Despite these widely held assumptions, we consistently describe patients who fail to abort automatic actions or fail to appropriately engage effortful processing as executively impaired or, in the clinical vernacular, as "frontal." Similarly, we frequently comment that the limitation of clinical assessment of EF lies in the fact that clinical situations are "structured." This means that we, the clinicians, are responsible for telling our patients to *turn their EF on*, yet if the mechanism that turns EF on is not executive, then the structure of the assessment setting would not present a problem for the assessment of EF.

To address these inherent inconsistencies, the EF conceptualization employed in this text assumes that *whereas some EF processes require a great deal of top-down control and effort, certain bottom-up automatic processes are also necessary so as to appropriately trigger controlled processes as needed.*

Definition and Model Used in This Book

To summarize what has been detailed thus far, this book makes the following assumptions: (1) EF is defined based on what functions contribute to its evolutionary purpose rather than on their presumed neuroanatomical underpinnings, (2) EF is a multifaceted construct, (3) to arrive at a comprehensive definition of EF, an integration of what is known both about healthy EF functioning and about EF dysfunction is necessary, (4) a model of EF that is intended for use in clinical practice must adhere to the level of analysis that is clinically meaningful, practical, and realistic, and (5) although some EF processes require a great deal of top-down control and effort, certain bottom-up automatic processes are necessary so as to appropriately trigger effortful processing as needed.

Given these assumptions, EF is defined for the purpose of this book as *an umbrella term that subsumes a set of higher-order top-down neurocognitive processes involved in planning, selection, and execution of actions that are purposeful and adaptive, goal-directed and future-oriented, and socially informed* (Cummings & Miller, 2007; Gazzaley, D'Esposito, Miller, & Cummings, 2007; Lezak et al., 2013), *and that are aided by a set of lower-order, automatic, bottom-up processes that serve to trigger top-down processing as needed or appropriate.*

Chapters 2 through 6 offer a detailed description of five subdomains of EF, as well as multiple elemental processes that contribute to each subdomain. Decisions about how finely to fractionate EF, on the one hand, and how densely to populate each subdomain with elemental processes, on the other, were based on what is known about typical patient presentations, as well as which elemental processes were deemed most key in contributing to clinical syndromes.

PART TWO

EXECUTIVE SUBDOMAINS AND THE ASSOCIATED SYNDROMES

This part of the book offers a conceptual analysis of the construct of executive functioning (EF), breaking it down into five subdomains (and the five associated syndromes that result from specific EF deficiencies). These are (a) the executive cognitive functions (dysexecutive syndrome), (b) meta-tasking (disorganized syndrome), (c) response selection (disinhibited syndrome), (d) initiation/maintenance (apathetic syndrome), and (e) social cognition (inappropriate syndrome).

For each subdomain, the construct is explained using concrete, everyday examples. When relevant, other related constructs are reviewed so as to further sharpen the reader's understanding of the broader literature. To maximize the clinical utility of the conceptual discussion of each subdomain, the neuroanatomical underpinnings of each subdomain and its elemental processes are reviewed, and the typical clinical presentations of each associated syndrome are described (including the typical performance on common measures of EF). Each chapter closes with an overview of typical etiologies of a given syndrome.

In reading these chapters, the reader should keep in mind that "pure" instantiations of these syndromes are relatively rare, as many patients present with some combination of several syndromes at the same time. Thus, the apparently discrete boundaries between syndromes are somewhat artificial; nevertheless, the hope is that this focused presentation will help sharpen the reader's conceptual understanding of each syndrome (and its neurocognitive underpinnings).

2

Executive Cognitive Functions and the Dysexecutive Syndrome

Defining the Construct

Although the term *executive cognitive functions* (ECFs), as opposed to *executive functions*, has been previously used by some authors (Amanzio et al., 2013; Blume, Marlatt, & Schmaling, 2000; S. W. Brown, Collier, & Night, 2013; Cicerone, Levin, Malec, Stuss, & Whyte, 2006; Fling et al., 2013; Grigsby, Kaye, Baxter, Shetterly, & Hamman, 1998; Haug, Havnen, Hansen, Bless, & Kvale, 2013; Marshall, Hendrickson, Kaufer, Ivanco, & Bohnen, 2006; Royall & Mahurin, 1996), it is not firmly established within the nomenclature of clinical neuropsychology and hence requires a definition. The term executive cognitive functions refers to a set of higher-order cognitive processes that allow one to engage in *reasoning, problem-solving, planning,* and *mental organization*. There are two important conceptual points to keep in mind when reading this chapter:

First, note that reasoning, problem-solving, planning, and mental organization represent entities that are truly "cognitive" or "mental." In other words, although ECFs set the stage for subsequent behaviors, they do not in and of themselves guarantee that a certain behavioral outcome will occur. For example, generating well-thought-out plans does not guarantee that those plans will eventually be executed because other processes, such as the abilities to initiate and sustain behavioral output, also play a role (Eslinger & Damasio,

1985; Goldstein, Bernard, Fenwick, & Burgess, 1993; Metzler & Parkin, 2000; Shallice & Burgess, 1991a). By the same token, an inability to generate a plan does not necessarily always mean that behavior will be ineffectual or disorganized because prior procedural learning or a plan generated by another individual may carry a person through the day without readily apparent glitches (Allain et al., 2005). Thus, there is some disconnect between the ECFs and behavioral outcomes.

Second, although it is tempting to consider reasoning, problem-solving, planning, and mental organization as neurocognitive components of ECFs, this chapter will argue that they are actually better thought of as the *products* of ECFs. This is because plans, reasoned solutions to problems, and organizational frameworks are all produced by a coordinated set of other, more discrete elemental processes. These are *goal-directed retrieval* of relevant information from long-term storage, *manipulation* of available information in *working memory*, and *flexible applications* (i.e., mental flexibility) of previously learned strategies (Hills, Mata, Wilke, & Samanez-Larkin, 2013; Moscovitch & Winocur, 2002; Shimamura, 2011; Shimamura, Stuss, & Knight, 2002). Let us consider each of these in turn.

Goal-Directed Retrieval of Information. Goal-directed retrieval refers to a conscious, purposeful mental search for important and relevant information within one's fund of semantic knowledge and/or within one's episodic memory. This retrieval needs to be self-cued and continuously monitored for consistency with the goal of a given search; as such, it is effortful and fundamentally different from effortless free association or mind wandering. Also inherent in this goal-directed process of retrieval is the inhibition of retrieval of irrelevant or undesired information. As such, goal-directed retrieval could be viewed as the ability to essentially control one's thoughts.

The importance of goal-directed information retrieval for planning, reasoning, and problem-solving has been demonstrated by an extensive body of research (A. D. Brown et al., 2014; Madore & Schacter, 2014; Schacter, 2012; Schacter, Benoit, De Brigard, & Szpunar, 2013) and becomes readily apparent when one carefully examines how it is that we go about planning, reasoning, and so forth. Consider, for example, that you intend to paint a room in your house. Before you begin, you engage in an effortful, goal-directed search in your semantic and episodic storages for your past experiences with painting a room, which allows you to generate a list of all the supplies you know are needed to accomplish the task (brushes, drop cloth, paint, etc.); additionally, you search your episodic memory for information about whether you have any of these items at home, as well as information about where in your house you might look for them (in the garage, in the basement, etc.). All this information is key for you to be able to begin the planning and organizing process.

Note that this purposeful search and retrieval is dissociable from the domain of memory itself, as there is a difference between engaging in a goal-directed and purposeful mental search and the ability to simply retrieve the correct information. Thus, if someone asked you where in your house you keep paint brushes, you may or may not be able to answer that question, depending on your memory abilities. In contrast, goal-directed retrieval that is key for ECFs relies not only on the ability to retrieve but also on the ability to generate the correct *questions* and to self-cue until all relevant information is gathered. Thus, although impairments in memory will interfere with optimal ECFs (Addis, Sacchetti, Ally, Budson, & Schacter, 2009), excellent memory functioning in and of itself is *not* sufficient for ECFs. Note that in clinical neuropsychology, this aspect of ECFs is assessed using various verbal fluency tests; by requiring retrieval of information from semantic networks, these tests are generally unconfounded by memory abilities per se.

Manipulation of Information in Working Memory. According to some theoretical accounts, working memory is thought to be so central to EF that it is viewed as being virtually synonymous with it (Baddeley & Della Sala, 1998; McCabe, Roediger, McDaniel, Balota, & Hambrick, 2010). For the purpose of this text, working memory is viewed as a more limited construct, one that is responsible for holding and manipulating information in mind.

Returning to our example of painting a room in your house, working memory will serve as temporary storage for all the relevant information that you have retrieved from permanent semantic and episodic storages, such as the fact that you will need brushes, drop cloth, paint, and so on, as well as which of those items you already own and which you still need to purchase. Working memory then allows you to manipulate all this information, combining and comparing the findings from your various searches, toward the goal of generating a plan. For the purpose of this discussion, being able to sequence information appropriately is considered to be subsumed under working memory, consistent with the common sequencing requirements of working memory tasks (e.g., letter-number sequencing; Wechsler, 2008).

Mental Flexibility. Mental flexibility allows flexible application of old ideas in new ways, abandoning old ideas that are no longer working in favor of new ideas, or abandoning old issues that have been addressed in favor of new issues that still need addressing. In other words, mental flexibility is the ability to fluidly move from one concept to another, one thought to another, one level of analysis to another, one perspective to another, or one perceptual mode to another. It is also the ability to generalize from the past to the future, or from the concrete to the abstract (Moscovitch & Winocur, 2002; Shimamura, 2002). Of note, although difficulties in abstract thinking (i.e., the inability to flexibly shift from a concrete level of analysis to the abstract level of analysis) do not in and of themselves preclude simple reasoning (Lezak et al., 2004, p. 569), concrete thinking is nevertheless likely to lead to problems in more complex types of reasoning tasks, especially as they relate to real-world problems.

On a neuronal level, mental flexibility is likely related to the ability of the neural networks to become flexibly engaged or disengaged (Cossart, Aronov, & Yuste, 2003). Consider, for example, the well-known drawing of a woman that can be seen from two different perspectives: one perspective allows one to see a young woman, whereas the other perspective allows one to see an old woman (see Figure 2.1).

Importantly, one can never see both images simultaneously. Rather, in order to perceive both, one needs to be able to flexibly "configure" one's perceptual networks so as to move back and forth between the two. Another well-known example from clinical neuropsychology is the need to shift between perceiving color, form, or number of items on the Wisconsin Card Sorting Test (Heaton, Chelune, Talley, Kay, & Curtiss, 1993); an example from cognitive neuroscience is extradimensional switching (Ozonoff et al., 2004; Yun et al., 2011). Regardless of the example, in order to switch from one perspective to the other, the perceptual network of one image needs to become disengaged in order for the perceptual network of the other image to become activated (Cossart et al., 2003; Hoshino, 2013). Note that these examples require flexibility in perceptual networks, but the same networks are activated during perceptual imagery (M. R. Johnson & Johnson, 2014) or thinking about percepts, as is typically done during planning and problem-solving (Addis & Schacter, 2013; Madore & Schacter, 2014).

The term *mental flexibility* (or *cognitive flexibility*) is used frequently in clinical neuropsychology. However, it is often poorly defined, referring to a potentially wide range of processes, including not only the ability to abandon old ideas in favor of new ideas or to activate multiple perspectives but also the ability to respond adaptively to changing contingencies or to flexibly move between two tasks. Although these various abilities share the notion of "change" or "shifting," they are not necessarily subserved by the same

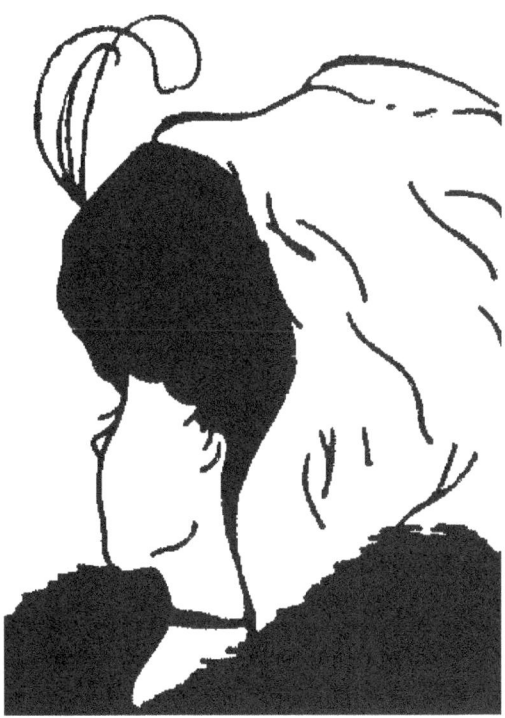

FIGURE 2.1 The figure illustrates the well-known "Young Girl/Old Woman" illusion. It is thought to originally date back to an anonymous postcard from the late 19th century, though many public-domain versions of this drawing exist. By engaging mental flexibility, one can exert top-down control over which of the two images (i.e., the young girl or the old woman) one perceives.

cognitive or neural substrates. In fact, the ability to recognize, and respond to, changes in contingencies represents a separate neurocognitive process related to contingency updating (covered in Chapter 4), and the ability to flexibly move among multiple tasks falls under the domain of meta-tasking (covered in Chapter 3). For the purpose of this chapter, we limit the meaning of the term mental flexibility to the ability to disengage one mental or perceptual set in favor of another set, independent of behavioral outcomes. Of note, the task-switching paradigm frequently used in cognitive psychology as a measure of cognitive control does in many cases tap into mental flexibility, as it requires fundamental mental and perceptual shifts, such as switching from perceiving the color of a stimulus to perceiving the stimulus shape.

Now, let us examine how mental flexibility contributes to ECFs. Consider again the example of your planning to paint a room in your house. You go to the store and gather most of the needed items, but you encounter a glitch: The store is fresh out of drop cloths. What to do? You now engage the same processes you engaged before, that is, goal-directed retrieval of information and manipulation in working memory, so as to begin to solve this problem. However, in addition to these processes, mental flexibility begins to play a role as you move from one level of analysis to another. That is, rather than retrieving information about the concrete supplies for painting (i.e., a drop cloth), you now shift to a more abstract level of thinking, retrieving information from the supraordinate category of items that *can cover a floor*. This memory search then yields the information about a stack of old newspapers in your garage that you were going to take to the recycling center. Armed with this new knowledge, you decide that you will cover the floor with the newspaper instead of a drop cloth. The product of these cognitive efforts is a solution to the problem that the store was out of drop cloths.

Summary of the Construct. The term executive cognitive functions refers to a set of elemental neurocognitive processes that generate *mental products* such as solutions to problems, plans, or organizational systems. The elemental processes that undergird these mental products include *goal-directed retrieval of relevant information, manipulation of information in working memory*, and *flexible application of information* to a question at hand. Importantly, intact ECFs do *not* guarantee execution of planned or organized actions, or achievement of goals. See Table 2.1 for an overview of the constructs discussed here, as well as their application to concrete real-world scenarios.

Other Relevant Constructs

Perseveration. The *INS Dictionary of Neuropsychology* defines *perseveration* as "persistence of the same response, even when it is shown to be inappropriate," that may involve "motor acts, speech, or ideas" (Loring, 1999, p. 125). Perseveration is often thought to imply poor mental flexibility. This is true to the extent that one defines perseveration as the inability to abandon old ideas (or old mental sets) in favor of new ideas (or new mental sets). This may manifest itself, for example, as an inability to make the mental switch from color to shape on the Wisconsin Card Sorting Test (Heaton et al., 1993).

However, perseveration typically manifests itself behaviorally rather than mentally. Specifically, perseveration may present as repetitive motor actions, such as persistent tapping with a hand, writing over previously drawn figures, or repeating letters when writing. This type of behavior is also known

Table 2.1 Overview of ECFs elemental processes, as they relate to mental products of ECFs in daily life scenarios

MENTAL PRODUCTS OF ECFs	EVERYDAY SCENARIO REQUIRING ENGAGEMENT OF ECFs	ELEMENTAL ECFs PROCESSES		
		GOAL-DIRECTED RETRIEVAL	MENTAL FLEXIBILITY	WORKING MEMORY
Reasoning	Solving a sudoku puzzle.	Retrieve previously learned strategies on how to solve the puzzle.	Flexibly move between examining columns, rows, and squares.	Hold in mind which numbers are in which columns and rows.
Problem-solving	Your car breaks down on an extremely rarely-traveled road many miles away from civilization with no cell phone reception.	Retrieve relevant information: • Current location, its distance from civilization, frequency of other traffic • Knowledge that cell phone reception may change in either direction	Examine apparently unrelated information, e.g.: • You've never unpacked camping equipment that's been in your car since a camping trip last summer Flexibly apply such information: • You can backpack your way out of this situation	Simultaneously examine all available information, including pros and cons for all possible solutions, to select the best solution.

(continued)

Table 2.1 (Continued)

MENTAL PRODUCTS OF ECFs	EVERYDAY SCENARIO REQUIRING ENGAGEMENT OF ECFs	ELEMENTAL ECFs PROCESSES		
		GOAL-DIRECTED RETRIEVAL	MENTAL FLEXIBILITY	WORKING MEMORY
Planning	You are in charge of organizing a birthday party for a coworker.	Retrieve relevant knowledge of what a party consists of • guests • food • location • decorations	Flexibly move between subgoals to allow interleaving of steps as needed to maximize efficiency.	Hold relevant information in mind and sequence steps appropriately.
Organization	You are charged with clearing your elderly aunt's cluttered attic so her house can be put on the market.	Retrieve relevant knowledge about • utility of attic items • ways of disposing of items • available services	Flexibly move between subgoals to allow interleaving of steps as needed to maximize efficiency.	Hold relevant information in mind and sequence steps appropriately.

as motor, or hyperkinetic, perseveration (Goldberg, 1986; Lamar et al., 1997; Suchy, Lee, & Marchand, 2013); it is likely related to poor ability to inhibit motor actions, rather than a deficit in ECFs, although the true neurocognitive and neuroanatomical underpinnings are still poorly understood (Suchy et al., 2013). Other examples of perseveration include reverting to a previously reinforced response set due to poor ability to maintain the current set, poor ability to inhibit prepotent response, a failure to register feedback or errors, or a failure to register emerging discrepancies between plans/expectations and reality.

Thus, it is important for clinicians to recognize that perseverative behaviors can result from impairments within several different subdomains of EF (e.g., response selection or set maintenance, in addition to ECFs) and could be linked to deficits in a variety of elemental processes (e.g., sensitivity to incentives, contingency updating, or discrepancy monitoring, in addition to mental flexibility; these are covered in Chapters 4 and 5). In other words, perseveration is a nonspecific sign of EF dysfunction and should not be rigidly interpreted as deficient mental flexibility; rather, qualitative aspects of performance and of the overall performance profile need to be considered.

Cognitive Decision Making. Cognitive decision-making is a deliberative process of arriving at decisions about future actions. Outside of clinical neuropsychology, it has been described as "thoughtfully-reflective decision-making (TRDM)" (Paternoster & Pogarsky, 2009; Paternoster, Pogarsky, & Zimmerman, 2011) and is purported to consist of four processes: (a) collection of information, (b) thinking of alternative solutions, (c) systematically deliberating over alternatives, and (d) retrospectively analyzing the effects of one's decisions (Paternoster & Pogarsky, 2009; Paternoster et al., 2011). In the context of this chapter, the reader can readily see the parallel between cognitive decision-making and reasoning, problem-solving, planning, and organization, that is, the mental products that fall under the umbrella of ECFs (De Bruin, Del Missier, & Levin, 2012; Del Missier, Mäntylä, & De Bruin, 2012). In other words, cognitive decision-making clearly relies on (a) search and retrieval of relevant memories or concepts, (b) manipulation of information in working memory, and (c) flexible application of solutions to the current situation. In fact, it is essentially synonymous with reasoning and should not be considered as a separate cognitive product (and even less so as a separate elemental process).

Emotion Regulation (i.e., Cognitive Reappraisal and Reinterpretation/Reframing). Emotion regulation refers to the ability to modulate how one feels.

For example, if another driver cuts in front of you, you may feel angry or affronted. To alter these uncomfortable feelings, you can re-evaluate the situation by placing it in a larger context and realizing that the relative importance or value of that situation is trivial compared with other, more highly valued aspects of your life. You can also reinterpret the situation by generating more benign (and therefore less anger-producing) reasons for why the other driver may have cut in front of you (maybe the other driver is running late getting to the airport, or maybe he is driving his child to a hospital).

It may appear somewhat counterintuitive to have a section on emotion regulation included in the chapter on ECFs, as emotions and cognitions are often viewed as separate processes. However, let us consider how one accomplishes cognitive reappraisal or reinterpretation. First, one needs to retrieve important information about the broader context, such as things that really matter in one's life, or what legitimate reasons there are that might cause someone to cut in front of other drivers. As mentioned earlier, inherently related to retrieval of desired information is also the *non*retrieval of undesired information, that is, clearing one's working memory of intrusive thoughts about rude or reckless drivers. Next, one compares the retrieved information with the situation at hand. Lastly, one mentally shifts so as to truly allow oneself *to perceive* the current situation in a new way.

This notion that ECFs play a key role in top-down regulation of how we feel is supported by several lines of empirical research. First, children's ability to regulate how they feel emerges in conjunction with the emergence of ECFs (Carlson & Wang, 2007; Liebermann, Giesbrecht, & Maller, 2007). Second, the ability to modulate one's feelings correlates with performances on measures of ECFs (Andreotti et al., 2013; McRae, Jacobs, Ray, John, & Gross, 2012; Schmeichel, Volokhov, & Demaree, 2008). Third, clinical populations that are known to be characterized by weaknesses in emotion regulation are also known to have weaknesses in ECFs (George, Kellner, Bernstein, & Goust, 1994; Martel, 2009; Ritchie & Lovestone, 2002). Lastly, there is considerable evidence that the neuroanatomical networks that subserve ECFs also subserve emotion regulation (Abler, Hofer, & Viviani, 2008; Kalisch, Wiech, Herrmann, & Dolan, 2006; Ochsner, Bunge, Gross, & Gabrieli, 2002; Ochsner & Gross, 2007, 2008).

Typical Presentation of the Dysexecutive Syndrome

Cognitive and Behavioral Changes in Daily Life. Patients with deficits in the ECFs subdomain present with a *dysexecutive syndrome* (Duffy, Campbell,

Salloway, & Malloy, 2001), which is characterized by reasoning that is erroneous or illogical; an inability to generate effective goals, plans, or solutions to problems; and actions that appear ineffectual or haphazard. Here, the reader may object, given that it was previously stated that the products of ECFs are inherently "mental." However, it is important to recognize that a deficient mental product can, and often does, lead to behaviors that reflect that product. Thus, for example, patients may become paralyzed by poverty of ideation and a concomitant inability to generate solutions, or alternatively may engage in purposeless, ill-advised, agitated, or perseverative actions. They may act without a plan, starting a task before having all the needed pieces in place, or acting in a haphazard fashion. Table 2.2 presents examples of patient behaviors in concrete, real-world scenarios. Note, however, that the permutations of how a given patient may behave in a given situation are virtually endless, and reactions of individual patients will also depend on the severity of the deficit, the specifics of a given context, patients' prior experiences, as well as temperament, personality traits, and strengths or weaknesses in other EF subdomains.

It also warrants mentioning that patients with right hemisphere lesions sometimes present with highly tangential and disorganized speech patterns, with paragraph-level structure being particularly poor (Al-Zahrani, 2003; Marini, 2012; Marini, Carlomagno, Caltagirone, & Nocentini, 2005). Although not typically considered an aspect of dysexecutive syndrome, deficits in ECFs can nevertheless be detected in such patients (I. Martin & McDonald, 2006). Also, it is worthwhile mentioning that ECFs elemental processes are closely linked with language. Thus, if the effective usage of language is disturbed, it follows that higher reasoning, problem-solving, planning, and organization would also be affected.

Personality Changes. To understand how dysexecutive syndrome can affect one's personality, it is important to understand how ECFs contributes to personality traits. There is considerable evidence that normal individual differences in ECFs are in part genetically determined (Anokhin, Golosheykin, & Heath, 2008; Anokhin, Heath, & Ralano, 2003; Fossella, Sommer, Fan, Pfaff, & Posner, 2003), and as such inherently contribute to the development of one's personality (P. G. Williams, Suchy, & Rau, 2009). A personality trait that is particularly strongly associated with ECFs is openness to experience (Clifford, Boufal, & Kurtz, 2004; Farsides & Woodfield, 2003; P. G. Williams, Suchy, & Kraybill, 2010). High openness to experience is usually assessed using the NEO Personality Inventory (P. T. Costa & McCrae, 1992).

Table 2.2 Examples of dysexecutive presentations in real-world scenarios

MENTAL PRODUCTS OF ECFs	EVERYDAY SCENARIO REQUIRING ENGAGEMENT OF ECFs	HYPOTHETICAL PATIENT ACTIONS
Reasoning	Solving a sudoku puzzle	• Becoming paralyzed, agitated, frustrated by a lack of ideas • Randomly placing numbers in boxes, using trial-and-error approach • Applying reasoning to easy aspects of the puzzle but becoming agitated and frustrated as subsequent steps in the solution become more demanding • Repeatedly (perseveratively) attempting the same approach that has failed in the past, in lieu of new ideas
Problem-solving	Running out of gas on a rarely traveled road with no cell phone reception	• Becoming paralyzed, agitated, frustrated by a lack of ideas • Walking away from the car without a plan or an idea what the ramifications of such an action might be • Walking away and returning to the car, walking haphazardly in different directions • Repeatedly (perseveratively) trying to use the cell phone, as if hoping the connectivity problem will resolve on its own.
Planning	Putting together a surprise birthday party for a friend	• Becoming paralyzed, agitated, frustrated by a lack of ideas • Ordering food before generating the guest list • Sending out invitations prior to determining the time and place of the party
Organization	Clearing out a cluttered attic so a house can be put on the market	• Becoming paralyzed, agitated, frustrated by a lack of ideas • Randomly moving objects from one place in the attic to another

Individuals with high openness are characterized by openness to or even deliberate pursuit of novel experiences, including trying new foods or new activities, traveling to new places, learning new skills, meeting new people, and so forth. Additionally, high openness is associated with being open to one's own *internal* experiences, that is, seeking insight about and understanding of one's own cognitive and characterologic strengths and weaknesses. Relatedly, individuals who are high on openness exhibit greater readiness to re-examine their social, political, or religious views (DeYoung, 2015; Jost, Glaser, Kruglanski, & Sulloway, 2003). High openness is associated with higher IQ, higher educational attainment, greater cognitive reserve, and lesser cognitive and functional decline in old age (Chamorro-Premuzic & Furnham, 2008; Chapman, Duberstein, & Lyness, 2007; Clifford et al., 2004; Farsides & Woodfield, 2003; Franchow, Suchy, Thorgusen, & Williams, 2013; Suchy, Williams, Kraybill, Franchow, & Butner, 2010; P. G. Williams et al., 2010).

Declines in ECFs are associated with decreases in openness, which in turn are associated with declines in willingness to try new experiences, meet new people, or travel to new locations, as well as increased rigidity in attitudes and behaviors (P. G. Williams, Suchy, & Kraybill, 2013; P. G. Williams et al., 2009) that is sometimes interpreted by clinicians as perseveration. Patients who experience declines in ECFs also tend to become increasingly critical of new things, such as new technologies (e.g., new cell phones), new dress styles, or new developments in one's city or neighborhood (e.g., a new mall, a new movie theater). These changes are likely to be more salient, or more striking, for individuals who were premorbidly high on openness. This is because decline in openness for such individuals may result in fundamental changes in attitudes. In contrast, for those who were less open over the course of their lives, declines in openness will more likely be perceived as a simple exaggeration of a previous personality trait.

In addition to decreases in openness to experience, patients with impairment in ECFs may have difficulty regulating their emotions, being prone to depressed mood or anger, and having difficulty reframing emotionally negative situations in more positive ways (Ochsner & Gross, 2008). Deficient mental flexibility has been linked to increases in rumination (Koster, De Lissnyder, & De Raedt, 2013), which may sometimes be interpreted by clinicians as perseveration. Once again, this is more salient for patients who were previously characterized by good emotional control, whereas those who had long-standing difficulties with emotion regulation are more likely to be seen as simply exhibiting an exaggeration of a premorbid trait.

Presentation During Assessment. The key feature of patients with deficits in ECFs is difficulty on tests of working memory and generative fluency, as well as reasoning (e.g., the category test, various card sorting tests, matrix reasoning tests, and the tower tests). Of note, because of the relatively simple reasoning demands of the Wisconsin Card Sorting Test, patients with high premorbid intelligence and educational attainment may perform well on this test (Heck & Bryer, 1986); in contrast, those with lower premorbid intelligence or those with more severe deficits will exhibit difficulties generating more than one sorting principle or switching from the first sorting principle.

Overall, however, virtually all classical tests of EF tap into multiple elemental processes of ECFs (see Table 2.3). For example, patients may exhibit difficulty on alphanumeric sequencing due to difficulties in holding information in mind and may require extra time due to the need to repeatedly rehearse the number or letter sequences from the start. Errors on this task tend to be characterized by generation of the wrong letter or the wrong number (rather than failing to switch between letters and numbers). Patients are also likely to exhibit difficulties on tests of verbal fluency, due primarily to retrieval problems, as well as to difficulties in generating an effective strategy. Similarly, design or figural fluency may be impaired, once again due to difficulties in generating a strategy or a plan.

In addition to poorer performances on measures of EF, patients are virtually certain to exhibit deficits on list-learning tests, particularly on encoding and retrieval/free recall portions. See Table 2.3 for an overview of the relationship of ECFs processes and EF tests. Note that multiple elemental processes contribute to performance on all tests; consequently, identification of a unique elemental deficit is generally not realistic.

Exceptions to the Rule. Although it is fairly clear that deficits in goal-directed retrieval, working memory, and mental flexibility can preclude one's being able to reason, solve problems, plan, and organize, it is also the case that many individuals fail to engage in normal planning, reasoning, problem-solving, and organization despite normal ECFs capacity. For example, many individuals with highly developed reasoning and problem-solving skills do not keep their desks organized or do not always plan effectively when it comes to their personal lives. In light of these exceptions, it is important to distinguish between the abilities themselves and the *willingness* or *desire* to employ them. A failure to plan, for example, could very well be a function of one's personality, value system, or even a deficit elsewhere in the executive system. In addition, some individuals with intact ECFs may be unable to

Table 2.3 Overview of the association between the elemental processes of ECFs and typical neuropsychological measures presumed to assess EF

	WORKING MEMORY	GOAL-DIRECTED RETRIEVAL	MENTAL FLEXIBILITY
Trail-Making (Switching Condition)	Hold rules in mind; hold sequences in mind.	N/A	Move flexibly between sequencing letter and numbers.
Verbal Fluencies	Hold rules in mind; hold in mind which words have already been generated.	Retrieve words according to rules.	Move flexibly to new "categories" of search (e.g., animals, furniture, etc. that begin with a given letter).
Design Fluencies	Hold rules in mind; hold in mind which designs have already been generated.	N/A	Move flexibly to new strategies (e.g., once finished with starting designs with top left dot, move to starting with top right dot).
Stroop Tests	Hold rules in mind.	N/A	Move flexibly between perceiving words vs. perceiving color of ink.
Wisconsin Card Sorting Tests	Hold currently correct principle in mind.	N/A	Move flexibly between perceiving/abstracting color, shape, or number.
Halstead Category Test	Hold currently correct principle in mind.	Retrieve semantic knowledge, such as understanding of quadrant labeling.	Move flexibly between perceiving/abstracting different aspects of the stimuli.
Tower Tests	Hold the sequence of steps in mind.	Retrieve strategy if previously exposed to a similar task.	Flexibly envision intermediate solutions.

execute their well-thought-out and reasoned plans. Once again, this may be due to problems in other aspects of EF, such as lack of motivation, an inability to inhibit other desired actions, or problems in meta-tasking; these will be discussed in more detail in Chapters 3, 4, and 5.

Neuroanatomy

Structures that subserve ECFs involve both cortical and striatal regions, as well as diencephalic (i.e., the thalamus) and hindbrain (i.e., the cerebellum) regions. Because it is becoming increasingly recognized that most cognitive abilities rely on *networks* (as opposed to discrete regions), this wide range of structures should not be surprising. In fact, all activities of the frontal lobes are dependent on "loops" that carry information from the cortex to the basal ganglia, then to the thalamus and back to the cortex. Similarly, the cerebellum is richly connected with virtually all cortical and subcortical areas of the cerebrum, with discrete aspects of the cerebellum contributing to discrete aspects of cognition. Cortico-cortical networks are also key for proper functioning of ECFs processes, as well as cortical and subcortical white matter tracts. Lastly, the right hemisphere more generally has been recognized at being important for perception of, or attention to, gestalt and the ability to keep the "big picture" in mind while engaging in more detail-oriented activities. The literature on the neuroanatomical underpinnings of individual elemental processes of ECFs is summarized in the following.

Working Memory. Much research supports the notion that the dorsolateral prefrontal cortex (DLPFC particularly Brodmann areas 46, 9, and 6) plays a key role in working memory. This has been demonstrated via single neuron recordings, functional imaging, and animal and human lesion studies (Edin et al., 2009; Goldman-Rakic, Leung, Stuss, & Knight, 2002; Nacher, Ojeda, Cadarso-Suarez, Roca-Pardinas, & Acuna, 2006; Naghavi & Nyberg, 2005). As detailed by Lichter and Cummings (2001), normal functioning of these cortical regions depends on normal connectivity with the dorsolateral head of the caudate nucleus, lateral dorsomedial globus pallidus internal, and ventral anterior and mediodorsal nuclei of the thalamus (which represent the *direct* cortico-subcortical pathways), as well as normal connectivity among dorsal globus pallidus external, lateral subthalamic nucleus, and globus pallidus/ substantia nigra complex (which represent the *indirect* pathways). It should also be noted that although hemispheric specialization for verbal versus spatial working memory has been demonstrated in cortical working memory substrates (Nagel, Herting, Maxwell, Bruno, & Fair, 2013), *bilateral* subcortical involvement may be necessary regardless of the nature of the manipulated material (Moore, Li, Tyner, Hu, & Crosson, 2013).

In addition to these frontal-subcortical connections, the cortico-cortical network involving the DLPFC and aspects of the parietal lobe is important for working memory (Edin et al., 2009; Naghavi & Nyberg, 2005). This network appears to be fairly widespread, involving posterior parietal cortex (including superior parietal lobule and intraparietal sulcus; Berryhill & Olson, 2008; Edin et al., 2009; Rottschy et al., 2012; Wendelken, Bunge, & Carter, 2008). Interestingly, some research suggests functional specificity of frontal versus parietal regions for various components of working memory processing, such that parietal regions have been implicated in the *storage and manipulation* of the working memory content, whereas the strength of the top-down control of the parietal cortex by the DLPFC has been implicated in working memory *capacity* (Edin et al., 2009; Koenigs, Barbey, Postle, & Grafman, 2009; Waechter, Goel, Raymont, Kruger, & Grafman, 2013). Consistent with the notion that manipulation of information occurs in the parietal lobe, lesion research has shown that problems with reasoning may be more strongly related to posterior parietal than frontal lesions (Waechter et al., 2013).

Although the frontal-subcortical and frontoparietal networks represent the most "classic" working memory substrates, research has also implicated the hippocampus for retrieval from working memory (Chein, Moore, & Conway, 2011) and the anterior and posterior cingulate cortex for maintenance of information in working memory (Chein et al., 2011; Harms, Wang, Csernansky, & Barch, 2013; Moore et al., 2013).

Given the complexity of the working memory network, it should not be surprising that working memory also relies on the integrity of white matter tracts connecting these regions, including superior longitudinal fasciculus, pathways connecting the medial temporal lobe and the frontal lobe, the uncinated fasciculus, the cingulum, and the corpus callosum (Charlton, Barrick, Lawes, Markus, & Morris, 2010; Østby, Tamnes, Fjell, & Walhovd, 2011; Treble et al., 2013).

Lastly, functional imaging research and lesion studies have consistently found that the cerebellum plays a role in working memory (Desmond, 2001; Justus & Ivry, 2001; Paquier & Mariën, 2005; Stoodley, 2012; Timmann & Daum, 2010). Although the exact location of cognitive substrates within the cerebellum is not well understood, some evidence implicates the ventral regions of the dentate nucleus and associated regions of the cerebellar cortex (Paquier & Mariën, 2005).

Goal-Directed Retrieval. Retrieval of relevant memories also relies heavily on the prefrontal cortex (Cabeza & Nyberg, 2000; Shimamura et al., 2002), particularly its ventrolateral and dorsolateral aspects (Gerlach, Spreng, Gilmore, & Schacter, 2011; Kostopoulos & Petrides, 2008; Suzuki, Tsukiura, Mochizuki-Kawai, Shigemune, & Iijima, 2009), as well as ventral posterior parietal cortex (important particularly for retrieval of episodic memories; Shimamura, 2011). These networks coactivate with the core components of the default mode network (Gerlach et al., 2011). Lastly, effective goal-directed memory retrieval also engages the medial temporal lobe (Gaesser, Spreng, McLelland, Addis, & Schacter, 2013). These same regions appear to be needed for effective performance of tests of verbal fluency (Costafreda et al., 2006; Pihlajamäki et al., 2000; Verma & Howard, 2012).

Mental Flexibility. Mental flexibility has been linked to networks that largely overlap with those that subserve working memory, namely, those involving DLPFC, posterior parietal cortex, the anterior cingulate cortex/medial prefrontal cortex, and the cerebellum (Cusack, Mitchell, & Duncan, 2010; DiGirolamo et al., 2001; Gold, Powell, Xuan, Jicha, & Smith, 2010; Hampshire, Gruszka, Fallon, & Owen, 2008; Imamizu, Kuroda, Yoshioka, & Kawato, 2004; Jimura & Braver, 2010; C. Kim, Johnson, & Gold, 2012; Philipp, Weidner, Koch, & Fink, 2013; Serrien & Sovijärvi-Spapé, 2013; A. B. Smith, Taylor, Brammer, & Rubia, 2004). This is consistent with cognitive research that shows that successful switching among tasks depends in large part on working memory (Vandierendonck, 2012). More discrete areas that have been implicated within these networks include DLPFC (or inferior frontal gyrus) in the *left* hemisphere (Gold et al., 2010; Hirshorn & Thompson-Schill, 2006), pre-supplementary motor area (pre-SMA; Crone, Wendelken, Donohue, & Bunge, 2006; Mansfield, Karayanidis, Jamadar, Heathcote, & Forstmann, 2011), and medial superior parietal lobule and intraparietal sulcus (Tamber-Rosenau, Esterman, Chiu, & Yantis, 2011). Lastly, some research has also implicated the temporal lobe (Barrett et al., 2003; A. B. Smith et al., 2004).

Much research examining the substrates of mental flexibility relies on various switching tasks that require participants to switch among perceptual sets, attentional sets, motor or response sets, task sets, or intentions and plans. Such tasks have also been used for mapping the time courses and substrates of different types of switches or different phases in the switching process, and the nuances of this research are beyond the scope of this chapter. Suffice it to say that this research has confirmed that the act of switching itself is *not* a unitary construct (Philipp et al., 2013; Rushworth, Passingham, & Nobre, 2005): Those aspects of switching that are *covert* (e.g., attention, perception) largely overlap with the working memory networks (consistent with the construct of *mental* flexibility described here), whereas those aspects of switching that are *overt* or behavioral (e.g., motor responses) rely on meta-tasking, response selection, and initiation (Kenner et al., 2010; Marklund & Persson, 2012; Philipp et al., 2013), described in Chapters 3, 4, and 5, respectively.

Given the overlap between the networks involved in working memory and in mental flexibility, one may wonder whether these two constructs are dissociable. One possible explanation for overlap may lie in the fact that all conscious mental activity is processed by working memory networks. Thus, switching among perceptual or cognitive perspectives requires that old information be cleared from working memory and new information be "loaded."

Typical Etiology of Impairments in ECFs

Given the fairly long list of structures presented here, it should be no surprise that ECFs can become compromised in a large number of disorders. Middle cerebral artery cerebrovascular accidents often result in cortical lesions involving either (or both) the dorsolateral convexity of the frontal lobes or the superior and lateral aspects of posterior brain regions (including posterior parietal and temporal regions). These same regions are also vulnerable to coup-counter coup injuries secondary to traumatic brain injury, or watershed lesions associated with hypoxic/anoxic events (Bigler, 2001; Hopkins & Bigler, 2008). Hypoxic/anoxic events of course also place metabolically demanding structures, such as the hippocampus and the basal ganglia, at risk (Hopkins & Bigler, 2008). Additionally, the basal ganglia and the thalamus, as well as white matter tracks that connect cortical and subcortical structures, are also vulnerable to the effects of small vessel disease (Makin, Turpin, Dennis, & Wardlaw, 2013; Werring et al., 2004). Lastly, large vessel disease can also affect the cerebellum.

In addition to acute events, neurodegenerative diseases (including dementias of old age, as well as younger-onset disorders such as multiple sclerosis), affect the relevant structures to differing degrees. Vascular dementia in particular is associated with dysexecutive syndrome, due to its obvious involvement of the networks and structures described in the earlier section on neuroanatomy, particularly involving the frontal lobes (Miralbell et al., 2012). However, even disorders that are less often associated with frontal lobe pathology, such as Alzheimer's disease, present with symptoms of the dysexecutive syndrome, in part due to problems with retrieval and mental manipulation of relevant information (Allain, Etcharry-Bouyx, & Verny, 2013; Oosterman, Oosterveld, Olde Rikkert, Claassen, & Kessels, 2012). Thus, disorganized, purposeless behavior is not uncommon in this patient population.

At the opposite end of the spectrum, many neurodevelopmental conditions are also associated with dysexecutive syndrome. In many such cases, simply just low intelligence is associated with deficits in ECFs (Danielsson, Henry, Rönnberg, & Nilsson, 2010). In others, ECFs are specifically targeted, such as in attention deficit hyperactivity disorder, where the ability to manipulate information in working memory represents a hallmark symptom (Dovis, Van der Oord, Wiers, & Prins, 2013; Kofler et al., 2014; Roodenrys, 2006).

Lastly, many neuropsychiatric conditions are associated with some limitations in ECFs. Arguably the most prominent among these is schizophrenia (Heinrichs, 2005; Royer et al., 2009), but other populations exhibit subtle weaknesses, including patients with depression and anxiety disorders (Christopher & MacDonald, 2005; L. S. P. de Almeida et al., 2012), as well as those with various personality disorders (Berlin, Rolls, & Iversen, 2005; Coolidge, Segal, & Applequist, 2009; Gvirts et al., 2012; V. Ø. Haaland, Esperaas, & Landrø, 2009; Hagenhoff et al., 2013; Hazlett et al., 2014; Lazzaretti et al., 2012; McClure et al., 2007; Mitropoulou et al., 2005). Some populations can be characterized by fairly circumscribed deficits in specific elemental processes, such as deficient mental flexibility among patients with obsessive-compulsive disorder (Gu et al., 2008).

Chapter Summary

Executive cognitive functions refer to a set of neurocognitive processes that together generate *mental products* such as solutions to problems, plans, or organizational systems. The elemental neurocognitive processes that subserve ECFs include *generative retrieval of relevant information, manipulation of information in working memory*, and *flexible application of information to a question at hand*. Deficits in ECFs present as a dysexecutive syndrome, which is characterized by impaired reasoning, failures to effectively plan, poverty of ideation, and behavioral disorganization. A range of brain regions/networks are implicated in the development of the dysexecutive syndrome, including both cortical and subcortical regions of the frontal lobes, superior parietal lobule or right parietal lobe more broadly, cortical and subcortical temporal lobe structures, and the cerebellum. Given the complexity of the networks that subserve ECFs, many brain insults, as well as neurodevelopmental, neurodegenerative, and neuropsychiatric conditions. are associated with compromised ECFs.

3

Meta-tasking and the Disorganized Syndrome

Defining the Construct

Meta-tasking (MT) refers to one's ability to carry out, in a coordinated manner, several *multistep* tasks in an interleaved fashion over the course of somewhat extended periods (involving completion of subgoals of one task interleaved with completion of subgoals of another task). If one is to understand the fundamental underpinnings of deficient MT, one needs to dissociate the intrinsically behavioral products of MT from the intrinsically mental products of the *executive cognitive functions* (ECFs; discussed in Chapter 2). By the same token, based purely on observing a patient's actions in daily life, deficits in ECFs (i.e., the dysexecutive syndrome) can sometimes be difficult to distinguish from apparent deficits in MT (i.e., the disorganized syndrome). This is because successful execution of any task also relies on availability of organized plans.

As an everyday example of MT, consider preparing a meal that consists of three courses: salad, main course, and dessert. To prepare the salad, you need to (a) mix the ingredients for the salad dressing and let the mixture sit in the refrigerator for at least 2 hours and (b) cut up the vegetables, but do this only once the rest of the meal is ready so as to ensure that the vegetables are not wilted. To prepare the main course, you need to (a) marinade the meat for 3 hours before putting the meat in the oven, (b) preheat the oven to 425 degrees 1 hour before dinner, and (c) bake the meat for 45 minutes, then serve hot. To prepare the dessert, you need to (a) prepare the cake batter, (b) preheat the oven to 350 degrees, (c) bake the cake for 30 minutes, and (d) then allow it too cool for at least an hour before applying the frosting. In this scenario, it is clear that you will not successfully complete the meal preparation if you focus on one course at a time. Rather, you need to interleave steps for each course in a staggered fashion to allow all the pieces to come together approximately at the same time. It is virtually impossible to accomplish this set of steps without a plan; thus, one employs ECFs, generating a plan for the correct sequencing and timing of the nine main steps needed for the preparation of this meal. Figure 3.1 shows how such a plan may look.

However, the plan alone does not guarantee successful execution: This is because there are ample opportunities throughout the course of the day (2:00 p.m. to 6:30 p.m.) to get caught up in other activities (as indicated by shaded rows in the figure). In the course of the other activities, one might, for example, forget to turn on the oven, or to put the cake or the meat into the oven, or to take the cake or the meat out of the oven, and so forth. In fact, skipping, forgetting, or poor timing of any one step along the way will derail the entire process. The elemental neurocognitive processes that are needed for effective plan execution and that make up the subdomain of MT are *event-based prospective memory*, *time-based prospective memory*, and *meta-monitoring*

Time	Other Activities	Salad	Main Course	Desert
2:00 PM			Apply marinade and put meat in fridge for 3 hrs.	
2:30 PM		Prepare salad dressing, put in fridge for 2 hrs.		
3:00 PM				
3:30 PM	*Waiting for meat and dressing to marinade...*			Turn oven to 350 Prepare batter
4:00 PM	*Waiting for oven to heat..*			Put cake in oven
4:30 PM	*Waiting for cake to bake..*		Turn oven to 425	Cake out of oven Let cool 1 hr
5:00 PM	*Waiting for oven to heat, cake to cool...*		Put meat in oven	
5:30 PM	*Waiting for meat to bake, cake to cool..*	Cut up veggies		
6:00 PM				Apply frosting
6:30 PM		Serve salad & dressing	Take meat out of oven & serve	Serve desert after dinner

FIGURE 3.1 The figure illustrates the need to interleave activities during the course of 4.5 hours while preparing a three-course meal. Shaded areas reflect periods of time when no progress can be made on the meal preparation itself, leaving room for other, unrelated activities.

(Logie, Law, Trawley, & Nissan, 2010; McAlister & Schmitter-Edgecombe, 2013). We will consider each of these in turn.

Event-Based Prospective Memory and "Branching." Event-based prospective memory refers to one's ability to spontaneously retrieve relevant information when a given context (or event) presents itself. In other words, when event-based prospective memory is intact, certain contexts should cue the recall of certain memories (such as recalling that when driving to a party one needs to stop at a store to pick up a bottle of wine). Using the meal preparation example, upon hearing the ding of a kitchen timer, one recalls the next step, that is, taking the meat out of the oven.

Another way of conceptualizing event-based prospective memory is to think of it as mental or behavioral branching. Branching refers to one's ability to carry out mental or behavioral tasks that rely on complex multistep sets of rules (e.g., "if . . . then . . ." rules). In branching, there is often a primary task that needs to be carried out (e.g., drive to a party), with the if-then rule invoked only occasionally or perhaps only once, so as to trigger execution of a secondary task (e.g., *if* driving past a liquor store on the way to a party, *then* pick up a bottle of wine).

As another example of event-based prospective memory, consider inheriting a house from your aunt and needing to clean out all her old possessions before putting the house on the market. You generate a plan for how to go about this large, multifaceted task, that is, you successfully engage your ECFs. To help you carry out the plan, you hire a helper and instruct him to start creating three piles: (a) old magazines, intended to be recycled, (b) old clothing, intended to be donated, and (c) old jewelry, intended to be sold to an antique dealer. Creating these piles is the primary task. However, you also warn your helper that *if* he comes across any old issues of the *New Yorker*, a blue scarf with a golden fringe, or a pair of diamond earrings, *then* those items should be put into a fourth pile of items that are intended to be kept. This fourth pile is a secondary task, as the if-then rule is invoked on only a handful of occasions.

Your helper energetically throws himself into opening up drawers, closets, and boxes stored in the attic, pulling out any magazines, clothing, and jewelry he can find and putting them into appropriate piles. He is proud of himself as he finds and sets aside diamond earrings and a blue scarf. However, he loses track of the fact that he was also supposed to be on the lookout for *New Yorker* magazines. This would be an example of a lapse in event-based prospective memory. In other words, encountering *New Yorker* magazines does not trigger the memory of the specific if-then rule you explicitly explained earlier. When you confront your helper about his mistakes, he exclaims, "Oh my gosh, you're right! It completely slipped my mind." Importantly, this is a failure in prospective memory only if your helper does in fact recall the rule when later confronted about his mistake (i.e., had your helper completely forgotten the rule existed, then his lapse would have been due to a error in the domain of memory, not EF).

This example illustrates that execution of a plan can fail even when the if-then rule is explicitly stated and stored in episodic memory. To make matters worse, we do not always explicitly state the rules when generating a plan for a project, particularly if we expect to execute the project ourselves—in other words, many such rules remain implicit, or even somewhat inchoate, in our mind, as we generally assume that we can access such rules as needed in the course of the day. Consider again our example of preparing a meal. The explicit plan for meal preparation outlined in Figure 3.1 helps you keep track of the timing and order of each step, but it does not explicitly list every if-then rule to be encountered. In other words, you implicitly understand that if the oven timer beeps, it is time to take the meat or the cake out of the oven. Because, as seen in the attic-cleaning example, it is possible to make mistakes even when the if-then rules are explicitly spelled out, then clearly a patient with MT deficits is even more likely to fail when the rules remain implicit in his or her mind.

For MT to be carried out properly, one not only needs to understand the rules at the outset but also, more important, needs to keep those rules in mind while engaging in other activities. There are two main types of failures in prospective memory. One type of failure is the one described earlier, wherein a person fully engages in the primary task, working efficiently and accurately, but loses track of all the if-then rules and thus makes mistakes on the secondary task. The other type of failure involves careful maintenance of the if-then rules in mind and frequently double-or triple-checking, at the expense of the primary task. In this scenario, mistakes on the secondary task may not occur; however, overall performance is slow and inefficient, and the primary task does not get completed on time. In contrast, a healthy person can quickly and efficiently work on the primary task, yet have the capacity to maintain an awareness of all the secondary tasks in the background and triggering the if-then rules only as needed.

Time-Based Prospective Memory and Time Estimation. Time-based prospective memory refers to the ability to remember to do something at a particular time or after a particular amount of time has elapsed. Time-based prospective memory has been shown to be dissociable from event-based prospective memory, both in terms of performance and in terms of the neuroanatomical substrates (Picton, Stuss, Shallice, Alexander, & Gillingham, 2006). In fact, patients with deficient time-based prospective memory may still exhibit normal event-based prospective memory and vice versa. The principal difference between the two is that there is less need for active maintenance of event-based prospective memory online, because presumably a stimulus in the environment will trigger the memory that needs to be recalled. In contrast, time-based prospective memory is fully self-maintained and self-initiated. In addition, time-based prospective memory requires normal capacity for time estimation. Importantly, time estimation itself is dissociable from time-based prospective memory and, as discussed later in this chapter, appears to be subserved by slightly different neuroanatomical network (Picton et al., 2006). However, for time-based prospective memory to be effective, time estimation would ideally also be intact.

Because time-based prospective memory is more prone to failures than event-based prospective memory, it is common for people to utilize various aids that essentially convert time-based prospective memory into event-based prospective memories. Timers represent the most typical example of such an aid: Once the timer beeps, we know what to do, assuming our event-based prospective memory is intact. However, not all situations lend themselves to conversion of a time-based prospective memory into an event-based prospective memory. As an example, consider once again that you are preparing a meal. You put the meat in the oven and are about to set the timer, and then the phone rings. You answer the phone; your sister is calling, eager to hear about your recent trip to the Bahamas. You, too, are eager to tell her about your trip. Chances are, you will say, "I don't have a lot of time right now, but let me at least tell you about . . ." Thus you begin to meta-task, interleaving your meal preparation with a phone conversation. The question is, do you maintain the notion of time in mind while talking with your sister, having a sense of how much time is passing by and periodically checking your watch to make sure you do not burn the meat? Or do you lose track of time, such that half an hour later you feel as though you've been taking for only a few minutes? Or do you fully lose track of the fact that you are supposed to check on the meat in 30 minutes? The answers to these questions speak to your strengths and weaknesses in time estimation and time-based prospective memory and will determine how successful you will be at completing this MT challenge. Importantly, as you can see, external aids are not always practically available in daily life, and opportunities for failures in multitasking are plentiful. To minimize the deleterious impact of momentary failures in prospective memory, meta-monitoring of all our activities needs to take place. This process is described in the following.

Meta-monitoring. *Meta-monitoring* refers to an active, conscious process whereby we maintain mental set and periodically refresh our awareness of the "big picture" of a given task (i.e., what have we completed? what remains to be done?), its implicit or explicit rules (e.g., have we followed all if-then rules?), and the time and space within which a task is to occur (i.e., are we on track?). For meta-monitoring to be successful, the ability to hold the big picture in mind is needed, as well as the ability to break the big picture into its component pieces. Additionally, one needs to be able to differentiate between what steps have actually been completed versus steps that have only been thought about—in other words, discrimination between *real* and *imagined* events. Lastly, the ability to estimate our own capacity to successfully monitor the big picture is also important: That is, we need to recognize if the big picture is beyond our cognitive capacity, in which case we may choose to engage in compensatory strategies, such as making lists or writing out explicit plans, which would allow us to check off steps that have been completed.

Although meta-monitoring certainly has an element of both time-based and event-based prospective memory, it differs in that it actively monitors simultaneously all the other processes and compares progress on a task or a series of tasks against a mental blueprint. Additionally, it detects deficiencies in other cognitive processes and recognizes the need for compensatory scaffolding. Table 3.1 provides an overview of how the elemental processes involved in MT relate to an everyday life scenario.

Summary of the Meta-tasking Construct. Meta-tasking refers to the ability to interleave several multistep tasks over a somewhat extended period, so as to accomplish some future goal. The elemental processes involved in meta-tasking are *event-based prospective memory* (aka branching), *time-based prospective memory* (including time estimation), and *meta-monitoring*, which involves top-down, purposeful comparison of the progress on each task with the "blueprint" of the overarching goal.

Other Relevant Constructs

Task Switching. *Task switching* refers to an experimental paradigm in which examinees continually switch between two mental tasks, such as switching between classifying stimuli according to either their shape or their color. The

Table 3.1 Overview of elemental processes of meta-tasking (MT) as they relate to everyday life scenario

REAL-LIFE SCENARIO	ELEMENTAL PROCESSES OF META-TASKING			META-MONITORING
	EVENT-BASED PROSPECTIVE MEMORY	TIME-BASED PROSPECTIVE MEMORY		
Preparing a meal for a party.	Effectively use events or stimuli to trigger memories, e.g.: • If timer dings, put meat in the oven. • If water boils, put pasta in. • If pasta is boiling over, reduce heat.	Effectively use elapsed time to trigger memories, e.g.: • If it's 4:00 p.m., turn oven on. • If the oven has been on for 15 minutes, it is likely preheated.		Monitor for mismatch between plans and outcomes. • If meat seems to be burning, take out of oven sooner than recipe suggested. Mentally check that all steps/courses are on track.
Ramifications of MT failures in the context of the above scenario.	Failing to recognize cues and thus skipping steps in the cooking sequence.	Failing to note passage of time and thus skipping steps in the cooking sequence.		Failing to recognize that plan needs adjustments. Failing to recognize if a step has been omitted.

cost of switching between such two tasks, relative to performing a single task without switching, is typically referred to as the "switching cost" (Gold et al., 2010; Meiran & Marciano, 2002; West & Travers, 2008). In the literature, the switching cost is sometimes purported to be a measure of cognitive control, and it does, in fact, invoke similar processes as those needed for performance of the Stroop test—that is, one relies on mental flexibility to perceptually reconfigure from shape to color and back to shape, as well as on working memory to keep in mind the task rules. However, task switching is not a good measure of MT because it generally does not require one to engage prospective memory, nor is there a requirement to engage in meta-monitoring because there is no overarching goal toward which the task itself is being completed.

Related to task switching, a new construct of "supertasking" has recently emerged in the literature (Medeiros-Ward, Watson, & Strayer, 2014; J. M. Watson & Strayer, 2010), purporting to reflect the ability to "multitask" without a decrement in performance. Once again, this construct simply measures the efficiency of the ECFs system, possibly in conjunction with the speed of processing, without demonstrating any relationship to prospective memory of meta-monitoring. Thus, readers need to be vigilant when reviewing literature on MT, especially if using the search term "multitasking," because this term can be associated with a variety of paradigms that do not relate to the construct as described in this chapter.

Typical Presentation of the Disorganized Syndrome

Cognitive and Behavioral Changes in Daily Life. Patients with *pure* disorganized syndrome are characterized by generally intact ECFs and normal performance on most or all traditional measures of EF, in the context of frequent executive lapses in daily life. In complex situations, the patients' actions can be notably disorganized, to the point of frustration and agitation and an overt inability to complete a task, or an inability to complete all aspects of a given set of tasks. In less complex daily situations, the patients' lapses are characterized by frequent instances of "forgetting to remember," losing track of time, chronic tardiness, and failing to initiate or complete tasks as intended. This is particularly troublesome in cases where patients manage their own medications or other disease-related regimens, such as glucose monitoring (Zogg, Woods, Sauceda, Wiebe, & Simoni, 2012). Importantly, once again, forgetting to remember needs to be dissociated from deficits in episodic memory, as among patients with a *pure* disorganized syndrome episodic memory should be normal.

In addition to general disorganization and tardiness, patients with disorganized syndrome are characterized by rule-breaking. Importantly, this deficit cannot be accounted for by the inability to learn or memorize the task rules. Among these patients, there is a marked disconnect between stated plans and goals and actual execution. Additionally, such patients exhibit a considerable disconnect between virtually intact cognition and grossly impaired execution. This presentation was first described as "strategy application disorder" (Shallice & Burgess, 1991a).

Because of their cognitive strengths, these patients represent a considerable challenge for clinicians, as test results often fail to detect deficits. This is particularly challenging when clinicians are asked to document a disability of a patient who is legitimately seeking compensation or a patient who exhibits deficits on the job but lacks insight. Similarly, these patients represent a challenge for family members, who may find it difficult to understand the disconnect between apparently intact cognition and impaired execution. An additional difficulty for family members lies in the fact that patients with disorganized syndrome often do not have the capacity to recognize their own cognitive limitations and therefore are prone to not following compensation strategies or other rehabilitation recommendations. This latter point is particularly relevant with respect to perceived personality changes, as described in the following.

Personality Changes. In general, individuals who are good at MT are often viewed as conscientious by trait. They tend to finish what they started, they remember to do what they promised they would do, they follow through with plans, keep good track of time, and therefore also tend to be on time. Consequently, a decline in MT abilities gives the appearance of a change in one's conscientiousness or, put differently, a change in one's priorities and a decline in caring about others. For example, it may appear that a patient has become selfish or inconsiderate, as the patient starts missing appointments, coming late to meetings, and forgetting to do what he or she had promised to do. It is important to explain to family and friends that this change is due to an impairment in EF rather than a decline in one's sense of morality, a change in feelings toward others, or a fundamental change in personality.

Additionally, patients with disorganized syndrome are often characterized by poor insight or limited awareness of their own cognitive deficits. Consequently, communicating with these patients about rehabilitation, compensatory strategies, or the need for supervision is challenging. For patients who were previously insightful and thoughtful, this deficit may appear as a dramatic and fundamental change in personality, and patients may be perceived as arrogant or narcissistic by family and health care practitioners.

Assessment Presentation. Patients with deficits in MT are likely to perform well on most typical tests of EF, but they may exhibit errors, rule-breaking, and failures to complete all tasks on multitasking measures (Frisch, Förstl, Legler, Schöpe, & Goebel, 2012). Experimental measures of multitasking have begun to emerge in recent years and include the Multitasking in the City Test (Jovanovski, Zakzanis, Campbell, Erb, & Nussbaum, 2012; Jovanovski, Zakzanis, Ruttan, et al., 2012), Day-Out Task (Schmitter-Edgecombe, McAlister, & Weakley, 2012), and Cooking Breakfast Task (Craik & Bialystok, 2006), to name a few. Although clinical versions of tests of multitasking have been available for some time and include the Six Elements Test and the Zoo Map Test from the Behavioural Assessment of the Dysexecutive Syndrome (BADS; B. Wilson, Alderman, Burgess, Emslie, & Evans, 1996), they are yet not commonly incorporated into typical assessment batteries in the United States, as only UK norms are available.

Aside from the dissociation between performances on typical tests of ECFs and MT, there may be some qualitative evidence of behavioral disorganization during performance of tasks that are less structured or that require self-cuing, such as the various tower tests or the Wisconsin Card Sorting Test. Overall, however, virtually no classical tests of EF strongly tap into the elemental processes of MT, and thus identification of MT deficits based purely on test scores is generally not realistic in a typical assessment situation. See Table 3.2 for an overview of the relationship of MT processes and EF tests.

Exceptions to the Rule. Although it is fairly clear that deficits in MT will lead to potentially debilitating impairment in daily functioning, there are many individuals who essentially *choose* to be somewhat disorganized in their daily life. For such individuals, the choice is potentially based on underlying personality traits, such as low conscientiousness or low agreeableness (as measured by the NEO Personality Inventory). Such individuals may be tardy simply because they prefer for someone else to have to wait rather than having to wait for others, or because they are unconcerned about the social stigma of being tardy. Importantly, when faced with serious consequences, such individuals demonstrate that they have the capacity for organized and timely task completion. Conversely, apparent MT deficits can be present in patients with a variety of other, lower-order deficits, such as patients with memory impairment, attentional deficits, and, of course, dysexecutive syndrome. Lastly, even though it was stated that patients with pure disorganized syndrome perform

Table 3.2 Overview of the association between the elemental processes of MT and typical neuropsychological measures presumed to assess EF

	EVENT-BASED PROSPECTIVE MEMORY	TIME-BASED PROSPECTIVE MEMORY	META-MONITORING
Trail-Making (Switching Condition)	N/A	N/A	Taxed if working memory is poor
Verbal Fluencies	N/A	N/A	N/A
Design Fluencies	N/A	N/A	N/A
Stroop Tests	Respond appropriately to boxes around stimuli in the D-KEFS Color-Word-Interference Switch condition	N/A	N/A
Wisconsin Card Sorting Tests	Know to switch when cued with "Incorrect" once the general principles of the test have been learned	N/A	N/A
Halstead Category Test	N/A	N/A	N/A
Tower Tests	N/A	N/A	N/A

normally on measures of EF, it is obviously possible for patients to exhibit both the dysexecutive syndrome and the disorganized syndrome simultaneously. Importantly, whereas patients with a pure dysexecutive syndrome will benefit from written plans or organizing structure provided by others, patients with a combination of dysexecutive and disorganized syndromes are less likely to benefit from such aids.

Neuroanatomy

The principal brain regions involved in MT are rostral prefrontal cortex (PFC), which is also known as frontopolar cortex, as well as lateral PFC (P. W. Burgess, Veitch, de Lacy Costello, & Shallice, 2000; Koechlin, Basso, Pietrini, Panzer, & Grafman, 1999; Koechlin, Ody, & Kounelher, 2003; Roca et al., 2011; Volle, Gonen-Yaacovi, de Lacy Costello, Gilbert, & Burgess, 2011). Importantly, some differences in localization exist with respect to the individual neurocognitive processes that contribute to MT, most notably a greater tendency to exhibit rule-breaking with left lateral/frontopolar lesions and a greater tendency for losing track of time and failing to actively monitor one's activity with the right lateral/frontopolar lesions (P. W. Burgess, Dumontheil, et al., 2008; P. W. Burgess, Gilbert, & Dumontheil, 2008). Additionally, subtle dissociations within the rostral cortex have been shown between the substrates for event-based prospective memory, time-based prospective memory, and time estimation (Picton et al., 2006; Volle et al., 2011).

Active meta-monitoring for discrepancies between one's actions and intended goals has also been related to activation in the temporoparietal juncture (Miele, Wager, Mitchell, & Metcalfe, 2011). Given that temporoparietal juncture represents at least one of several substrates implicated in crystallized intelligence, this finding is consistent with research that shows an association between intelligence and insight about, or awareness of, the accuracy of one's own performance (Suchy, Kraybill, & Franchow, 2011). Because meta-monitoring requires active maintenance of multiple task rules in mind, at least some contributions from working memory can also be expected. Thus, functional imaging research has repeatedly demonstrated that maintaining set rules, especially in situations when attention is divided between two or more tasks, is subserved in part by the left dorsolateral prefrontal cortex (G. C. Burgess et al., 2010; Fassbender, Foxe, & Garavan, 2006; Fassbender et al., 2004; Santangelo & Macaluso, 2013).

Lastly, although the frontal regions outlined here have been confirmed as necessary for MT via lesion studies (Volle et al., 2011), contributions from other regions are likely. Specifically, there is some evidence that cerebellar lesions may be associated with deficit in prospective memory (Hetherington, Dennis, & Spiegler, 2000), and functional imaging research has implicated contributions of the precuneus, the parietal lobe (BA 7, 40), and the anterior cingulate cortex (BA 32) to MT (P. W. Burgess, Gonen-Yaacovi, & Volle, 2011). Clinical evidence for the importance of these regions for MT is sparse, but at least one case study has reported MT deficits following a right temporoparietal stroke (Lazar, Festa, Geller, Romano, & Marshall, 2007).

Typical Etiology of Impairments in MT

Given the neuroanatomy of MT, it is not surprising that the disorganized syndrome, most notably deficits in prospective memory, can be associated with traumatic brain injury (Shum, Levin, & Chan, 2011). Neoplasms involving the frontopolar regions may represents the "cleanest" examples of the disorganized syndromes, as in such patients other brain regions can be fully intact, resulting in the starkest dissociation between intact cognition and impaired MT. However, children with a history of a posterior fossa tumors and focal radiation have been shown to have a deficit in prospective memory, pointing to the need to consider damage to other brain regions as possible etiology as well (Hetherington et al., 2000). Similarly, MT has been shown to be impaired in individuals with HIV (J. C. Scott et al., 2011). In addition to acute events, neurodegenerative diseases, in particular frontotemporal lobar degeneration, Alzheimer's disease, Parkinson's disease, and mild cognitive impairment, are all associated with pervasive deficits in prospective memory (A. Costa, Caltagirone, & Carlesimo, 2011; A. Costa, Carlesimo, & Caltagirone, 2012; Kliegel, Altgassen, Hering, & Rose, 2011; Roca et al., 2013; Spíndola & Dozzi Brucki, 2011).

At the opposite end of the spectrum, neurodevelopmental conditions are also associated with differing degrees of difficulties in MT. Most notable among these is attention deficit hyperactivity disorder (ADHD), wherein deficits in prospective memory (Kerns & Price, 2001; Zinke et al., 2010) and meta-monitoring (R. C. K. Chan et al., 2006; Siklos & Kerns, 2004) have been found, as well as autism spectrum disorders, including both Asperger's syndrome (Hill & Bird, 2006) and high-functioning autism (Mackinlay, Charman, & Karmiloff-Smith, 2006; Rajendran et al., 2011). Lastly, consistent deficits in MT in general (Laloyaux et al., 2014) and prospective memory in particular (Ordemann, Opper, & Davalos, 2014) have been identified in schizophrenia.

Chapter Summary

Meta-tasking refers to the ability to execute several multistep tasks in an interleaved fashion over somewhat extended periods. Elemental processes of MT include *time-based prospective memory, event-based prospective memory*, and *meta-monitoring*. Deficits in MT result in the disorganized syndrome, which is characterized by pervasive difficulties with successful completion of complex daily activities (e.g., preparation of a complex meal), tardiness, forgetfulness, and rule-breaking. Neuroanatomically, the frontopolar cortex and lateral prefrontal cortex (bilaterally) are most often implicated, although contributions from more posterior brain areas have been suggested by both functional imaging and lesion studies. Typical clinical populations include persons with traumatic brain injury, neoplasm involving frontopolar cortex, dementias, ADHD, autism spectrum, and schizophrenia.

4

Response Selection and the Disinhibited Syndrome

Defining the Construct
Response selection (RS) refers to one's behavioral response in situations that allow for (or even invite) multiple potential behavioral outcomes. To understand the construct of RS, one needs to appreciate the central difference between this aspect of *executive functioning* (EF) on the one hand and the *executive cognitive functions* (ECFs; discussed in Chapter 2) on the other. Specifically, whereas the products of ECFs are inherently "mental," the products of RS are inherently "behavioral." Thus, as was already mentioned in Chapter 2, ECFs and RS are mutually dissociable, such that individuals with perfectly intact ECFs may still select inappropriate responses, and vice versa.

When thinking about RS, one may be tempted to equate it with *decision-making*, as every behavioral choice creates at least the impression that a conscious decision has been made. However, the purely cognitive (and somewhat abstract) process of cognitive decision-making (as described in Chapter 2) is not nearly sufficient for us to adaptively accomplish the many behavioral choices we are faced with on a daily basis. The following explains why.

The purely cognitive decision-making that relies on ECFs can effectively precede an action *only* in situations that afford time for such a deliberative process to take place (Paternoster & Pogarsky, 2009; Paternoster et al., 2011). However, in most situations, we are inherently driven to act. For example, a dieter may be driven to eat a cookie offered by a coworker at an office party.

In order to decide deliberatively whether to eat the cookie or not, the dieter would need to consider whether cookies are allowed on his diet plan or not, and, if so, whether the caloric content of this particular cookie would be in line with the expected caloric intake for the day. This deliberation process (or one's capacity to engage in this process) is, of course, rendered moot *unless* it occurs *prior to* taking and eating the cookie. And herein lies the paradox: The behavioral "choice" to *not* eat the cookie (or at least to *delay* eating it) needs to occur *before* the deliberative, cognitive decision-making process can take place.

Despite this apparent paradox, we clearly make many perfectly appropriate behavioral choices throughout each day without pausing to deliberate prior to each, or, conversely, we appropriately pause as needed in order to allow deliberation to take place. How is that possible? That is, how do we know at any given moment whether to pause (i.e., inhibit and deliberate) on the one hand or to *not* pause (i.e., release the desired action) on the other? This question, to pause or to not pause, is at the heart of what RS is all about. In other words, the principal purpose (and challenge) of RS is not to rigidly inhibit every single action (if that were the case, we could simply call it "inhibition"), nor is it to come up with the best and most reasoned decision for each situation (if that were the case, we could simply call it "cognitive decision-making"). Rather, the core purpose of RS is to appropriately *select* when to *passively release* a given motor program, allowing our body to do its thing (i.e., eat the cookie), versus when to *actively inhibit* such an action from taking place (and maintain the inhibition until the release of the action is appropriate or until a new, more appropriate action is put into place). Because these choices need to occur rapidly, they rely, at least in part, on implicit, preconscious, bottom-up neurocognitive processes that include *threat sensitivity, contingency updating*, and *discrepancy detection*. In turn, these processes together trigger the more conscious, effortful, top-down process of *response inhibition*. Let us consider each in turn.

Threat Sensitivity. Threat sensitivity refers to one's ability to (a) *detect* and (b) *learn from* punishing or otherwise undesirable environmental cues or outcomes. This means that first and foremost one needs to be able to implicitly recognize cues that signal danger to oneself or others. Note that because sensitivities to social versus nonsocial threats seem to be mutually dissociable (South et al., 2008), this chapter focuses only on sensitivity to nonsocial threats, such as snakes or spiders, whereas the ability to detect, understand, and learn from social threats is covered in more detail in Chapter 6, which discusses social cognition.

Assuming normal ability to detect and recognize nonsocial threats, encounters with such stimuli are associated with autonomic and hormonal cascades that facilitate changes in sympathetic activation (i.e., increase arousal), as well as certain behavioral responses (e.g., startle) and certain cognitive responses (e.g., increase in vigilance, attention, and possibly speed of processing; Phelps, Fiske, Kazdin, & Schacter, 2006). These responses occur rapidly and thus facilitate rapid behavioral inhibition. In contrast, when threatening stimuli are not normally detected or recognized, adaptive autonomic, behavioral, and cognitive responses do not take place, allowing a release of behavioral choices that may appear foolish, impulsive, or reckless, as is typical of individuals who are disinhibited or impulsive (Huebner et al., 2008; Marsh et al., 2008).

A second key aspect of threat sensitivity is the ability to *learn* the associations between stimuli and punishing consequences, a cognitive process known as *fear conditioning*. The importance of fear conditioning should be self-evident: Whereas some stimuli (e.g., snakes) signal threat inherently (Ohman & Mineka, 2001), the punishing properties of other stimuli (e.g., guns) need to be learned from experience (whether direct or vicarious). Importantly, although our experiences with different threatening objects certainly result in explicit memories (assuming a normal episodic memory), effective fear conditioning requires that learning take place on an *implicit* level. This implicit-level learning is fully dissociable form explicit (episodic) learning (Phelps, 2004), and, in fact, neither episodic memory nor conscious experience of aversion or pain is either necessary or sufficient for fear conditioning to take place (Fischman & Foltin, 1992; Leterme, Brun, Dittmar, & Robin, 2008; Phelps, 2004; Wyvell & Berridge, 2000). These implicit memories then trigger changes in autonomic and cognitive arousal (Adolphs et al., 2005), which in turn facilitate appropriate behavioral choices. Once again, however, individuals with deficient fear conditioning fail to experience the appropriate autonomic and hormonal cascade during encounters with threats and consequently fail to trigger the inhibitory mechanisms needed for selection of the most adaptive responses. Importantly, as alluded to earlier, individuals who have intact episodic memories of punishing circumstances in the context of impaired fear conditioning may explicitly and genuinely express their desire to avoid behaviors that would result in future punishment yet fail to inhibit such behaviors when opportunities present themselves.

Contingency Updating. *Contingency updating* refers to a rapid, preconscious process that updates or reverses previously learned associations based on a given context. Although contingency updating is inextricably dependent on normal threat sensitivity, it also considers broader contexts and integration of a broader array of both threatening and inviting cues, as well as more targeted allocation of attentional resources (Cox, Andrade, & Johnsrude, 2005; Grossberg, Bullock, & Dranias, 2008). Importantly, this process involves not only the implicit coding of the *valence* of likely outcomes but also implicit computations of the *probability* that a given outcome will occur, as well as crude implicit *cost-benefit* analysis (Rolls, 2004; Windmann et al., 2006). If the aggregate of continuously updated valence coding, heuristic probability computation, and cost-benefit analysis suggests a suboptimal outcome, the inhibitory mechanism is triggered so that one may begin to engage in a more deliberative decision-making process or, alternatively, simply move on to the next readily available and previously reinforced action.

Discrepancy Detection. *Discrepancy detection* refers to an automatic process whereby the external environment and one's own actions are continuously compared against the mental set of goals, plans, or expectations. Like contingency updating, discrepancy detection occurs at an implicit, preconscious, highly heuristic level, and it is this bottom-up monitoring process (as opposed to a top-down, deliberate meta-monitoring described in Chapter 3) that is relevant here. Consistent with this notion, EEG research has shown that the brain can detect discrepancies or errors without, or prior to, conscious awareness, as evidenced by a robust error-related negativity that occurs within 100 milliseconds of a response (O'Connell et al., 2007; Orr & Hester, 2012); in contrast, for conscious error awareness to take place, a closely related yet distinct electrophysiological response known as *error positivity* appears to be necessary (Orr & Hester, 2012). When a discrepancy is detected, an inhibitory mechanism is triggered and a corrective action can take place.

Inhibition. Response inhibition is principally behavioral, and it literally means stopping a motor output from taking place. Response inhibition is triggered by automatic processes reviewed earlier, that is, when a threat is detected, when contingencies or probable outcomes are negative, or when a discrepancy or error is signaled. Given its reliance on these systems, it should not be surprising that inhibition of motor output is also intimately linked to processing of emotional information (Kalanthroff, Cohen, & Henik, 2013).

Because inhibitory control can be deployed *after* a behavioral response has been released, it needs to be faster (approximately 200 milliseconds) than initiation of a new response (i.e., reaction time, approximately 250 milliseconds; Logan & Irwin, 2000). When interrupting a response that has already been initiated, inhibition may be overtly evident, as overt interruption of an initiated action can be observed. However, much inhibition occurs *covertly*, that is, much inhibition either prevents a given action from occurring altogether or delays a release of such an action. Thus the act of inhibiting is often not directly evident or observable; rather, it is often only the absence of inhibition that is overtly apparent.

Interestingly, although behavioral inhibition is generally considered to be a conscious and potentially effortful process, research suggests that it may in some situations be deployed without a conscious awareness (G. Hughes, Velmans, & De Fockert, 2009). Regardless of the intentionality of the initial deployment of inhibition, it is important to note that inhibition is the point at which intentional, effortful, goal-directed control of behavior begins. In fact, much research has demonstrated that even simple motor actions, if delayed by inhibitory control for as little as 2 seconds, become intentional and effortful and begin to rely on neuroanatomical networks that are distinct from those involved in automatic output (McIntosh, Pritchard, Dijkerman, Milner, & Roberts, 2001; Milner et al., 2001; Rossetti et al., 2005). In other words, inhibition is a point at which automatic action ends and effortful executive control of behavior begins. For a review, see Rossetti and Pisella (2003).

To illustrate how RS processes manifest themselves in daily life, consider, for example, arriving at an intersection as the stoplight changes to yellow. You have an important meeting to get to, and you are running late; also, on your front seat, you have a box of doughnuts that you are bringing to the meeting. You have less than a second to decide whether to step on the brake or proceed through the intersection. Considerations are multiple and complex: On the one hand, it is technically illegal to proceed through the intersection as long as it is safe for you to stop; you are a prosocial person who doesn't really want to break the laws of traffic; plus, if you were to be stopped by a police officer, you would be delayed even further; and so on. On the other hand, stopping may cause the box of doughnuts to fly off the seat; stopping would also further delay you for your meeting; plus, you live in a city where yellow lights are fairly long (and the red lights are *very* long), and so most motorists tend to not stop unless they see the light change from green to yellow from more than a hundred yards away. Bottom line: There is a lot to consider and only a little time in which to consider it. Fortunately, in situations such as this, *rapid heuristic calculations* of the odds of good versus bad outcomes will take place, as well as the analysis of the relative costs and benefits of either action. Although you are aware of some aspects of this process, many of the underlying computations take place preconsciously, and depending on the result of these largely implicit calculations, the inhibitory mechanism will be either triggered or not triggered.

To further illustrate the dynamic contributions of *implicit discrepancy detection*, consider that the preceding scenario takes place while you are out of town, driving to a professional meeting. While you are driving a rental car, a green light turns to yellow as you approach an intersection. Your initial behavioral choice (based on contingencies and probabilities learned in your hometown) may be to proceed through the intersection, and so you continue driving at your cruising speed. As you approach the intersection, however, you notice that all cars to the left and right of you are slowing down and stopping. This observation is not in line with your expectation. At this point it behooves you to respond to the discrepancy between your erroneous expectation (i.e., that the yellow light will be long, allowing you and others to easily drive through) and the reality (i.e., that you are the only person who seems to believe that the yellow light will be long). Ideally, in this scenario, the discrepancy detection system triggers the inhibitory system, and you will stop. Lastly, note that deliberative decision-making is not necessary while you are waiting for the light to turn back to green because an automatic behavioral choice is readily built into this context.

Table 4.1 provides an overview of how the elemental processes involved in RS relate to daily life scenarios.

Summary of the RS Construct. Overtly, response selection refers to a behavioral choice that often involves active inhibition of a prepotent (i.e., previously reinforced) response. Covertly, the choice to inhibit is often based on implicit processes, including *incentive sensitivity, contingency updating*, and *discrepancy detection*, as well as the effortful, top-down process of *inhibition* or delay of action. If the choice is to inhibit, the resulting "pause" in action may be filled with a deliberative decision-making process, as described in Chapter 2, or with another, more benign or more appropriate action that readily presents itself. Alternatively, another action may be effortfully initiated; processes needed for execution of such actions are covered in Chapter 5.

Other Relevant Constructs

Emotion Regulation (Expressive Suppression). As already discussed in Chapter 2, emotion regulation involves modulation of how one *feels*. However,

Table 4.1 Overview of elemental processes of response selection (RS) as they relate to everyday life scenario

REAL-LIFE SCENARIO	ELEMENTAL PROCESSES OF RESPONSE SELECTION			
	THREAT SENSITIVITY	CONTINGENCY UPDATING	DISCREPANCY DETECTION	INHIBITION
Driving on a country road where you normally enjoy letting your car coast downhill. This time, you are caught in a snowstorm.	Experience physiologic and cognitive arousal in response to the threat of inclement weather.	Update contingency: Coasting normally feels rewarding, but under the circumstances it could result in an adverse/punishing outcome.	Notice cars in the snowbanks and recognize conditions are worse than you expected.	Avoid coasting. Slow down.
Ramifications of RS failures in the context of the above scenario.	Fail to experience any concern about the weather.	Seek to experience the joy of coasting downhill.	Notice cars in the snowbanks but fail to note that this is unexpected.	Go at your regular speed. Coast downhill.

there is a second aspect to emotion regulation: modulation of how one *acts*. In recent literature, this aspect of emotion regulation has been referred to as *expressive suppression*. Expressive suppression is ubiquitous in daily life, as reflexive manifestations of our feelings constantly emerge in the form of facial expressions, tone of voice, verbalizations, and posture and gestures. However, daily social life dictates that we modulate these reflexive responses by suppressing them or replacing them with deliberate approximations of different, more socially appropriate feelings. For example, when feeling angry, we may suppress an angry facial expression and substitute it with a posed smile. Much research suggests that our ability to engage in expressive suppression is related to the elemental process of inhibition, and that our ability to employ expressive suppression at appropriate times is related to the elemental process of discrepancy detection, as well as various aspects of social cognition as discussed in Chapter 6. Not surprisingly, then, research also shows that expressive suppression relies on the same neuroanatomical networks as RS (Abler et al., 2008; Blair, 2001; Falkenbach, Poythress, & Creevy, 2008).

Typical Presentation of the Disinhibited Syndrome

Cognitive and Behavioral Changes in Daily Life. Patients with the disinhibited syndrome are characterized by impulsive responses in situations where a more reasoned approach would be preferred, or where simple inhibition of one response in favor of another would be appropriate. Because deficient inhibition is also typically associated with deficient contingency updating, patients may present as extremely perseverative, repeating again and again a response that had been previously reinforced but subsequently became inappropriate; similarly, because discrepancy detection is typically deficient, patients may have difficulty noticing even gross mistakes or may appear as though they are not registering even explicit error feedback (Fellows & Farah, 2003). Importantly, it is not the case that patients with the disinhibited syndrome necessarily cannot generate reasonable goals or plans; rather, they *fail to inhibit* inappropriate responses, at times thus preventing the reasoning process from taking place. Alternatively, patients may have previously generated plans in mind and have every intention of following through with those plans, but once in the presence of previously reinforced stimuli they may engage in actions that are grossly inconsistent with their stated goals. Such actions are reminiscent of behaviors exhibited by addicts, who often state their desire to abstain from a substance but then use the substance anyway if it is available.

In such situations, patients may quite genuinely express exasperation, making statements such as "Why did I do that?" or "I don't even know how that happened," demonstrating that behaviors and actions "get away" from them. These maladaptive behaviors may occur due to an inability to inhibit a previously reinforced behavioral response, or a failure to even attempt to inhibit that response due to deficiencies in threat sensitivity, discrepancy detection, or contingency updating.

Less frequently, patients with extreme deficits in inhibitory control or those in acute phases of recovery from an injury may also present with magnetic apraxia (also known as environmental dependency syndrome) or with echolalia and extreme mirroring. Although discrete failures within the RS system are, in theory, dissociable, in reality many patients who present with the disinhibited syndrome will exhibit deficits in several or all elemental components of the RS system due to close proximity and/or overlap of the networks subserving these processes. From a behavioral standpoint, however, those with spared discrepancy detection will be characterized by impulsive errors followed by attempts at self-correction.

Personality Changes. Given the difficulties described earlier, inherently prepotent responses (i.e., various emotionally driven actions, such as expression of anger) tend to be insufficiently inhibited, leading to anger outbursts, irritability, or other emotionally driven behaviors, regardless of whether the context renders such behaviors inappropriate or insensitive. In addition to overtly emotional behaviors, patients may become excessively driven by rewards, due to deficient sensitivity to threats or punishments. This can lead to compulsive buying or gambling, compulsive sexual acting out, or compulsive overeating. Additionally, patients may fail to learn from the consequences of their actions, such that actions that were reinforced in one situation are applied in other situations where the reinforcing valence should have reversed. As a result of these behaviors, patients may be perceived as reckless or foolish, irritable and angry, inflexible and stubborn, insensitive and inconsiderate, and, of course, impulsive. All these characteristics, especially if inconsistent with premorbid style, are likely to be perceived by others as a fundamental change in personality.

Assessment Presentation. Patients with deficits in RS are most likely to exhibit impulsive errors on tasks that require inhibition of prepotent responses, such as reading the words rather than naming the color of ink on the Stroop test, or sequencing numbers rather than switching between numbers and letters on Trails B. Because frequent errors invariably slow down performance on timed tests, these patients' scores may appear to be characterized by slow speed. However, careful observation of these patients along with examination of errors and other qualitative aspects of performance should clearly differentiate them from those whose performance is legitimately slow. Specifically, despite test scores suggesting a slow performance, these patients work fast and maybe even appear eager to generate quick responses. As mentioned earlier, examination of the types of errors these patients make will reveal a tendency to choose a prepotent, automatic response over an effortful, novel response. Alternatively, patients may appear to disregard rules, such as generating proper names or words that begin with the correct sound but the wrong letter on tests of verbal fluency. These patients may also exhibit elevations on various perseverative scores, such as repeating previously generated responses on tests of figural fluency, filling the stimulus page rapidly with invalid designs. On the Wisconsin Card Sorting Test, they may exhibit occasional losses of set due to reverting to a previously reinforced sorting principle, as well as high numbers of perseverative responses. Whereas patients whose RS is globally impaired may appear oblivious to making such errors, those with primarily impaired inhibition (in the context of normal discrepancy detection) will place the cards incorrectly, only to exclaim virtually immediately that their response was wrong.

Overall, however, error-free performance on virtually all classic tests of EF relies not only on intact RS but also on good ECFs, making these tests rather nonspecific with respect to EF subdomain, let alone identification of deficits within specific elemental processes. Of note, no classic tests assess threat sensitivity, and contingency updating is also somewhat inadequately tapped. See Table 4.2 for an overview of the relationship of RS processes and EF tests.

Exceptions to the Rule. Although it is fairly clear that deficits in behavioral inhibition, threat sensitivity, contingency updating, and error detection lead to disinhibited, inappropriate responding, it is also the case that many individuals engage in apparently foolish, inappropriate behavioral choices *on purpose*. In other words, many individuals with the capacity to make good choices nevertheless choose to do what they fully understand at the time to be foolish or inappropriate. For example, people engage in illegal activities or extramarital affairs, or in actions that are dangerous and likely to lead to bodily harm. It is still possible, or perhaps even likely, that many such individuals have *slight imbalances* in the contingency updating system or may

Table 4.2 Overview of the association between the elemental processes of RS and typical neuropsychological measures presumed to assess EF

	THREAT SENSITIVITY	CONTINGENCY UPDATING	DISCREPANCY DETECTION	INHIBITION
Trail-Making (Switching Condition)	N/A	N/A	Monitor for errors.	Inhibit responding to letters or numbers that logically follow.
Verbal Fluencies	N/A	N/A	Monitor for errors.	Inhibit responding based on phonemic similarities (e.g., inhibit saying "phone" when the letter is "F").
Design Fluencies	N/A	N/A	Monitor for errors.	Inhibit repeating previously generated design.
Stroop Tests	N/A	N/A	Monitor for errors.	Inhibit reverting to prepotent response.
Wisconsin Card Sorting Tests	Register feedback; only severe deficits are relevant.	Update based on feedback.	Monitor for errors.	Inhibit reverting to previously reinforced principle.
Halstead Category Test	Register feedback; only severe deficits are relevant.	Update based on feedback.	Monitor for errors.	Inhibit reverting to previously reinforced principle.
Tower Tests	N/A	N/A	Monitor for errors.	Inhibit responding prior to having a plan in place.

have an unusually strong proclivity to respond to rewards while not being adequately sensitive to punishments. However, such proclivities, in and of themselves, do not represent an executive deficit—rather, they reflect normal temperamental variability or normal individual differences.

Neuroanatomy

The neuroanatomical substrate of RS is composed of multiple regions within the ventral and medial convexities of the frontal lobes (Rolls, 2004), as well as temporal regions and the anterior insula (Ullsperger, Harsay, Wessel, & Ridderinkhof, 2010). More specific associations of those regions with elemental processes of RS are reviewed in the following.

Threat Sensitivity. The most central structure for threat sensitivity is the amygdala. The amygdala represents the trigger mechanism that affords rapid communication between the external world on the one hand and the body and the brain on the other. Specifically, the amygdala is hardwired to detect emotionally (and socially, addressed in Chapter 6) salient information through all sensory modalities. What makes the amygdala so important for appropriate behavioral choices and, in fact, survival is that it has the capacity to bypass the slow processing in sensory cortical areas (de Gelder, Vroomen, Pourtois, & Weiskrantz, 1999, 2000; Morris, de Gelder, Weiskrantz, & Dolan, 2001), delivering instead relevant emotional information rapidly and directly to subcortical emotional control centers, which in turn trigger a cascade of reflexive motor as well as autonomic and hormonal responses (Berntson, Bechara, Damasio, Tranel, & Cacioppo, 2007; Ohman, 2002, 2005). Importantly, the amygdala has the capacity to learn the associations between emotional outcomes and stimuli that were previously neutral, resulting in rapid reflexive motor and physiologic responses to stimuli whose threatening qualities have been learned (or conditioned; Adolphs et al., 2005; Bechara, Tranel, Damasio, & Adolphs, 1995; LeDoux et al., 2002). In addition, rich reciprocal connections between the amygdala and the orbitofrontal cortex allow for more sophisticated learning of associations between complex behaviors and rewarding or punishing consequences (Cox et al., 2005; Grossberg et al., 2008). For a review of the literature on the role of the amygdala as an emotional trigger, see Suchy (2011, pp. 43–69).

Contingency Updating. With respect to contingency updating, the ventral frontal cortex (orbitofrontal cortex, including ventrolateral and ventromedial regions) represents the central substrate (Kringelbach & Rolls, 2004). It is generally agreed that more rostral areas of the orbitofrontal cortex play a role in coding contingencies that are more abstract (e.g., monetary rewards or punishments, praise or disapproval), whereas more caudal orbitofrontal areas code contingencies that are more concrete (e.g., food, touch, pain). Similarly, rostral areas code contingencies for responses that are expected to occur farther in the future, whereas caudal areas code responses that are more immediate. Thus, relative ranking takes place in terms of relevant priorities, as well as probabilities of likely outcomes. However, there is some disagreement with respect to the organization of the ventral frontal areas as they relate to the *valence* of the coded information. In general, two opposing theoretical accounts have been described: (a) the valence hypothesis and (b) the somatic marker hypothesis. For a review, see Rolls (2004) and Windmann and colleagues (2006).

The valence hypothesis suggests that coding of rewards takes place in the medial orbitofrontal cortex, and coding of punishments takes place in the lateral orbitofrontal cortex. This conceptualization is supported by functional imaging studies that have found greater medial activation in response to rewards, and greater lateral activation in response to punishments (Grabenhorst, Rolls, Margot, da Silva, & Velazco, 2007; Ursu & Carter, 2005). Additionally, individuals with greater capacity for experiencing pleasure in response to pleasurable stimuli exhibit stronger activation in the medial orbitofrontal cortex (Harvey, Pruessner, Czechowska, & Lepage, 2007). In contrast, at least one study found equal medial orbitofrontal activation during delivery of both rewards and punishments (Dillon et al., 2008). However, it is not clear whether activation during incentive delivery necessarily translates into learning.

In contrast to the valence hypothesis, the somatic marker hypothesis (Bechara, Damasio, Damasio, & Anderson, 1994; Bechara, Damasio, Tranel, & Damasio, 1997) proposes that the substrate for learning from punishment is in the ventromedial prefrontal cortex. This hypothesis posits that the brain codes associations between behaviors and physiologic outcomes (or "somatic markers") of such behaviors. Thus, for example, if a particular behavior leads to a negative outcome, which in turn is associated with intense physiologic arousal, then future initiation of the same behavior will reactivate the same arousal pattern, which in turn will facilitate the decision about aborting such a behavior. Importantly, detection of these physiologic changes may take place implicitly and without conscious awareness, allowing rapid "gut feeling" types of decisions in lieu of lengthy deliberation (Bechara & Damasio, 2005; Bechara, Damasio, Tranel, & Damasio, 2005). This "gut feeling" approach to making behavioral choices has come to be known as *emotional decision-making*.

In support of the somatic marker hypothesis, behavioral and autonomic deficits in implicit coding of negative consequence have been demonstrated among patients with ventromedial, but not other cortical, damage (Bechara et al., 1994; Bechara, Damasio, & Damasio, 2000). However, more recent research suggests the possibility that the ventromedial prefrontal cortex damage in the right, but not the left, hemisphere alone is sufficient for such deficits (L. Clark, Manes, Antoun, Sahakian, & Robbins, 2003; Tranel, Bechara, & Denburg, 2002). Additionally, similar decision-making deficits can be found among individuals with bilateral amygdala damage (Brand, Grabenhorst, Starcke, Vandekerckhove, & Markowitsch, 2007; Weller, 2007), and some research has shown that emotional decision-making is also disrupted by lesions in the dorsolateral or dorsomedial prefrontal convexities (Fellows & Farah, 2005; MacPherson, Phillips, Della Sala, & Cantagallo, 2008). Lastly, some research has shown that other cognitive domains, such as memory (Premkumar et al., 2008) and attention (Loesel & Schmucker, 2004), may contribute to emotional decision-making. In sum, despite the theoretical elegance of the somatic marker hypothesis as it relates to "gut decisions," the neuroanatomical substrates of somatic markers have yet to be definitively determined.

Discrepancy Detection. There are at least two systems that appear to contribute to effective detection of discrepancies between expectations and outcomes. One such system seems to rely on the integrity of the von Economo neurons and the fork neurons that form what some have called the "salience network" (Menon & Uddin, 2010). This network includes the anterior insula, the anterior cingulate gyrus, and the inferior frontal gyrus, primarily in the right hemisphere (Allman et al., 2010). These neurons exist only in highly social species and have therefore been hypothesized to play a role specifically in the detection of socially relevant discrepancies (Butti, Santos, Uppal, & Hof, 2013). There is in fact considerable evidence that selective degeneration of these neurons has a deleterious impact on the ability to maintain social and interpersonal appropriateness (E.-J. Kim et al., 2012). An additional discussion of the ramification of the social role of these neurons is presented in Chapter 6 on social cognition. However,

Chapter Summary

Response selection refers to one's ability either to inhibit an inappropriate response before it takes place or to stop a response that has already been initiated. The elemental processes that constitute RS include *threat sensitivity*, *contingency updating*, and *discrepancy detection* (all of which are largely implicit), as well as *inhibition* (which is typically a conscious, effortful process). Deficits in RS present as the disinhibited syndrome, which is characterized by impulsivity. The networks that subserve these elemental processes greatly overlap and include primarily the right inferior frontal gyrus, the right anterior insula, the anterior cingulate gyrus, and the amygdala. The most typical populations that are characterized by deficit in RS include persons with acquired injuries (primarily TBI), neurodegenerative disorders (primarily frontotemporal lobal deterioration [behavioral variant]), and ADHD.

5

Initiation/Maintenance and the Apathetic Syndrome

Defining the Construct

Initiation and Maintenance (I/M) of effortful cognitive and behavioral acts is exactly what it sounds like: It is one's ability to initiate behavioral and mental actions in a top-down fashion, as well as one's ability to continuously refresh one's mental set and thereby sustain behavioral or mental output. As was the case with response selection (RS; discussed in Chapter 4), it is once again important to dissociate I/M from executive cognitive functions (ECFs; discussed in Chapter 2), such that individuals with perfectly intact ECFs may still fail to initiate and follow through with appropriate behaviors (and vice versa). Importantly, however, the output of I/M can be both mental and behavioral, in that I/M is responsible for being the driving force not only behind externally observable actions but also behind exertion of *mental* effort. Thus, patients with deficits in I/M may fail to initiate planning or reasoning processes and consequently, in practical terms, may appear to exhibit symptoms of the dysexecutive syndrome. As was the case with RS, I/M elemental processes include both the effortful top-down control that is classically executive (i.e., the top-down *initiation* and *maintenance*) and a set of more implicit bottom-up processes that allow I/M to take place (collectively referred to later as *effort mobilization*).

Initiation. Initiation refers to an elemental cognitive process that takes place just prior to motor output. It is assumed that this process involves planning of a motor or verbal sequence, as well as integration of the emerging plan with stored representations or other prior knowledge. Initiation is sometimes referred to as "motor planning," "action planning," or "motor programming," which creates the impression that a deficit in this process has purely motor ramifications. However, much research has demonstrated that initiation and planning of motor output (particularly complex motor sequences) is highly correlated with EF (Kraybill & Suchy, 2008, 2011; Kraybill, Thorgusen, & Suchy, 2013; Suchy, Kraybill, & Larson, 2010), and that this correlation is particularly high for the latencies that directly precede motor output (Suchy & Kraybill, 2007). Additionally, the length of these action planning latencies is related to the magnitude of the so-called motor readiness potential, which in turn is correlated with EF, above and beyond simple motor or processing speed (Euler et al., 2015). When initiation is catastrophically impaired, the result is the complete inability to initiate action. When initiation is partially compromised, longer than usual delays occur prior to each motor or verbal output, and shorter response sequences may be bundled into each output, resulting in slower performance overall (Verwey, Abrahamse, Ruitenberg, Jiménez, & de Kleine, 2011).

To illustrate how slowed initiation may impact the speed of performance overall, consider two checkout clerks as they move grocery items from the conveyor belt across the scanner and into a bag. One clerk completes the task in half as much time as the other clerk, and yet by casual observation the slower clerk does not appear to be slacking off or moving his hands more slowly. However, a closer inspection of how the clerks approach the task provides some insight. The faster clerk picks up each item with his right hand and in a single smooth motion moves the item across the scanner, into his left hand, and into the bag. Furthermore, as soon as each item leaves the right hand, that hand initiates the next movement, already picking up the next item while the left hand is placing the previous item into the bag. This illustrates a highly efficient initiation process, such that multiple motor programs are loaded and released simultaneously, and each program contains multiple steps that are smoothly coordinated with one another. In contrast, the slower clerk picks up an item, briefly pauses, scans the item, briefly pauses, switches hands, briefly pauses, places the item in the bag, briefly pauses, picks up the next item with his right hand, and so on. Clearly, the slower clerk is not taking time to chat with coworkers, answer text messages, or engage in any other extraneous activity that would slow down his performance. Rather, this clerk's initiation ability is limited, such that only very brief motor programs can be loaded at a time. Readers may notice that the performance of the slower clerk is somewhat similar to that of some individuals with untreated inattentive attention deficit hyperactivity disorder (ADHD), especially those characterized by sluggish cognitive tempo, or patients with Parkinson's disease, as well as the performance of patients with more severe types of brain dysfunction.

Maintenance. Maintenance refers to the ability to *persist* with a behavioral output over a period of time. Other terms that have been used in this context are "persistence" or "vigilant attention." Importantly, maintenance is a more focused, or more discrete, process than the overarching meta-monitoring described in Chapter 3 (meta-tasking). That is, maintenance simply requires that a single attentional, cognitive, or behavioral set be continuously refreshed in the absence of external cues or prodding. As such, maintenance is closely related to, or possibly virtually synonymous with, the ability to sustain attention as assessed via continuous performance tasks. Research suggests that the ability to maintain attention relies on "refresh" cycles that last less than 10 seconds (Langner & Eickhoff, 2013), and it is the ability to continually and repeatedly refresh the set that allows maintenance across extended periods. Individuals with severely compromised maintenance may completely fail to refresh their mental set and thus be unable to sustain any action beyond a few seconds. Such failures are readily evident on simple tasks such as reciting the alphabet, wherein a patient's performance begins to slow down after the first few letters and shortly thereafter stops altogether; such severity would be typical, for example, of patients suffering from a delirium. Lesser impairments are characterized by more gradual slowing in performance and by losses of set (typically characterized by errors of omission or commission) that become evident over periods that span minutes rather than seconds; this level of impairment would be seen, for example, among patients with ADHD.

Effort Mobilization. Effort mobilization is an implicit characteristic that supports initiation and maintenance of actions (Matthews et al., 2010), just as the implicit elemental processes of threat sensitivity, contingency updating, and discrepancy monitoring described in Chapter 4 support RS. Effort mobilization refers to one's inherent tendency to move through the environment and to act upon or interact with objects or stimuli. In other words, effort mobilization is the intrinsic desire to "collect data" from the environment by interacting with it, whether physically or mentally; it is why animals explore new territory, even when not searching for food or mates; it is why humans play physical games or solve mental puzzles.

Effort mobilization has been described by different researchers as "behavioral activation" (Salamone, Correa, Farrar, & Mingote, 2007; Salamone,

Cousins, & Snyder, 1997), "psychomotor sensitization" (T. E. Robinson & Berridge, 2000), "energization" (Stuss, 2011; Stuss & Alexander, 2008), or simply "wanting" (Berridge & Kringelbach, 2008) and is thought to undergird the intention to move (Desmurget, 2013). Interestingly, effort mobilization can be heightened implicitly and without conscious awareness. It could also be said that effort mobilization is the energy that is responsible for boredom, that is, the energy that drives us to find something to do, either physically or mentally or both. Excessive effort mobilization, then, will present as agitation, whereas deficient effort mobilization will present as apathy.

Of note, effort mobilization is inextricably linked to sympathetic activation (Gendolla, 2012; Silvia, Nusbaum, Eddington, Beaty, & Kwapil, 2014), with some overlap in neuroanatomical underpinnings for both processes (Critchley, 2009). Additionally, effort mobilization is virtually inextricably linked to reward sensitivity, as sensitivity to rewards is what drives one to pursue goals that are expected to have rewarding consequences and to maintain response sets that are rewarding or adaptive. Reward processing can occur on an unconscious level and as such can have implicit impact on immediate physiology and effort mobilization (Gendolla, 2012; Silvia, Kelly, Zibaie, Nardello, & Moore, 2013; Wyvell & Berridge, 2000), or it can reach consciousness and can contribute to cognitive decision-making, as described in Chapter 2 (Pas, Custers, Bijleveld, & Vink, 2014). As rewards become more remote or more abstract, greater top-down effort is needed to initiate and sustain a given activity. For example, it is more difficult (or effortful) to initiate and sustain studying toward a remote goal of graduation, or to initiate and sustain an exercise routine toward a remote goal of becoming fit, than it is to initiate and sustain a brief activity toward a more immediate goal, such as getting food when hungry. As such, effort mobilization drives behaviors in patterns that parallel principles of operant conditioning. Effort mobilization can be influenced, or manipulated, in a top-down fashion via the ECFs system, such that one can purposefully search for and retrieve memories of remote goals (which are associated with remote, or delayed, rewards).

Effort mobilization appropriately fluctuates, such that fatigue following vigorous physical or mental activity leads to declines in effort mobilization, resulting in the prepotent desire to do nothing, or "veg." Importantly, effort mobilization is necessary for maintenance (or persistence) of actions or thoughts over time, especially if no external prompts are conspicuously present.

Table 5.1 provides an overview of how the elemental processes involved in I/M relate to daily life scenarios.

Table 5.1 Overview of elemental processes of initiation/maintenance (I/M) as they relate to everyday life scenarios

REAL-LIFE SCENARIO	ELEMENTAL PROCESSES OF INITIATION/MAINTENANCE		
	INITIATION	MAINTENANCE	EFFORT MOBILIZATION
Sorting family laundry into piles by person (e.g., self, spouse, children) and type (e.g., socks, underwear, outerwear).	Effectively initiate and chunk movements. • Remove two matching socks in one smooth movement. • Remove two or more items that belong to one person in one smooth movement.	Effectively maintain mental set. • Persist with the task without stopping or becoming distracted. • Keep track of the sorting principles.	Initiate and persist with the task, while maintaining appropriate tempo.
Ramifications of I/M failures in the context of the above scenario.	Reach for one item at a time and laboriously reinitiate search for new items after an item is removed.	Stop attending to the sorting principles and mistakenly make a single pile, or several piles sorted by the wrong principle.	Unable to muster the effort for task performance. Fail to initiate, or stop shortly after initiation.

Summary of the I/M Construct. Initiation/maintenance refers to the ability to initiate and maintain mental and behavioral actions. The elemental processes involved in I/M are *initiation, maintenance,* and *effort mobilization*. Whereas initiation is responsible for efficient planning and chunking of motor output, maintenance is responsible for continually refreshing the mental set approximately every 10 seconds so as to persist with a given task. Effort mobilization provides the energy that drives or motivates behavioral and mental output.

Other Relevant Constructs

Motivation. When thinking about various elements of I/M, one may be tempted to equate it with *motivation*, and this would be a fairly appropriate analogy to draw, as long as one understands that motivation is not the same as "desire." In other words, one may believe oneself to be very motivated to achieve a goal (i.e., *desiring* that goal) but not be motivated to actually engage in the behaviors that are needed toward the achievement of that goal. Thus, for example, it is possible for a person to deeply desire to lose weight and be physically fit, yet never initiate a diet or engage in an exercise routine due to lack of motivation.

Sluggish Cognitive Tempo. *Sluggish cognitive tempo* is a recently identified construct that is likely related to, or possibly synonymous with, diminished I/M. It is marked by slow motor and cognitive processing speed, poor ability to sustain attention, low arousal, and difficulties with initiation and persistence (Jacobson et al., 2012). Sluggish cognitive tempo is sometimes associated with ADHD-inattentive type, but many studies have shown that it is distinct from ADHD (Burns, Servera, del Mar Bernad, Carrillo, & Cardo, 2013; S. Lee, Burns, Snell, & McBurnett, 2014; Willcutt et al., 2014). Unfortunately, much research on sluggish cognitive tempo has examined cognition only via self-report, though a handful of studies of cognition in this population point to slow speed of processing, slow motor speed, and attentional difficulties (Barkley, 2014; Bauermeister, Barkley, Bauermeister, Martínez, & McBurnett, 2012; Becker & Langberg, 2014; Bernad, Servera, Grases, Collado, & Burns, 2014; Watabe, Owens, Evans, & Brandt, 2014). Interestingly, unlike ADHD, sluggish cognitive tempo is associated with relatively lesser reward sensitivity (Becker et al., 2013), which further supports its likely relationship to the construct of I/M.

Task-Rule Maintenance. Many activities, particularly meta-tasking, require active maintenance of multiple task rules in mind. This construct relies on somewhat different neuroanatomical substrates than I/M and requires top-down rehearsal of rules in verbal working memory. Functional imaging research has repeatedly demonstrated that maintaining set rules, especially in situations in which attention is divided between two tasks, is subserved by the left dorsolateral prefrontal cortex (G. C. Burgess et al., 2010; Fassbender et al., 2006; Fassbender et al., 2004; Santangelo & Macaluso, 2013), consistent with its reliance on verbal rehearsal. This is distinct from the more right hemisphere–dominant substrates for maintenance/attentional vigilance (see the "Neuroanatomy" section later in this chapter).

Typical Presentation of the Apathetic Syndrome

Cognitive and Behavioral Changes in Daily Life. The key feature of patients with the apathetic syndrome is slowness of output, apparent lack of motivation, and a lack of persistence. In less severe cases, this may simply present as the patient being cognitively slower than previously. In daily life, such patients appear to get less work done, and they fail to initiate and complete tasks, especially if not prompted. Patients may verbalize intentions and plans, but these may never come to fruition. Patients' personal space or workspace may be disorganized, in part because they may make repeated attempts to initiate new tasks but then fail to complete them. Other times, patients may appear to make erratic responses that are not consistent with obvious contingencies, such as abandoning a successful, reinforced response in favor of another, apparently random behavior (Hornak et al., 2004).

In extreme cases, a complete lack of initiation can occur, resulting in abulia or akinetic mutism (Marin & Wilkosz, 2005). These patients may appear mute and exhibit sparse volitional motor function, but they will track environmental stimuli and exhibit normal arousal. They may initiate certain automatic responses, such as joining in singing an overlearned song or in reciting the alphabet. Similarly, they may attempt to catch, or at least deflect, a ball that is thrown at them. However, when simply asked to do something, they will generally not respond in any way, as though they are not processing or hearing the request.

Personality Changes. Patients with apathetic syndrome are often described as unmotivated or "lazy." This may be seen by others as a fundamental change in personality, especially if the patient was premorbidly highly motivated or driven to succeed. Motivation is a driving force that is, on the one hand, strongly rooted in the biology of all species and, on the other, mistakenly viewed by humans as something we can control, something that gives us character and moral fiber, or something that we can talk our children, spouses, or friends into. Unmotivated people are sometimes judged harshly and angrily by others and are chastised in a manner that clearly blames them for their plight. For this reason, family members often believe that a decrease in motivation represents not only a change in personality but also possibly a willful refusal to participate in worthwhile pursuits, such as rehabilitation regiments or job searches. It is important to educate family members about the distinction between willful refusal and a brain-based deficit. After all, although no one would tell their child or their spouse to "get your act together and become smarter," people feel quite comfortable demanding that their loved ones become more motivated and "apply themselves." It may be helpful to use cognition as an analogy when explaining these issues to family.

In addition to being viewed by family as unmotivated or lazy, patients with apathetic syndrome may sometimes be viewed as being depressed or as "not being as fun" as they used to be. Thus, for example, a patient who was premorbidly seen by others as "the life of the party" is not interested in joining social gatherings or is slow to participate and is socially minimally interactive. Similarly, a quick-witted person may become "slow-witted," with little interest in initiating conversations, let alone entertaining others with funny stories or jokes.

Assessment Presentation. The key feature of test performance among patients with apathetic syndrome is slow performance across the board on all timed measures (Stuss, 2011). Additionally, on tasks that require that performance be sustained for a period of time, such patients' speed of performance further decreases with time. In patients with moderate deficit, this decline in speed can be evident fairly quickly and does not necessarily require that a given task span an extended period, such as is done, for example, with continuous performance tests. In fact, gradual decline in performance speed can become evident even on measures of fluency, color-word interference, or digit symbol coding. In more severe cases, patients will exhibit complete lack of persistence, stopping performance within seconds rather than just slowing down. Alternatively, patients may sometimes continue to respond but lose mental set even when a given response has been repeatedly reinforced. Importantly, errors are characterized not by deficient reasoning but by a failure to pursue rewards or failures in favoring rewards over punishments.

Because patients with apathetic syndrome are characterized by a ubiquitous deficit in performance speed across virtually all types of tasks, it may be difficult to distinguish them from patients with poor processing speed. However, a careful examination of performance profile along with behavioral observations is likely to provide useful clues. Specifically, patients with poor processing speed are likely to perform equally poorly throughout the day, whereas patients with initiation and maintenance deficits may fluctuate more in their speed, often performing faster early on in a task and slowing down as the task progresses. Also, unlike patients with poor processing speed, patients with deficits in initiation and maintenance are likely to require more prompting and redirecting throughout testing sessions.

With respect to overall test profile, tests of fluency (both verbal and nonverbal) and color-word interference often exhibit the lowest scores (G. Robinson, Shallice, Bozzali, & Cipolotti, 2012; Stuss, 2007). Additionally, on the Wisconsin Card Sorting Test and on the Halstead Category Test, these patients may exhibit frequent losses of set, while exhibiting no difficulty identifying the correct sorting principle. Importantly, unlike the reversion to a prior mental set exhibited by patients with impaired response selection, the losses of set associated with the apathetic syndrome are more likely to appear nonsensical, erratic, or random. See Table 5.2 for an overview of the association between the elemental processes of I/M and typical neuropsychological measures presumed to assess EF.

Exceptions to the Rule. Although it is fairly clear that deficits in I/M can result from structural and metabolic brain insults, some individuals without any brain abnormalities may appear "unmotivated" by choosing lifestyles that prioritize leisure activities, or social and family activities, over career achievements or financial pursuits. This may be viewed by some as a sign of "laziness" or a "lack of motivation," but it should not be mistaken for apathetic syndrome. In fact, although such individuals may be uninterested in (or apathetic about) career-related pursuits, they may keep "busy" reading, spending time in conversations with family, or playing games with friends. It should also be noted that there are cultural differences in the degree to which career versus family and leisure are prioritized.

Neuroanatomy

Initiation. Initiation of motor output relies on a network that includes the anterior cingulate gyrus, the rostral medial prefrontal cortex, and the supplementary motor area (Hoffstaedter et al., 2014; Volle et al., 2012). Presupplementary motor area was further found to relate to chunking of output sequences (Ruitenberg, Verwey, Schutter, & Abrahamse, 2014). Initiation

Table 5.2 Overview of the association between the elemental processes of initiation/maintenance (I/M) and typical neuropsychological measures presumed to assess EF

	INITIATION	MAINTENANCE	EFFORT MOBILIZATION
Trail-Making (Switching Condition)	Rapidly initiate response.	Persist with task.	Maintain fast tempo throughout task.
Verbal Fluencies	Rapidly initiate response.	Persist with task.	Maintain fast tempo throughout task.
Design Fluencies	Rapidly initiate response.	Persist with task.	Maintain fast tempo throughout task.
Stroop Tests	Rapidly initiate response.	Persist with task.	Maintain fast tempo throughout task.
Wisconsin Card Sorting Tests	N/A	Persist with task and maintain the most recently reinforced sorting principle.	N/A
Halstead Category Test	N/A	Persist with task and maintain the most recently reinforced classification principle.	N/A
Tower Tests	N/A	Persist with task and maintain the logic of sequencing of move.	N/A

appears to be heavily dependent on dopamine, with initiation differences evident among medicated and unmedicated patients with Parkinson's disease (Tremblay et al., 2010). Of note, the neuroanatomical distinction between initiation and effort mobilization is somewhat blurred depending on a given research paradigm; for example, initiation related to reinforcement has been linked to reward-sensitive striatal regions (Schlund, Magee, & Hudgins, 2012), covered under effort mobilization.

Maintenance. A recent extensive review that integrated the results of a meta-analysis of functional imaging research with the literature review of lesion studies identified a complex network of regions that are important for continually refreshing mental set (Langner & Eickhoff, 2013); the network proposed by this study was largely right hemisphere–dominant and included the dorsomedial and ventromedial prefrontal cortices, the anterior insula, the intraparietal sulcus, the temporoparietal junction, the cerebellar vermis, thalamus, putamen, and midbrain. Other studies that have focused on dissociating the networks needed for maintenance of stable task sets from the networks needed for other potentially confounded processes reported the importance of medial superior frontal gyrus (Wilk, Ezekiel, & Morton, 2012), caudal premotor cortex (Stelzel, Kraft, Brandt, & Schubert, 2008), dorsal anterior cingulate gyrus and medial superior frontal cortex, and anterior insula and frontal operculum (Dosenbach et al., 2007).

Effort Mobilization. Neuroanatomical networks that subserve effort mobilization are inextricably linked to the substrates for reward sensitivity, most notably the mesolimbic dopaminergic system, including ventral striatum (nucleus accumbens; Faure, Reynolds, Richard, & Berridge, 2008; Fuchs, Ramirez, & Bell, 2008; Salamone et al., 2007; Volle et al., 2012). The network further includes the anterior cingulate gyrus, supplementary motor area, anterior insula, and the thalamus (Burke, Brünger, Kahnt, Park, & Tobler, 2013; Cho et al., 2013; Knutson et al., 2014; Mutschler, Reinbold, Wankerl, Seifritz, & Ball, 2013; Pessoa, 2009).

Typical Etiology of Impairments in I/M

Initiation/maintenance is often affected among patients with focal lesions involving the superomedial frontal structures, most typically as a result of a space-occupying lesion, an injury, or a cerebrovascular accident (CVA) involving the anterior cerebral artery or anterior communicating artery (Tibbetts, 2001). In most severe cases, a complete inability to engage in volitional action or speech occurs (known as *akinetic mutism*), typically associated with bilateral damage to the anterior cingulate cortex (Nicolai, van Putten, & Tavy, 2001; Tibbetts, 2001). Less frequently, akinetic mutism has been associated with bilateral thalamic or mesencephalic infarctions (Alexander, 2001; Cavanna et al., 2009), as well as bilateral globus pallidus infarctions (Mega & Cohenour, 1997). Additionally, akinetic mutism is also a common presentation of the final stages of Creutzfeldt-Jakob disease (Iwasaki, Mimuro, Yoshida, Kitamoto, & Hashizume, 2011; Kowalczyk et al., 2013; Satoh et al., 2007) and has been reported in patients suffering from anoxia and carbon monoxide poisoning (Rozen, 2012; Tengvar, Johansson, & Sörensen, 2004), multiple sclerosis (T. F. Scott, Lang, Girgis, & Price, 1995), toxicity related to certain pharmacologic treatments (Sierra-Hidalgo et al., 2009), and bilateral epileptiform discharges (Nicolai et al., 2001).

In contrast to akinetic mutism, less severe cases of apathetic syndrome may simply be characterized by a lack of initiation without prompting, sometimes referred to as *amotivational syndrome*, or difficulty sustaining attention. This less severe presentation can be seen in a wide range of patients, including those with infarctions within the basal ganglia (Quattrocchi & Bestmann, 2014; Rochat, Van der Linden, et al., 2013), moderate to severe traumatic brain injury (Larson, Kelly, Stigge-Kaufman, Schmalfuss, & Perlstein, 2007; Zoccolotti et al., 2000), and/or dysfunction in the dopaminergic systems (Adam et al., 2013). Additionally, apathetic syndrome is commonly seen among patients suffering from neurodegenerative disorders, including Parkinson's disease (Czernecki et al., 2002), Alzheimer's disease (Cook, Fay, & Rockwood, 2008), vascular dementia (Sparto et al., 2008), and frontotemporal lobar dementia (Chow et al., 2009). Importantly, gait freezing (or problems initiating gait) among patients with Parkinson's disease appears to be related to the same I/M system, specifically problems with motor planning/initiation (Knobl, Kielstra, & Almeida, 2012). Lastly, right hemisphere prefrontal and premotor lesions secondary to CVAs are associated with high frequency of motor impersistence, as well as more general problems with initiation and maintenance of motor output (Seo et al., 2009).

Interestingly, although initiation of movement is thought to be a hallmark symptom of Parkinson's disease, research suggests that slow initiation in these patients is related to cognitive processes that take place prior to response output (Stelmach, Teasdale, & Phillips, 1992), consistent with the conceptualization of initiation in this chapter. For example, patients with Parkinson's disease who are off medication fail to plan motor sequences several movements at a time (Tremblay et al., 2010), reminiscent of the example of the slow checkout clerk earlier in this chapter.

In addition to neurological conditions, neurodevelopmental and neuropsychiatric conditions can also be associated with I/M deficits. Most notable among these is ADHD-inattentive or combined type (Klimkeit, Mattingley, Sheppard, Lee, & Bradshaw, 2005; O'Driscoll et al., 2005; O'Brien, Dowell, Mostofsky, Denckla, & Mahone, 2010) and schizophrenia (Faerden et al., 2009; Grootens et al., 2009), both of which tend to be associated with difficulties with initiation and maintenance; and major depressive disorder, which tends to be associated with impaired reward sensitivity and effort mobilization (Shankman et al., 2013; Silvia et al., 2014). Lastly, reward sensitivity and associated I/M difficulties can be seen among individuals who are under acute and chronic stress (Berghorst, Bogdan, Frank, & Pizzagalli, 2013; B. D. Nelson et al., 2013).

Chapter Summary

Initiation/maintenance refers to a subdomain of EF that controls the effectiveness, speed, and maintenance of motor output and associated mental processes. The elemental processes that subserve I/M include *initiation, maintenance*, and *effort mobilization*. Deficient I/M results in an apathetic syndrome, which is characterized by sluggish behavioral and mental output, inadequate chunking of actions into a single motor program, and an inability to sustain actions across time. The neuroanatomical underpinnings of I/M are quite complex, including most notably the supplementary motor area, anterior cingulate cortex, distributed attentional network (relying primarily on the right hemisphere), and mesolimbic dopamine system. Typical populations characterized by the apathetic syndrome include patients who have suffered an infarct affecting medial frontal structures and those who have neurodegenerative disorders or ADHD.

6

Social Cognition and the Socially Inappropriate Syndrome

Defining the Construct

Social cognition (SC) is not always considered to fall under the EF umbrella. Yet, when considering the evolutionary purpose of EF, one cannot ignore the fact that EF in animals (primitive as it may be) is virtually always related to appropriate response selection (RS) within the context of social situations. An additional examination of the animal world reveals that the most consistent correlate of brain size is not only performance on animal analogues to EF tasks but also the degree to which a given species engages in social behavior (Dunbar, 1998; Reader & Laland, 2002). Similarly, in human children, there appears to be a link between SC and the development of EF (Aro, Laakso, Määttä, Tolvanen, & Poikkeus, 2014; Hensler et al., 2014; Zelazo, Chandler, & Crone, 2010), such that SC and EF begin to jointly emerge in early childhood (S. T. Baker, 2009). Thus, SC and EF have likely evolved in tandem, both phylogenetically and ontogenetically. Translated into intraspecies functioning, individuals who do not receive the proper socially relevant signals fail to engage EF processes as needed and therefore, for all intents and purposes, are executively impaired.

Concretely, SC refers to one's ability to understand social norms, to comprehend complex social situations, to be aware of one's impact on others, and to be able to act in socially appropriate ways. Although passive understanding of social norms certainly relies in part on crystallized knowledge or familiarity with a given culture, successful application of such norms depends on elemental emotional processes, including (a) emotional self-awareness and (b) emotional communication. Impairments in either one of these processes is likely to result in behaviors that are socially inappropriate or calloused, and decisions that may be viewed by others as insensitive, inconsiderate, or impulsive. Note that although additional elemental processes could be included under the umbrella of SC, a full examination of all aspects of emotional processing is beyond the scope of this chapter (for a more detail treatment, see Suchy, 2011, Chapters 2–6).

Emotional Self-Awareness. Emotional self-awareness refers to an explicit, conscious knowledge of one's own feelings. It relies on two related but distinct neurocognitive processes. The first is *interoceptive awareness*, or the ability to detect physiologic processes or changes within one's own body, such as racing heartbeat, increased perspiration, or flushing cheeks. The second is *feeling awareness*, or the ability to detect, understand, and talk about one's own feelings. This means that individuals with good feeling awareness not only can detect when they are anxious, angry, or happy but also can reflect on the sources of such feelings and link these feelings to appropriate verbal labels so as to describe them to others. In general, individuals with better interoceptive awareness tend to experience their feelings more intensely and also tend to be more aware and have a better understanding of what they are feeling (Heims, Critchley, Dolan, Mathias, & Cipolotti, 2004; Pollatos, Gramann, & Schandry, 2007; Pollatos, Kirsch, & Schandry, 2005). An exception to this rule are individuals with alexithymia, which is characterized by (a) an inability to be aware of, understand, or talk about one's own emotions while (b) being keenly aware of one's own physiologic reactions, but misinterpreting associated bodily sensations as signs of physical illness rather than emotions (Connelly & Denney, 2007). In other words, alexithymic individuals have poor feeling awareness in the context of normal or even superior interoceptive awareness. For more on alexithymia, see the section on typical presentation of the inappropriate syndrome later in this chapter.

Emotional Communication. Emotional communication is a complex construct that can be examined along at least two orthogonal axes. These are (a) the *mode* of emotional communication (i.e., paralinguistic vs. linguistic vs. situational) and (b) the *direction* of emotional communication (i.e., receptive vs. expressive; for a review, see Suchy, 2011, pp. 112–115; see Table 6.1).

Although the paralinguistic mode of emotional communication is fairly self-explanatory, the linguistic and situational modes warrant further explanation. First, regarding the linguistic mode of emotional communication, the

Table 6.1 Emotional communication matrix

DIRECTION	EMOTIONAL COMMUNICATION MODE		
	PARALINGUISTIC	LINGUISTIC	SITUATIONAL (AKA SOCIAL AWARENESS)
Receptive	The ability to *understand* affective expression in • Tone of voice • Facial expression • Gestures • Posture	The ability to *understand* emotional content in • Figures of speech • Connotative language • Allusions	The capacity to *understand* • Social norms • Social interactions • Emotional experiences of others (empathy)
Expressive	The ability to *generate* affective expression in • Tone of voice • Facial expression • Gestures • Posture	The ability to *express* emotional content by way of • Figures of speech • Connotative language • Allusions	The capacity to *produce* behaviors/verbalizations that are consistent with social norms

important issue here is *not* whether a person understands and uses emotional words or content (e.g., using the words *sad, angry, happy*, etc.) but whether a person can *glean* emotion when it is only implied, or *produce* statements that imply emotion. Put differently, the question is whether a person can communicate about emotions indirectly. Thus, for example, the statement "She was left all alone" may imply sadness, loneliness, or disappointment, without actually having to say the words *sad*, or *lonely*, or *disappointed* (Karow, Marquardt, & Marshall, 2001).

In contrast to the verbal messages subsumed under linguistic communication, the situational mode of emotional communication essentially refers to *social awareness*, that is, our ability to understand social norms, to comprehend social interactions, and to have insight into emotional experiences of others (i.e., emotional and cognitive empathy), regardless of whether language is involved. As mentioned earlier, understanding of social norms is in part a function of crystallized knowledge (such as knowing when to say "please" or "thank you"), and these aspects of social norms are typically explicitly taught to us from early childhood. Other aspects of social norms are learned implicitly through daily interactions, such as the appropriate duration of eye contact or the appropriate physical proximity during a conversation. In contrast, some aspects of social awareness are inherent and fairly universal (although they still interact with social norms to some extent), such as understanding the feelings of others during tragic or joyous events.

Note that the focus of this chapter is *not* on people's strengths and weaknesses in social awareness as a function of prior social exposure or prior explicit learning. Rather, this chapter focuses on one's neurocognitive *capacity* for social awareness, that is, the capacity to acquire and flexibly adjust one's understanding of social norms, as well as one's capacity for comprehension of social scenarios and one's capacity for empathy. Of note, empathy itself is not a unitary construct, such that the ability to cognitively understand the emotional ramifications of a given situation have been termed *cognitive empathy*, whereas the ability to feel how others feel has been termed *emotional empathy* (A. Smith, 2006). Importantly, both behavioral and neuroanatomical research has shown that the two types of empathy are dissociable (Dziobek et al., 2008; Shamay-Tsoory, Aharon-Peretz, & Perry, 2009; Shamay-Tsoory et al., 2003).

As mentioned earlier, SC and its components (i.e., self-awareness and emotional communication) play an important role in EF, in that they represent an important source of signals and cues that fine-tune RS, as discussed in Chapter 4. The reader may recall that Chapter 4 presented a scenario in which a driver arrived at an intersection and needed to make a choice between running the yellow light or stopping. In such a scenario, a multitude of signals and cues entered into implicit calculations that ultimately fed into the selection of a response, that is, stopping versus going. One can easily translate this scenario into one wherein traffic lights are replaced by social signals. For example, just as in the original scenario in Chapter 4, you could be driving to an important meeting, running late. This time, however, you have a passenger—a colleague with whom you carpool to work. Suddenly, your colleague's cell phone rings. He answers the phone and, unbeknownst to you, receives the news of his fathers' death. In this scenario, many aspects of SC immediately begin to come into play. See Table 6.2 for an overview of SC processes that will contribute to your subsequent actions.

Summary of the SC Construct. Social cognition refers to the ability to understand one's own feelings as well as those of others, and the ability to understand and adhere to social norms. Elemental processes that contribute to SC include *linguistic, paralinguistic*, and *situational modes of emotional communication*, as well as *emotional self-awareness*. Different modes of emotional communication allow one to comprehend indirect or nonverbal emotional messages and to respond to them in a socially appropriate manner. Connotative language, facial expressions and prosody, and the ability to be empathic are all examples of emotional communication and fall under this category. Emotional self-awareness allows one to have insight about one's own feelings, which is necessary for modulation of behavior and adherence to social norms.

Other Relevant Constructs

Humor and Sarcasm. Although humor and sarcasm processing is somewhat beyond the scope of the present topic, it is nevertheless clear that the ability to comprehend humor and sarcasm relates, among other things, to the ability to detect incongruities (Y.-C. Chan et al., 2013; Samson, Hempelmann, Huber, & Zysset, 2009) that are often social in nature. Additionally, humor and sarcasm comprehension are related both to general intelligence and to executive functioning (EF) (Kipman, Weber, Schwab, DelDonno, & Killgore, 2012; Tsoi et al., 2008), relying on broad networks that overlap to some extent with networks that are important for various aspects of EF (Bartolo, Benuzzi, Nocetti,

Table 5.2 Overview of elemental processes of social cognition (SC) as they relate to everyday life scenario

REAL-LIFE SCENARIO	ELEMENTAL PROCESSES OF SOCIAL COGNITION				
	EMOTIONAL COMMUNICATION				EMOTIONAL SELF-AWARENESS
	PARALINGUISTIC MODE	LINGUISTIC MODE		SITUATIONAL MODE	
You are driving to an important meeting. A passenger in your car receives a phone call that informs him that his father passed away.	Detect paralinguistic signs of distress, such as signs of concern in the tone of voice. In return, express empathy via nonverbal cues.	Detect emotionally relevant statements in your passenger's phone conversation that are not necessarily concrete or explicit, such as him asking, "Is mom doing okay?" Verbally express empathy and concern, such as, "Is everything okay at home?"		Understand that your passenger is in distress (cognitive empathy) and momentarily experience sadness for his loss (emotional empathy). Understand that your passenger may need to be driven back home so he can start making arrangements.	Recognize your own empathic reaction, as well as other emotional reactions, such as potential frustration over missing the meeting. Modulate these reactions to maintain socially appropriate demeanor.
Ramifications of SC failures in the context of the above scenario.	Not notice anything is wrong. Keep driving and conversing as if nothing had happened.	Not able to "read between the lines," and thus remaining oblivious to the actual content of the phone conversation. Keep driving and conversing as if nothing happened.		Failing to appreciate the ramifications of the situation (sadness/grief, need to go back home to start making arrangements, etc.).	Failing to understand one's own feelings, resulting in irritability and anger evident in tone of voice and facial expression.

Baraldi, & Nichelli, 2006; Kipman et al., 2012; K. K. Watson, Matthews, & Allman, 2007). Thus, it is generally worthwhile to assume that patients with deficits in EF in general and in SC in particular may also exhibit deficits in humor and sarcasm comprehension. This may also explain why individuals with deficits in SC may engage in inappropriate humor.

Theory of Mind. *Theory of mind* (ToM; Premack & Woodruff, 1978) refers to our ability to understand that other people around us have their own internal mental worlds. In other words, we understand that other people have thoughts, feelings, knowledge, and memories, and that these are distinct from our own thoughts, feelings, knowledge, and memories. It is this understanding that allows us to make judgments about what others do or do not know, and to gauge our own ability to judge whether we understand the other person's mind. Theory of mind also allows us to understand that others do not have access to our thoughts. Thus, for example, rather than accosting another person with the statement, "That was a great movie," we first explain that we saw a particular movie, followed by a question about whether the other person saw that same movie as well, and then within that context proceeding to share our experience of the movie.

Properly functioning ToM is important for normal interpersonal and social functioning, and at least some evidence suggests that there are networks that are uniquely devoted to performance of ToM tasks (Bach, Happé, Fleminger, & Powell, 2000). Consequently, ToM is often classified as a component of SC. However, there is also some evidence that the ability to perform ToM tasks may rely in large part on other EF subdomains and elemental EF processes already described throughout this book, such as executive cognitive functions (ECFs) and/or working memory, as well as inhibition (Carlson, Moses, & Breton, 2002; Fahie & Symons, 2003; Jha, 2012; Mutter, Alcorn, & Welsh, 2006; Ogawa & Koyasu, 2008; Ting et al., 2006). For this reason, although the construct of ToM has utility in assessment of SC, it is not included in this chapter as a separate core elemental process.

Emotion Regulation. Different aspects of emotion regulation (i.e., cognitive reappraisal and expressive suppression) have already been discussed in Chapters 2 and 4, respectively, as these emotion regulation strategies rely on ECFs and inhibition, respectively. However, both of these strategies also rely on some aspects of SC. Specifically, in order to engage in emotion regulation, one needs to have adequate emotional self-awareness, so as to recognize that emotion regulation needs to take place. In addition, because expressive suppression primarily serves the purpose of maintaining social appropriateness, it is intimately linked to social awareness, such as understanding social expectations and norms. Thus, although one's sheer capacity to engage in expressive suppression is independent of social awareness, the answers to the questions of when, how, or whether one implements expressive suppression depend on how well one understands social norms.

Typical Presentation of the Socially Inappropriate Syndrome

Cognitive, Behavioral, and Personality Presentation in Daily Life. There are a number of ways in which deficits in SC interfere with other EF subdomains. With respect to emotional self-awareness, emotionally unaware individuals cannot adequately consider their own feelings when deliberatively making decisions or when weighing the pros and cons of various actions. Thus, their plans or courses of action may appear poorly reasoned, counterintuitive, or even self-destructive. Along the same lines, unaware individuals cannot appropriately alter their facial or other nonverbal expressions to make them be in line with desired plans and goals, because, once again, they lack insight about how they feel (Connelly & Denney, 2007). Thus, they may behave in a hostile manner when it would benefit them to be polite, or may communicate amusement when it would behoove them to appear somber; such inappropriate behaviors are typically interpreted by others as reflecting poor emotional and behavioral control, callousness, or a lack of prosocial sentiment. Interestingly, poor cognitive and behavioral control appears to be comorbid with poor emotional self-awareness (rather than just being exacerbated by it), as individuals with poor self-awareness also perform more poorly on measures of EF (Xiong-Zhao, Xiao-Yan, & Ying, 2006). In light of these findings, it should not be surprising that individuals with poor emotional self-awareness tend to have lower educational and occupational achievement (Jin, Mai, & Ding, 2001; Lunazzi de Jubany, 2000).

Unawareness of one's own feelings also precludes patients, virtually by definition, from engaging in emotion regulation, as described in Chapter 2. Consequently, unaware individuals cannot take steps to alter their feelings or their mood (because there is nothing to alter as far as they are concerned), which places them at an increased risk for developing psychiatric disorders, including depression, anxiety, eating disorders, and substance abuse disorders (Abbate-Daga et al., 2013; Guilbaud et al., 2002; Henry, Phillips, Crawford, Theodorou, & Summers, 2006; Henry, Phillips, Maylor, et al., 2006; Karukivi, Vahlberg, Pölönen, Filppu, & Saarijärvi, 2014; Mangelli, Semprini, Sirri,

Fava, & Sonino, 2006; Porcelli et al., 2013) and possibly even psychosomatic illnesses (Kojima, 2012).

A particular type of poor emotional self-awareness is *alexithymia*, which is a syndrome characterized by poor feeling awareness in the context of normal or even superior interoceptive awareness (Connelly & Denney, 2007; Stone & Nielson, 2001). This combination of keen sensitivity to physiologic states along with the inability to understand that such states may be related to emotions places individuals at a particular risk for somatization (Porcelli et al., 2013). This is particularly relevant to neuropsychology when somatization is comorbid with, or even masquerades as, a neurologic condition or insult. For example, alexithymia has been shown to be a factor in psychogenic seizures (R. J. Brown et al., 2013), postconcussive complaints (Wood, Williams, & Kalyani, 2009), dizziness (von Rimscha et al., 2013), and fibromyalgia and other pain conditions (A. Landa, Bossis, Boylan, & Wang, 2012; Tuzer et al., 2011). It has been suggested that whereas primary alexithymia represents a heritable personality trait, secondary alexithymia may result from a brain insult (Messina, Beadle, & Paradiso, 2014). More on the latter can be found in the section on etiology of impairments in SC later in this chapter.

In addition to impaired emotional self-awareness, impaired paralinguistic communication and social awareness will clearly interfere with adaptive interpersonal functioning, as well as with other aspects of EF. In particular, the inability to understand social and interpersonal cues via tone of voice, facial expressions, or indirect verbalizations interferes with the normal ability to rapidly respond behaviorally to emotional feedback, which in turn interferes with adaptive RS as described in Chapter 4. Consequently, patients may appear impulsive, especially in social situations or in situations where past social disapproval should have been noted and utilized for future adaptation of behavior. Such situations in particular may create the impression of patients willfully disregarding rules or wishes of others. In more extreme cases, patients' behaviors may be grossly out of line with social norms, such as engaging in public sexual acts, theft, or physical aggression.

Clearly, although some of the presentation in daily life may appear to be cognitive, such as an apparent deficit in planning or reasoning, the majority of behaviors among such patients are interpreted as changes in personality. For example, individuals who were premorbidly caring, empathic, and thoughtful of others are viewed as suddenly being calloused, reckless, or even psychopathic. Regardless of the interpretation, there is a common thread of behaviors that are apparently self-destructive: Patients may be angry and argumentative, suspicious and accusatory, or depressed and rejecting. Due to a lack of awareness and a lack of emotional communication, they place the blame for their physical or psychological discomfort on others, pushing their supports away and "burning bridges" with the very people who are in a position to provide help, including not only family and friends but also health care providers (Kovarsky, Schiemer, & Murray, 2011).

Assessment Presentation. Although the socially inappropriate syndrome cannot be detected by traditional measures of EF, problems in SC can be measured using some nontraditional tests, such as the Social Cognition subtests of the WAIS-IV Advanced Clinical Solutions (Pearson, 2009) or the Awareness of Social Inference Test (TASIT; S. McDonald, Flanagan, & Rollins, 2002). Additionally, patients' inappropriateness may become apparent via behavioral observations. For example, patients may engage in socially inappropriate verbalizations or attempts at humor, may inappropriately express anger and frustration, or may blame the examiner for the length of the examination. Sometimes, a patient may behave more like a "cranky" child than an adult or may present with some version of a temper tantrum. Patients with more severe impairment may engage in grossly inappropriate acts, such as touching themselves sexually during the session or mouthing objects.

Exceptions to the Rule. It is fairly clear that deficits in SC have an impact on patients' functioning, but one should not assume that all patients who are behaving inappropriately have sustained a neurologic insult. Inappropriate behavior may sometimes be a function of a person's personality, familial or cultural background, "antiestablishment" mentality, attention getting, or an inherent lack of concern for rules and for the welfare of others. Thus, it is important for clinicians to establish that inappropriate behavior represents a change from premorbid functioning.

Neuroanatomy

Emotional Self-Awareness. As mentioned earlier, emotional self-awareness relies on two separate processes: interoceptive awareness and feeling awareness. These two processes are mutually dissociable not only behaviorally but also neuroanatomially. With respect to interoceptive awareness, the right anterior insula and the right frontal operculum are involved in processing of a variety of interoceptive signals, including heartbeat (Critchley, 2009; Critchley, Wiens, Rotshtein, Ohman, & Dolan, 2004; Hoelzel et al., 2008; Pollatos et al., 2007), respiratory rate (Cameron & Minoshima, 2002), and skin temperature/perspiration (Davis, Pope, Crawley, & Mikulis, 2004;

Fredrikson et al., 1998), all of which are affected by changes in autonomic activation associated with emotional experiences.

Regarding feeling awareness, it appears that the signals from the anterior insula and operculum are further processed and interpreted in a distributed network that includes the dorsolateral prefrontal cortex, anterior and posterior cingulate cortex, and pons and cerebellum (Karlsson, Naaanen, & Stenman, 2008; Mantani, Okamoto, Shirao, Okada, & Yamawaki, 2005; Moriguchi et al., 2007), as well as the general integrity of the right hemisphere (Larsen, Brand, Bermond, & Hijman, 2003) and the corpus callosum (Tabibnia & Zaidel, 2005). For a comprehensive review, see Wingbermühle, Theunissen, Verhoeven, Kessels, and Egger (2012) and Messina and colleagues (2014).

Paralinguistic Mode. Although paralinguistic communication could be divided into more discrete categories based on the medium (facial, prosodic, postural, etc.) and the direction (receptive vs. expressive), the relevant networks largely overlap, and a detailed discussion of slight differences in neuroanatomy of individual subcategories is beyond the scope of this chapter. See Suchy (2011, pp. 119–122) for a more comprehensive review. On the whole, it appears that the most important structures for paralinguistic communication (both expressive and receptive) are the right orbitofrontal, frontal-opercular, and anterior cingulate cortices, as well as the basal ganglia and the thalamus (Blonder et al., 2005; Heilman, Leon, & Rosenbek, 2004; Hornak et al., 2003; Karow et al., 2001; Kipps, Nestor, Acosta-Cabronero, Arnold, & Hodges, 2009; T.-W. Lee, Josephs, Dolan, & Critchley, 2006; Ross & Mesulam, 2000).

The reader may notice an anomaly in the functional organization of paralinguistic communication, such that (unlike other sensory/receptive processing) *comprehension is localized anteriorly.* This anomaly likely reflects the close interaction between receptive and expressive aspects of emotional and social processing. Specifically, it has been suggested that our understanding of the emotional expressions relies in part on our ability to implicitly mirror those expressions, interpreting the associated feelings as we experience them. This notion is consistent with several prominent theories, including embodied emotions (Niedenthal, 2007; Niedenthal, Winkielman, Mondillon, & Vermeulen, 2009) and mirror neuron theory (Ginot, 2009; Pineda, Moore, Elfenbeinand, & Cox, 2009; Shamay-Tsoory et al., 2009).

Lastly, paralinguistic communication is also dependent on the integrity of the amygdala. Specifically, the amygdala and the orbitofrontal cortex together become reliably activated in response to paralinguistic cues such as emotional faces, prosody, and emotional postures, and damage to the amygdala (and/or connections of the amygdala with the orbitofrontal cortex) leads to impairments in paralinguistic communication (Atkinson & Adolphs, 2005; R. L. C. Mitchell & Ross, 2013; Whalen et al., 2013). Interestingly, although the amygdala is known to respond to emotionally salient stimuli in general, the ability to detect emotional stimuli in general appears to be distinct and dissociable from the ability to detect stimuli that have uniquely social significance (South et al., 2008).

Linguistic Mode. Although deficits in emotional linguistic communication clearly have a deleterious impact on social functioning, this area is greatly understudied. The sparse research that does exist is highly inconsistent. In general, both left and right hemisphere temporal lobe structures have been implicated in receptive processing (Beaucousin et al., 2007; Dietrich, Hertrich, Alter, Ischebeck, & Ackermann, 2008), and primarily the right hemisphere has been implicated in expressive processing (Borod, Bloom, Brickman, Nakhutina, & Curko, 2002).

Situational Mode (aka Social Awareness). Social awareness appears to rely on several distributed networks that have both theoretical and empirical associations with this construct. These are von Economo neuron networks, the mirror neuron system, and ToM networks.

Von Economo neurons are large neurons that are unique to humans, great apes, elephants, and some large marine mammals. They are presumed to serve the function of rapid communication among distant brain regions in large brains. These neurons are located primarily in the anterior insula and anterior cingulate gyrus; they send projections to multiple regions of the prefrontal cortex but primarily the orbitofrontal cortex (Allman et al., 2010). Because of the involvement of the anterior insula and cingulate cortex network in error detection in general, and in the detection of socially relevant error signals in particular, it is believed that these neurons play a role in our ability to rapidly alter our behavior in response to social disapproval, distress in others, guilt and embarrassment, and prosocial feelings and actions. Consequently, these neurons are thought to facilitate social awareness, toward the end of rapid intuitive social decision-making (Allman, Watson, Tetreault, & Hakeem, 2005; Brüne et al., 2010; Butti et al., 2013; Cauda et al., 2013; Craig, 2009; E.-J. Kim et al., 2012; G. Miller, 2010; Santos et al., 2011; Seeley et al., 2006; Seeley et al., 2012; Triarhou, 2006; Viskontas, Possin, & Miller, 2007).

The mirror neuron system[1] has been shown to play an important role in one's implicit tendency to imitate both simple actions and complex behavioral patterns observed in others (Heyes, 2011; Kanakogi & Itakura, 2010). The core aspects of this system include the inferior frontal gyrus and somatosensory cortex, as well as occipital, parietal, and temporal regions that play a role in visual processing (Rizzolatti & Craighero, 2004; Rizzolatti, Craighero, & Fadiga, 2002). Much evidence suggests that this system is important not only for imitation of gross motor action but also for imitation of subtle emotional displays evident in facial expressions, tone of voice, and posture (Kircher et al., 2013; Pfeifer & Dapretto, 2009). Thus, not surprisingly, the mirror neuron system is important for SC in general, and for paralinguistic communication and cognitive and emotional empathy in particular (Baird, Scheffer, & Wilson, 2011; Hooker, Verosky, Germine, Knight, & D'Esposito, 2010).

Similarly, ToM appears to be important for one's ability to understand not only what others know or what they might be thinking but also how or what they are feeling. Not surprisingly, then, much functional imaging research has shown that this network becomes activated when one is experiencing or processing cognitive empathy (H. Walter, 2012). The ToM network consists of medial prefrontal and medial orbitofrontal cortices, anterior paracingulate cortex, superior temporal gyrus, and temporoparietal juncture (Carrington & Bailey, 2009); however, lesion studies suggest that only medial orbitofrontal cortex is necessary for cognitive empathy to take place (Shamay-Tsoory et al., 2009).

Typical Etiology of Impairments in SC

Given the fairly heterogeneous networks and processes involved in SC, there is a wide range of populations that exhibit deficits in this subdomain. Importantly, some populations exhibit deficits in some discrete aspects of SC, such as only deficient understanding of certain emotions (e.g., poor understanding of anger but normal understanding of happiness) or deficient emotional empathy in the context of normal cognitive empathy. Full

---

[1] Although there is some controversy about the existence of actual mirror neurons in humans, the neuroanatomical networks that are associated with the mirror neuron construct have been consistently identified. This review is not intended to endorse, or refute, the existence of mirror neurons per se, but rather to identify networks that are associated with imitation, especially as it relates to emotional processing.

coverage of the specific patterns of deficits found in specific populations is beyond the scope of this chapter. For a more comprehensive review, see Suchy (2011, Chapters 3–7). In the following, only the most salient issues are highlighted.

First, research has repeatedly demonstrated fairly global impairments in SC among patients with traumatic brain injury, particularly those with ventral frontal lesions (Koponen et al., 2005; S. McDonald, 2013; Wood & Williams, 2007; Wood et al., 2009). Studies examining discrete deficits in SC have fairly consistently found poor facial affect recognition (Radice-Neumann, Zupan, Babbage, & Willer, 2007) and poor cognitive and emotional empathy (Shamay-Tsoory et al., 2004).

Second, SC is deficient in a variety of neurodevelopmental disorders. The most prominent among these are autism spectrum disorders (ASDs), which are characterized by deficits across many aspects of SC, most notably deficits in recognition of facial and prosodic affect and deficits in empathy (Hubbard & Trauner, 2007; Humphreys, Minshew, Leonard, & Behrmanna, 2007); of note, emotional empathy appears to be less impaired than cognitive empathy (Dziobek et al., 2008). Social cognition deficits in this population likely involve both abnormalities in the amygdala and abnormalities within distributed cortical networks that subserve ToM and the mirror neuron system (Hornak et al., 2004; Kenemans et al., 2005; Tsuchida, Doll, & Fellows, 2010).

In addition to ASD, deficits in receptive paralinguistic communication are present among individuals with attention deficit hyperactivity disorder (Boakes, Chapman, Houghton, & West, 2008; Da Fonseca, Seguier, Santos, Poinso, & Deruelle, 2009; Ibáñez et al., 2011) and in children and adults with Down syndrome (Kasari, Freeman, & Hughes, 2001; Wishart, Cebula, Willis, & Pitcairn, 2007), fragile X syndrome (Hagan, Hoeft, Mackey, Mobbs, & Reiss, 2008; Hessl et al., 2007), and fetal alcohol syndrome (Monnot, Lovallo, Nixon, & Ross, 2002), as well as in women and girls with Turner syndrome (Geuze, Vermetten, & Bremner, 2005; Mazzola et al., 2006; Skuse, Morris, & Dolan, 2005). Lastly, agenesis of corpus callosum is associated with severe reduction in von Economo neurons, with as much as 90% reduction among patients with complete agenesis and 50% reduction in those with partial agenesis, which likely explains these patients' social/interpersonal problems and the high rates of alexithymia (Badaruddin et al., 2007; L. K. Paul et al., 2006).

Third, SC deficits are apparent in a number of neurodegenerative disorders. From among these, frontotemporal lobar degeneration (FTD) represents the best-known example of impaired SC, including impairments in facial and prosodic affect recognition and cognitive empathy (Fernandez-Duque & Black, 2005; Lough et al., 2006; Snowden et al., 2008). Although it is generally believed that such deficits are unique to the frontal variants of FTD, patients with the temporal variant (e.g., semantic dementia) are also affected, with deficits in cognitive and emotional empathy being particularly pronounced (Rankin, Kramer, & Miller, 2005). Additionally, the behavioral variant of FTD is characterized by targeted degeneration of von Economo neurons, especially early on in the disease process, likely explaining these patients' gross deficits in social awareness, self-awareness, and empathy (Seeley et al., 2006). In fact, research suggests that as much as 75% of von Economo neurons degenerate early in the disease process (E.-J. Kim et al., 2012; Seeley et al., 2007). Given that von Economo neurons play a role in detection of socially relevant discrepancies, it should not be surprising that patients with FTD are also impaired at sarcasm detection (Kipps et al., 2009). In contrast, although patients with Alzheimer's disease do exhibit some losses of von Economo neurons, this reduction is proportionate to their overall neuronal loss (Seeley et al., 2007); consequently, they do *not* exhibit notable deficit in comprehending sarcasm until much later in the disease (Kipps et al., 2009).

In addition to FTD, patients suffering from other dementias, including Alzheimer's, vascular, Parkinson's, and Huntington's dementias, as well as amyotrophic lateral sclerosis, exhibit impairments in self-awareness and/or paralinguistic communication (Bogdanova & Cronin-Golomb, 2013; Dujardin et al., 2004; Lavenu & Pasquier, 2004; Rankin, Baldwin, Pace-Savitsky, Kramer, & Miller, 2005; Snowden et al., 2008; Zimmerman, Eslinger, Simmons, & Barrett, 2007). Importantly, mild SC deficits can begin to emerge early in some diseases, predating the onset of other cognitive symptoms. This is particularly true for amyotrophic lateral sclerosis (particularly the bulbar variant; Zimmerman et al., 2007) and Parkinson's disease (with deficits unrelated to the severity of motor symptoms; Dujardin et al., 2004).

Fourth, neuropsychiatric conditions are, virtually by definition, characterized by deficits or weaknesses in SC. For example, paralinguistic communication weaknesses are commonly reported among patients with schizophrenia (Addington & Addington, 1998; Shamay-Tsoory, Shur, Harari, & Levkovitz, 2007), mood disorders (Bozikas, Tonia, Fokas, Karavatos, & Kosmidis, 2006; Weniger, Lange, Rather, & Irle, 2004), and substance abuse disorders (Foisy et al., 2005; Kornreich et al., 2001; Monnot et al., 2002; Monnot, Nixon, Lovallo, & Ross, 2001; Philippot et al., 1999; Uekermann, Daum, Schlebusch, & Trenckmann, 2005). In addition to Axis I disorders, individuals with personality disorders also exhibit weaknesses in SC. Most notable among these are individuals with antisocial personality disorder (especially those capable of committing heinous crimes), who exhibit impairments in empathy (Kirsch & Becker, 2007) and paralinguistic communication (Carr, Iacoboni, Dubeau, Mazziotta, & Lenzi, 2003; Dolan & Fullam, 2006; Hastings, Tangney, & Stuewig, 2008; Kosson, Suchy, Mayer, & Libby, 2002; McCown, Johnson, & Austin, 1986; McCown, Johnson, & Austin, 1988; Suchy, Whittaker, Strassberg, & Eastvold, 2008).

Lastly, individuals with bilateral amygdala calcification secondary to Urbach-Wiethe disease exhibit deficits in detection and comprehension of socially and emotionally salient stimuli (including recognition of facial affect), memory for such stimuli, and difficulties learning from incentives (Brand et al., 2007; Hurlemann et al., 2007; Siebert, Markowitsch, & Bartel, 2003). To a lesser degree, patients with a history of prolonged febrile seizures in childhood or patients with epilepsy who have undergone anterior temporal lobectomy may also exhibit milder forms of these deficits (Cendes et al., 1993; Gloor & Aggleton, 1992).

Chapter Summary

Social cognition refers to one's ability to appropriately respond to social cues and to generate behaviors that are socially appropriate. The elemental processes that subserve SC include *emotional self-awareness*, as well as three types of *emotional communication* (linguistic, paralinguistic, and situational). Deficits in SC present as the inappropriate syndrome, which is characterized by poor responsiveness to social and interpersonal cues. Patients with severe deficits may engage in behaviors that are grossly inappropriate; less impaired patients may simply appear to be disregarding rules or the wishes of others and may engage in actions that appear self-destructive or counter to stated goals. Deficits in SC are not always correctly identified, and patients' inappropriate actions sometimes alienate their social support network or health care professionals. Neuroanatomical networks that subserve SC are highly distributed and include primarily the amygdala and its connections with the orbitofrontal cortex, cortical networks that subserve the theory of mind and the mirror neuron system, and von Economo neurons; in general, the right hemisphere plays a dominant role. Due to the highly distributed nature of these networks, many patient populations are characterized by some degree of impairment in SC; however, the most prominent examples include persons with traumatic brain injury, autism spectrum disorders, agenesis of corpus callosum, behavioral variant FTD, schizophrenia, substance abuse, and psychopathy/antisocial personality disorder.

PART THREE

CLINICAL ASSESSMENT OF EXECUTIVE FUNCTIONS

This part of the book covers the challenges in clinical assessment of executive functioning (EF), with a particular focus on providing guidance for how to *apply* the information provided in previous chapters *to interpretation of clinical data*. In other words, the next three chapters examine the familiar clinical tools utilized in a typical clinical practice through the theoretical lens of EF subdomains and the associated clinical syndromes. The first chapter of this part offers an overview of how to extract diagnostically useful information about EF from patient records, interviews, and behavioral observations and how to align such information with the syndromes described previously. The second chapter reviews the challenges associated with formal assessment of EF, including important psychometric characteristics (and limitations) of typical EF measures, and threats to construct validity that also represent a threat to valid clinical interpretations. The third chapter then offers some guidance for clinicians on how to deal with the various challenges of EF assessment, as well as guidance on how to integrate test data with other clinical information. This chapter also introduces the Contextually Valid Executive Assessment (ConVExA) model, which offers a framework for interpretive considerations, as well as a roadmap for future directions in EF research. The reader should know that this part is not intended to provide a cookbook, step-by-step approach to assessment and interpretation, nor does it offer laundry lists of tests or procedures. It is assumed that readers already possess solid general clinical skills and are therefore able to incorporate the information presented here into their current clinical practices.

7

Gathering Background Information

Assessment of executive functioning (EF) poses many challenges that have been well described in the literature. Among the most frustrating aspects of EF assessment is the fact that the structured clinical setting and the standardized test administration procedures do not allow for adequate generalization of patients' functioning to an unstructured, nonstandardized environment. Consequently, as compared with other neurocognitive domains, EF assessment relies rather heavily on background information gathered from patients' records and interviews, as well as casual observation of soft signs of EF dysfunction. This chapter offers some guidance on how to get the most out of available background information and behavioral observations, and how to align such information with the various EF syndromes.

Records Review

Gathering and reviewing records represents an inherent aspect of any neuropsychological evaluation (Heilbronner, Sweet, Morgan, Larrabee, & Millis, 2009). In cases of suspected EF deficits, a review of records can play an extremely important role, as some aspects of EF dysfunction are not readily detectable with standardized tests alone. Ideally, to the extent possible, records would be obtained and reviewed prior to the scheduled appointment with a patient, to allow follow-up or clarification questions during the interview, both with the patient and, if possible, with a collateral source. The types of records that are particularly useful include (a) school and/or work records,

(b) medical/psychiatric records, and (c) legal/criminal records. Table 7.1 provides an overview of the kind of information that is typically available from different types of records.

In reviewing the records, the clinicians should focus on gleaning information about the following: (a) the highest premorbid level of EF ability, (b) the time course of EF decline/change, and (c) the type, frequency, and severity of EF difficulties in daily life.

Records Reflecting Highest Premorbid Level of EF Ability. School and work records are particularly useful for determining the highest premorbid level of EF. Records reviewed for this purpose should encompass time *prior* to the onset of symptom through the present. To determine how well a patient functioned premorbidly, available job performance evaluations need to be considered in the context of the complexity of a given job. Additionally, in some cases simply the fact that one achieved and maintained a high-level position is a sufficient indicator of good premorbid abilities. Table 7.2 provides an overview of major job categories and associated EF-dependent duties.

Table 7.1 Overview of record types

RECORD SOURCE	RECORD INFORMATION
Work/Personnel File	• Application form, résumé, letter of interest, etc. • Test results (if testing was required by employer) • Regular (often yearly) evaluations of performance • Promotions/demotions/termination • Incident reports • Disciplinary actions/remediation plans • Exit interview summary
School	• Report cards/transcripts • Performance on standardized tests (sometimes including national, regional, and school-specific norms) • Attendance • Incident reports • Remediation plans • Termination/transfer if relevant

Table 7.1 (Continued)

RECORD SOURCE	RECORD INFORMATION

Medical/Psychiatric	• Inpatient
	  ○ Admission and discharge summaries
	  ○ Emergency room reports
	  ○ Physician notes
	  ○ Nursing (and other allied professions) notes
	  ○ Test results (e.g., neuroradiology, blood work)
	  ○ Procedure summaries (e.g., surgery)
	• Outpatient
	  ○ Office visit summary
	  ○ Letters/reports to referring physicians
	  ○ Test results (e.g., neuroradiology, blood work)
	  ○ Outpatient procedure summaries (e.g., surgery)

Legal/Criminal	• Law enforcement agencies (police, sheriff, highway patrol, etc.)
	  ○ Incident reports
	  ○ Traffic offenses
	  ○ Arrests
	  ○ Charges
	  ○ Investigations/interviews
	• Department of corrections (jail/prison)
	  ○ Convictions/sentences
	  ○ Sentencing
	  ○ Admission/processing/orientation records
	  ○ Work records
	  ○ Conduct records/incident reports
	  ○ Release record
	• Attorney
	  ○ Depositions

Importantly, different jobs place different demands on the various *subdomains* of EF. For example, it is virtually impossible to complete graduate training in clinical psychology without a high degree of initiative, an ability to sustain pursuit of long-term goals, organizational and meta-tasking abilities, and good social awareness. Similarly, individuals in managerial jobs typically require a high level of social skills and the ability to plan activities for others;

Table 7.2 Job categories and associated EF-dependent job duties

JOB TYPE	JOB REQUIREMENTS
Executive/Senior-Level Officials and Managers (e.g., CEO, COO, CFO, chief information officers, chief human resources officers, chief marketing officers, chief legal officers, management directors and managing partners)	• Formulate, plan, and direct policies. • Develop strategy and provide the overall direction of enterprises or organizations for the development/delivery of products or services. • Follow the parameters put forth by boards of directors or other governing bodies. • Plan, direct, or coordinate activities with the support of subordinate executives and staff managers.
First/Mid-Level Officials and Managers (e.g., vice presidents and directors; group, regional, or divisional controllers; treasurers; human resources, information systems, marketing, and operations managers)	• Oversee and direct the delivery of products, services, or functions at group, regional, or divisional levels of organizations. • Receive directions from the executive/senior level management. • Lead major business units. • Implement policies, programs, and directives of executive/senior management through subordinate managers and within the parameters set by executive/senior level management.
Managers (e.g., first-line managers; team managers; unit managers; operations and production managers; branch managers; administrative services managers; purchasing and transportation managers; storage and distribution managers; call center or customer service managers; technical support managers; and brand or product managers	• Directly report to middle managers. • Direct and execute the day-to-day operational objectives of officials and managers to subordinate personnel. • In some instances, directly supervise personnel.

Table 7.2 (Continued)

JOB TYPE	JOB REQUIREMENTS
Professionals (e.g., agents; business managers; analysts; scholars/scientists; financial/insurance agents; attorneys; medical personnel; general contractors; small business owners)	• Exercise discretion, judgment, and personal responsibility. • Apply an organized body of knowledge that is continually changing/evolving. • Make new discoveries and interpretations. • Improve data, materials, and methods.
Technical and Clerical (sales workers; administrative assistants; data managers; carpenters; plumbers; repair; cable installers, etc.)	• Carry out tasks, methods, procedures, and/or computations that are laid out in either published or oral instructions and covered by established precedents or guidelines. • May require a high degree of technical skill, care, or precision.
Unskilled	• Carry out tasks that are laid out in either written or oral instructions.

individuals in various professional positions require a great deal of initiation/maintenance, so as to sustain pursuit of long-term goals in the absence of a supervisor acting as the driving force; and individuals in jobs that require efficient maneuvering through hectic, busy work environments require a strength in meta-tasking. Table 7.3 provides an overview of how different EF subdomains relate to different job duties. Note that Tables 7.2 and 7.3 only provide a starting place. Follow-up questions in the interview will likely further refine where you might expect a given patient was prior to onset of symptoms.

Importantly, job or school records often only provide an indication of the *lowest necessary* level of premorbid functioning for good job performance. Thus, although one can assume that low average performance on EF measures represents a decline for a patient who was previously the CEO of a company, one should *not* assume that low average performance reflects an appropriate level of functioning for a patient who engaged in unskilled labor prior to symptom onset. Consider, for example, an undocumented immigrant who simply never had the opportunity for a higher educational and occupational

Table 7.3 Matching EF subdomains with common EF-dependent job duties

EF SUBDOMAIN	JOB-RELATED DUTIES AND CAPACITIES
ECT	• Planning and organization of complex projects to be executed by others, generating solutions for problems (e.g., directors, CEOs) • Planning one's own activities in the absence of existing organizing structure imposed by a boss (e.g., graduate students; small-business owners)
MT	• Completing multiple tasks at once (e.g., administrative support staff; nurses; graduate students) • Efficiency in a hectic or busy environment (e.g., administrative support staff; nurses; graduate students; emergency room physicians)
RS	• Exercising good judgment/choices in hectic and busy environment (e.g., nurses, physicians) • Adaptively learning from experience (e.g., physicians; small-business owners; directors)
I/M	• Initiative/motivation and the ability to sustain pursuit of one's own long-term goals in the absence of existing demands by a supervisor (e.g., graduate students; small-business owners)
SC	• Understanding societal rules (all jobs requiring interaction with the public) • Ability to engage in social/emotional give-and-take with others (e.g., sales; public relations) • Insight about one's own emotions and one's impact on others (e.g., public relations office; health care professionals)

attainment prior to symptom onset. Thus, once again, supplementing records with a detailed interview is key for gathering useful information about premorbid level of functioning.

Records Reflecting Time Course of EF Decline/Change. In some patients, the onset of impairment is straightforward, such as in cases of traumatic brain injury or a stroke. In other patients, onset is more insidious, and determining the time course of the illness is key for diagnostic decision-making. In such cases, legal and medical records are particularly useful for gleaning the timing of symptom onset, as well as objective evidence of change/decline. Legal records will contain any legal infraction or an incident that comes to the attention of law enforcement agencies. Thus, for example, a sudden onset of repeated traffic violations, minor car accidents, or aggressive outbursts may offer a fairly solid timeline of a patient's onset of symptoms, and this evidence may predate reported difficulties in school or at work. Similarly, medical records will detail every encounter of the patient with medical personnel. Thus, once again, sudden onset of accidental injuries, as well as hospital admissions due to episodes of confusion, psychosis, or emotional dysregulation, may provide a good window of the patient's onset of decline.

In contrast to legal and medical/psychiatric records, work/school records may, or may not, provide a good picture of the initial onset and course of decline. On the one hand, in most jobs, employees are reviewed regularly (often yearly) by supervisors, and written records of such reviews are kept. Similarly, work or school records may sometimes contain documentation of absences, tardiness, or other types of infractions, as well as documentation of a remediation plan and the employee's or student's successes or failures in fulfilling such a plan. All such records may prove helpful in trying to discern the history of a patient's EF decline. On the other hand, in some work or school settings, the initial infractions may be dealt with informally, and an official record may not exist. In such situations, official records of problems may only begin to appear when the employer, supervisor, or faculty committee come to recognize that a problem is intractable, persistent, or serious enough to warrant demotion or dismissal. Unfortunately, it is sometimes only at this point that a "paper trail" begins to emerge, often with the goal of protecting the employer or educational agency from lawsuits. In such cases, a decline in functioning may have lasted for a year or longer before the first official mention of a problem appears in the employee's or student's file.

Records Reflecting the Type, Frequency, and Severity of EF Difficulties in Daily Life. Because EF is a multifaceted construct, the *types* of difficulties patients with EF impairments exhibit in daily life are also multifaceted. Table 7.4 offers an overview of issues that may be found in patient records and their relationship to different EF syndromes.

Note that some symptoms appear similar across different syndromes. In order for a clinician to make helpful recommendations, however, it is important to identify which subdomain of EF is at the root of the patient's symptoms. As an illustration, consider the following example.

Table 7.4 EF deficits evident in patient records

SYNDROME	WORK/SCHOOL RECORDS	LEGAL RECORDS	MEDICAL/PSYCHIATRIC RECORDS
Dysexecutive	• Unable to generate plans, solve problems, coordinate job components • Poor judgment	• Work-related offenses, such as not following through with a contract due to *poor planning*	• Depression
Disorganized	• Unable to complete assignments and follow through with plans • Taking too long • Making mistakes • Tardiness	• Work-related offenses, such as not following through with a contract due to *poor organization* • Traffic accidents and moving violations	• Mania, agitation • Personal injury due to inability to multitask (e.g., stove catching on fire) • Dehydration, electrolyte imbalance
Disinhibited	• Making impulsive decisions and impulsive mistakes • Emotional outbursts • Poor judgment	• Traffic accidents and moving violations • Aggression, assault, destruction of property	• Mania, agitation • Personal injury due to impulsive mistakes • Emotional outbursts, aggression
Apathetic	• Unable to complete assignments or follow through with plans • Taking too long • Making mistakes • Tardiness	• Work-related offenses, such as not following through with a contract due to *apathy*	• Abulia and apathy • Depression • Dehydration, electrolyte imbalance
Inappropriate	• Emotional outbursts • Lability • Inappropriate/insensitive jokes, comments • Poor judgment	• Arrests for public urination, masturbation, etc. • Inappropriate sexual advances	• Public urination, masturbation, etc. • Inappropriate sexual advances

A patient is a general contractor who has begun to experience difficulties completing jobs and, as a result, has begun to experience financial difficulties. The situation came to a head when a client sued him for taking a deposit for a major remodel of a home but then not completing the job. Based on other clinical signs, you determine that this patient is suffering from a progressive decline in EF. However, it would be instructive to determine why this patient has been unable to complete jobs in his role as a general contractor. There are several options:

> Scenario 1: The patient may he suffering from *dysexecutive syndrome*, finding it difficult to coordinate or organize the various components of a job and failing to generate appropriate plans. For example, the patient may simply make arrangements for the kitchen to get painted prior to placing an order for having the old sink taken out. Similarly, the patient may be unable to solve problems when something goes wrong. For example, if one of the subcontractors has to cancel due to illness, the patient may become immobilized and fail to generate an alternative solution.
>
> Scenario 2: The patient may be suffering from *disorganized syndrome*. Thus, the patient may generate an initial plan for how the job should be completed. However, when it comes time to executing the plan, the patient does not follow through, completing some, but not all, requisite tasks or completing tasks out of order. For example, the patient may fail to place all the requisite work orders or to follow through with his subcontractors to make sure each step of the remodel is getting completed as planned.
>
> Scenario 3: The patient may be suffering from *apathetic syndrome*. Thus, he simply fails to take steps toward getting the job started, let alone completed. In other words, the patient may *think about* getting the job done but instead watches TV at home or sits in his office doing nothing.

Although on the surface the final outcome is the same, that is, the job is not getting done, understanding the underlying cause will inform recommendations for potential compensatory strategies, as well as recommendations for the level of independence the patient may be able to handle. In fact, it is also important to determine that the patient's inability to get the job done is a change from premorbid level of functioning, rather than simply a reflection of the patient's long-standing antisocial or psychopathic tendencies. A careful review of records would aid with the latter differential.

In addition to considering the types of problems and the underlying causes, it is important to consider the severity and frequency of problems. Specifically, if the patient's difficulties have resulted in documented problems at work, multiple encounters with the legal system, or multiple hospital admissions, a lack of supervision is bound to result in serious consequences. If, on the other hand, the patient's difficulties are limited to not being able to handle complex tasks at work due to a mild dysexecutive syndrome, then simply stepping down from a high-responsibility position may be the only intervention that is needed for the time being.

Interview With Patient and Collateral Sources

As stated earlier, a review of records represents a starting point for a clinician. To place the information from the patient's records into a proper context, an in-depth interview with the patient and at least one collateral source would ideally take place prior to selection of a testing battery. Interviews with both a patient and a loved one can shed further light on the premorbid level of functioning, the course of EF difficulties, and the nature and severity of current symptoms.

Interviewing About the Premorbid Level of EF Ability. Although work or school records provide a good starting point for understanding the patient's premorbid level of functioning, supplementing such records with an interview is crucial. First, an interview will allow the clinician to gather information about the degree to which the patient's occupational or educational achievements matched his or her native abilities. For example, in the course of an interview, it may become apparent that the patient's high occupational achievement was in part a function of much scaffolding provided by a spouse or a parent. Additionally, it may become clear that the patient struggled with his job throughout his life, always coming home exhausted and unable to participate in any additional executively demanding home activities. In the same vein, the patient may have brought work home and solicited help from family members in order to complete job responsibilities in a timely manner. In sum, such a patient may have maintained the appearance of competence at work (reflected in work records), yet was always functioning somewhat marginally, just barely keeping up with job demands. In such situations, even a relatively mild decline in EF is bound to lead to a considerable decline in work performance, one that may become evident in work records; importantly, in such situations, it may appear that a drastic and clinically relevant decline in EF occurred, when in reality perhaps even normal age-related changes in EF or changes in the patient's family situation could explain the apparent drastic declines in functioning. In contrast, another patient may have always handled her high-level job easily, typically coming home still full of energy and ready to embrace additional challenges. In this latter case, a mild decline in EF may be associated with no discernible change in performance at work but instead be evident at home, such that the patient may begin to exhibit fatigue and hesitance or unwillingness to face executively demanding challenges. These examples illustrate why it is important for the clinician to ask questions that will solicit information about the patient's premorbid capacity relative to objective educational or occupational achievement.

Second, the clinician should inquire about the actual level or complexity of a given job, as well as how competitive one needs to be in order to secure a particular position. This is because in some cases an identical job title may be associated with different degrees of complexity. For example, being selected to serve as the CEO of a major international company is considerably more competitive then becoming the CEO of a smaller, home-run business. Similarly, with respect to educational achievement, different schools require different scores for entrance exams, as well as different levels of achievement for passage. For example, there is a sizable difference in the admission requirements for Harvard Law School versus those for a regional third-tier law school.

Third, aside from school or job, daily life may provide many insights into a patient's premorbid EF ability. For example, was the patient organized and efficient in paying bills, preparing meals, planning travel, or organizing parties? Was the patient able to initiate and complete large projects? Was the patient capable of independently dealing with nuisances such as a broken water pipe, a leaking roof, or a broken appliance? Was the patient able to step up in emergencies, such as an illness of a loved one? Did the patient like to explore new things, such as new travel destinations, new recreational activities, or new technologies? For an overview of questions about premorbid functioning, see Table 7.5.

Interviewing About the Time Course of EF Decline/Change. When trying to understand the onset and the course of a patient's EF difficulties, the clinician should carefully match information available in the records with the interviewee's recall of the symptom onset and progression. For example, when the interviewee is uncertain about the order of events or their time frame, a clinician may facilitate the process by asking the interviewee to try

Table 7.5 Interview: Gathering information about premorbid functioning and course of decline

	TOPICS TO INQUIRE ABOUT

Premorbid Functioning	• Objective difficulty/complexity of prior jobs/course work
	• Subjective difficulty/complexity of prior jobs/course work
	• Enjoyment of or pursuit of new experiences, such as
	  ○ meeting new people
	  ○ traveling to new destinations
	  ○ trying new foods, new restaurants, new theaters, etc.
	  ○ picking up/learning new hobbies, sports, skills
	  ○ new technologies, such as cell phone upgrades, new computer etc.
	• Prior experience and ease vs. difficulty with
	  ○ meal preparation
	  ○ shopping
	  ○ bill paying
	  ○ cleaning/homemaking
	  ○ remodeling/repair projects around the house
	  ○ yard care, etc.
	• Prior experience and ease vs. difficulty with
	  ○ Planning/organizing events, parties, trips
	  ○ Solving unexpected problems, such as leaking roof or leaking pump, plugged toilet, bills lost in the mail, etc.

Course of Decline	• Did all symptoms appear at once or did they emerge gradually over time? • If symptoms did not emerge at once, could it be that there was a lack of opportunity for some of the symptoms to be observed previously? • Which symptoms were the first to appear? • How frequently were symptoms observed (daily, weekly, etc.)? • Were there symptoms that were not noticed at first, but in retrospect represented unusual behaviors/actions?

to recall when certain events occurred relative to other known events that are documented in the patient's records. Additionally, interview information can supplement much needed context for the purely factual information in the records. For example, it would be important to find out whether difficulties at work coincided with a major stressor, such as an illness or the death of a loved one. See Table 7.5 for an overview of sample questions to be asked in a clinical interview about the course of change in cognition.

Interviewing About the Type, Frequency, and Severity of EF Difficulties in Daily Life. When inquiring about EF symptoms, it is best to first ask the patient and/or the collateral source an open-ended question, simply asking them to describe what changes they have noticed. In this portion of the interview, the clinician needs to be vigilant to follow up descriptions of problems with clarifying questions to ensure that the exact nature of the patient's difficulties is correctly communicated. For example, if the patient reports that he has been forgetful, it is important to follow up with questions that will clarify whether the patient has difficulty with encoding, retrieving, and retaining information, or whether the forgetfulness simply reflects poor prospective memory. Similarly, when a patient complains of not being able to get things done, it would be important to clarify whether this is caused by disorganization (disorganized or dysexecutive syndrome), a failure to initiate (apathetic syndrome), or being easily distracted by other competing activities (disinhibited syndrome).

After the initial unstructured questioning and clarifying follow-up questions, it is helpful for the clinician to ask more systematically about other potential areas of EF difficulties as they relate to individual EF syndromes. As always, interview questions should focus not just on the nature of symptoms but also on the time course and the broader context in which symptoms began to emerge (e.g., stress, a major loss, a major change). Table 7.6 provides a list of sample questions a clinician may use to gain further insight into a patient's symptoms, as well as mapping those symptoms onto different EF syndromes.

Behavioral Observations and Pathognomonic Signs

Problems with EF sometimes become evident even prior to the patient's arrival for an evaluation. Patients with EF deficits, especially those with disorganized or disinhibited syndrome, may repeatedly reschedule or miss their appointment due to double-booking themselves with other activities or mistakenly marking the appointment on the wrong date or the wrong time slot in their

Table 7.6 Interview: Gathering information about the type of EF difficulties

SYNDROME	SAMPLE QUESTIONS
Dysexecutive	• Have you noticed changes in the ability/willingness to come up with plans for travel, holiday parties, home improvement projects, etc.? • Have you noticed changes in the ability/willingness to generate solutions in emergencies, such as when encountering plumbing problems, or when someone close to you becomes ill and needs help?
Disorganized	• Have you noticed a change in the ability to be on time for appointments or meetings with others? • Have you noticed a change in the ability to complete tasks, even when you start out with a good plan? • Have you noticed a change in the ability to complete tasks by deadlines, even when you are spending a great deal of time working on them?
Disinhibited	• Have you noticed an increase in making impulsive decisions and impulsive mistakes? • Have you noticed a change in the ability to show good judgment? • Have you noticed a change in the ability to control/hide emotions, anger, or frustration?
Apathetic	• Have you notice a change in motivation? • Have you noticed a change in energy levels? • Have you noticed a change in the ability to start projects? • Have you noticed a change in the ability to stick with projects through completion?
Inappropriate	• Have you noticed a change in the ability to judge what is or is not appropriate (OR Have people around you been complaining, perhaps unfairly, about some of your actions or behaviors)? • Have you noticed a change in the ability to behave appropriately (OR Have you done some things that people around you feel are inappropriate)? • Have you noticed a change in the ability to be sensitive to feelings of others (OR Have people around you been mentioning that you have been insensitive to their feelings, and is this a change from how things used to be)?

planner. Similarly, such patients may also arrive late for their appointment. Patients with disorganized syndrome in particular are prone to arriving late, in some cases even if arriving with a companion, as these patients' meta-tasking deficits often derail not only their own actions but also plans and actions of those around them.

Depending on the nature and severity of patients' EF difficulties, however, behavioral signs of EF deficits may or may not be evident per casual observation. Patients who have mild disorganized, dysexecutive, or apathetic syndrome in particular may appear executively intact per casual observation within the structured setting of a testing session. However, with increasing severity of symptoms, telltale signs of a dysfunction may begin to emerge.

Dysexecutive and Disorganized Syndromes. In addition to arriving late, patients with disorganized syndrome may fail to bring requested items, such as reading or hearing aids or a list of medications. They may also be observed to become discombobulated if given multiple forms to fill out while in the waiting room. However, once in the structured context of discrete testing instructions, such patients tend to be compliant, cooperative, and appropriately engaged in testing.

Disinhibited Syndrome. The most obvious sign of a disinhibited syndrome is the patient's tendency to begin responding prior to questions being fully asked or to begin to work on a task before the instructions are fully read. Such patients are prone to needing multiple and repeated reminders to wait for the examiner to tell them to begin. In more severe cases, these patients may reach over to the examiner's side of the testing table for a pencil or for other testing materials, or may repeatedly rummage through their pockets for a cell phone or other objects. Such patients may at times also unexpectedly stand up and leave the room to use the restroom or to satisfy some other random urge. Additionally, they may perseverate on an idea or an action. For example, a patient may repeatedly reach for his or her cell phone, or may repeatedly raise a subject he or she wants to discuss or a question he or she seeks an answer to. In severe cases, echolalia and utilization behaviors (i.e., magnetic apraxia) may also be present. With such patients, examiners need to be constantly on their toes, and the testing session is more reminiscent of an evaluation of a child even if the patient is an adult: In other words, constant supervision is key, and never letting a patient out of one's sight (or at least peripheral vision) is necessary.

Apathetic Syndrome. Mild symptoms of apathetic syndrome may not be readily apparent per casual observation, as the structure of the testing session and the built-in prompts associated with many tests (e.g., "keep going") tend to preempt any blatant problems with initiation or maintenance of behavior. However, patients with more severe deficits may exhibit EF difficulties even in the context of a structured testing session. For example, a clinician working with such a patient may find herself needing to provide more prompts than is typical, repeatedly reminding the patient to "keep going" and to "go as quickly as you can." It is sometimes readily apparent that such patients begin a task at a reasonable pace following the examiner's initial prompt but then noticeably slow down as the task proceeds. Of course, if the initiation/motivation deficits are severe, patients may not respond at all—such patients are not appropriate for formal testing, and only informal behavioral/qualitative evaluation may be possible.

Inappropriate Syndrome. There is virtually no limit to the types of inappropriate behaviors that patients with this syndrome may engage in. Unlike the other syndromes, in this case the structure of the testing session does not shield the patient, and even mild deficits may become apparent in the course of the interview and testing. Mild deficits are most likely to present as inappropriate comments, such as remarks that are inappropriately casual or familiar, or remarks that are sexual in nature. Such patients may at times perseverate on an inappropriate topic and repeatedly return to it, regardless of the fact that the examiner repeatedly and obviously tries to steer away from it.

As a cautionary note, however, clinicians need to consider the patient's background and prior levels of comfort with personal disclosures or observance of societal norms. For example, a higher level of education tends to be associated with greater comfort discussing sexual matters or disclosing personal information. Such disclosures still need to be situationally appropriate, though, such as in response to questions. The rule of thumb is that if the clinician feels uncomfortable, the comment was probably inappropriate. If, on the other hand, a comment would be acceptable (albeit not typical), then it is important to consider the possibility that the patient simply has an unusual interpersonal style.

As the severity of the deficits increases, the severity of inappropriateness increases as well. In these cases, patients may engage in grossly inappropriate behaviors, such as beginning to masturbate in the middle of a session, lick or mouth objects, or reach to grope the examiner.

Chapter Summary

When assessing EF, test data are rarely sufficient for determining the level of functioning or for differentiating among EF syndromes. Thus, additional information about the patient's functioning outside of the testing session is needed. Sources of such information include (a) medical/psychiatric, educational/occupational, and legal records, (b) interview with the patient (and collateral sources if possible), and (c) behavioral observations. Information gathered in this manner can help with the determination of (a) the highest level of premorbid functioning, so as to ascertain that a change has taken place; (b) the onset and time course of EF difficulties, so as to facilitate linking dysfunction with etiology; and (c) the type and severity of EF difficulties, so as to determine which EF syndrome explains the patient's difficulties. Fine-grained understanding of the nature of the patient's difficulties not only contributes to differential diagnosis but also helps with generation of relevant and useful recommendations.

8

Challenges in the Use of Standardized Tests of Executive Functions

Hierarchical Structure of Cognition

It is a well-recognized fact that cognition is organized in a hierarchical fashion (Stuss, Picton, & Alexander, 2001), such that *higher-order processes* (such as executive functioning [EF]) depend on *lower-order processes* (such as perception, language, and speed of processing). Thus, for example, effective problem-solving can only occur if one has the capacity to perceive the problem (or comprehend a communication about the problem), and it can only occur at the speed at which one processes new information as it is introduced in the environment. Similarly then, performance on measures of EF also relies on lower-order processes, as one needs to comprehend the test instructions and perceive the stimuli and then physically (motorically, orally, etc.) perform the task, often under time constraints. The lower-order processes that are needed for performance of a particular EF test are often referred to as *component processes*. Thus, when interpreting test results, clinicians need to be aware that disruptions in lower-order component processes can mimic disruption in the higher-order processes. Fortunately, some tests of EF have been developed in such a fashion so as to allow adequate disambiguation of component and executive processes. The best-known examples of this include various trail making tasks, as well as various versions of the Stroop color- word interference tests. Such tests often offer normative data for contrast scores or other types of scores that are presumed to separate component and executive processes.

Unfortunately, many tests of EF do not provide built-in controls for component processes, leaving clinicians to their own devices in terms of using heuristics for controlling for lower-order abilities. In such cases, a thoughtful comparison of performances on tests of EF versus other neurocognitive domains is key. For example, although measures of verbal fluency represent a typical staple for most clinical evaluations of EF, such tests should actually be interpreted as measures of language if performed by patients with primary speech problems, and as measures of memory retrieval for patients with severe memory retrieval deficits. Consequently, it is always important to administer multiple measures of EF and to select such measures in a manner so as to rely on a range of component processes. Table 8.1 offers an overview of the component processes that play a role in performing classic tests of EF.

In addition, it is well recognized that EF is not a unitary construct. Consistent with this notion, this book describes five different EF subdomains, with each EF subdomain itself consisting of several *elemental processes* (see Chapters 2 through 6). Because of this notion, it is customary for clinicians to interpret each measure of EF individually, with the goal of disambiguating problems with individual EF subdomains. For example, it is typical for clinicians to interpret deficits on the Stroop color-word interference tests as reflecting problems with inhibition, and deficits on the alphanumeric sequencing tests as deficits in mental flexibility. However, these interpretations assume that a single elemental process is reflected in any given test. Unfortunately, that is not the case.

Consider, for example, the processes needed for performance of the alphanumeric sequencing condition of the various versions of the trail making test (e.g., Trails B). In addition to the component processes (i.e., visual perception and scanning, sequencing of numbers and letters, and speed of processing), several elemental *executive* processes also need to be online. These are (a) working memory, so as to hold in mind sequences of letters and numbers; (b) inhibition, so as to avoid following a number with a number or a letter with a letter; (c) effort mobilization, so as to work quickly and persist with the task; (d) discrepancy detection, so as to catch mistakes; and (e) mental flexibility, so as to mentally shift between sequencing letters and numbers.

Similarly, on the Stroop color-word interference tests, the required elemental processes are (a) mental flexibility, (b) inhibition, and (c) effort mobilization. The first elemental process, mental flexibility, is frequently overlooked in interpretations of performance on this test. However, consider that in order to perform the test, the examinee needs to abandon the mental set of *reading*

Table 8.1 Component processes needed for performance of classic tests of EF

COMPONENT PROCESSES	TESTS							
	TRAIL MAKING (SWITCHING)	STROOP (COLOR-WORD)	VERBAL FLUENCY	DESIGN FLUENCY	WCST	HALSTEAD CATEGORY	TOWER
Speed	+	+	+	+	N/A	N/A	+
Attention	+	+ Greater attention needed in D-KEFS switching condition	+ Greater attention needed in D-KEFS switching condition	+ Greater attention needed in distractor or switching conditions	+ Greater sustained attention needed for categories 4–6	+	+
Visual Perception	+ Greater visual scanning demand in D-KEFS than in Army Beta	+	+	+	+	+	+
Visual-Spatial Abilities	N/A (or very minimal)	N/A	N/A	+	+ Configuration of figures on cards in lieu of "number"	+	+
Language	+ Instructions; rote sequencing	+ Instructions; reading	+ Instructions; expression	+ Instructions only	+ Instructions only	+ Instructions only	+ Instructions only
Memory Retention	+ Instructions only	+ Instructions only	+ Instructions only	+ Instructions only	+ Instructions; previous principles (cat 4–6)	+ Instructions; previously employed principles	+ Instructions; previously employed principles

and mentally "reconfigure" so as to allow oneself to *perceive the color of ink*. In fact, one cannot perceive both the meaning of the word and the color of ink simultaneously, just as one cannot simultaneously perceive both the young woman and the old woman depicted in Figure 3.1. This is also why patients with limitations in mental flexibility have difficulty even just comprehending the instructions for this task. Only if mental flexibility is adequate for a person to comprehend, and then perform, the task do additional elemental processes such as inhibition and effort mobilization become relevant.

Unfortunately, not much research exists that analyzes the discrete elemental processes (or even subdomains) needed for completion of any given EF measure, and the preceding examples are based on an integration of *indirect* research evidence and clinical experience. One exception is nonverbal (i.e., design or figural) fluency, which has been examined in more depth in several studies. Specifically, research has directly demonstrated the contributions of I/M (especially initiation) and ECFs (especially mental flexibility, as well as generation of strategies) to performance (Gardner, Vik, & Dasher, 2013; Kraybill & Suchy, 2008; Suchy, Kraybill, et al., 2010).

Given these complexities of typical clinical tasks, it is unrealistic to think that any one of our measures could clearly separate EF subdomains, let alone EF elemental processes. Although there are some experimental tasks that do, to some extent, isolate elemental processes, these generally do *not* lend themselves to clinical use, simply because the observed effects are small and only emerge over a large number of trials and a large number of study participants. In other words, the effects are not large enough to be of use in clinical decision-making. For these reasons, test scores alone are generally not sufficient for differential diagnosis of EF subdomains; rather, clinicians need to integrate test scores with behavioral observations, background information, and qualitative aspects of test performance in order to determine which subdomain principally contributed to impaired scores. For an overview of elemental EF processes needed for performance of typical EF tests, see Table 8.2.

Reliability

Challenges in Measuring Reliability of EF Tests. Reliability refers to the degree to which a test performance is repeatable. In other words, reliability tells us how much of a given score reflects an actual ability, and how much of it is due to error. It is well recognized that reliability of EF tests tends to be lower when compared with other cognitive domains, and this has been

Table 8.2 Elemental EF processes needed for performance of classic tests of EF

SUBDOMAIN	ELEMENTAL EF PROCESSES	TESTS							
		TRAIL MAKING (SWITCHING)	STROOP (COLOR-WORD)	VERBAL FLUENCY	DESIGN FLUENCY	WCST	HALSTEAD CATEGORY	TOWERS
ECFs	Working memory	+	+	+	+	+	+	+
	Goal-directed retrieval	N/A	N/A	+	+	+ Prior principles	+ Prior principles	+ Prior strategy
	Mental flexibility	+	+	+	+	+	+	+
MT	Event-based prospective memory	N/A	+ Switch condition	N/A	N/A	+ Switch when cued	N/A	N/A
	Time-based prospective memory	N/A	N/A	N/A	N/A	N/A	N/A	N/A
	Meta-monitoring	N/A	N/A	N/A	N/A	N/A	N/A	N/A

(continued)

Table 8.2 (Continued)

SUBDOMAIN	ELEMENTAL EF PROCESSES	TESTS							
		TRAIL MAKING (SWITCHING)	STROOP (COLOR-WORD)	VERBAL FLUENCY	DESIGN FLUENCY	WCST	HALSTEAD CATEGORY	TOWERS
RS	Threat sensitivity	N/A	N/A	N/A	N/A	+ Register feedback	+ Register feedback	N/A
	Contingency updating	N/A	N/A	N/A	N/A	+ Update principle	+ Update principle	N/A
	Discrepancy detection	+	+	+	+	+	+	+
	Inhibition	+	+	+	+	+	+	+
I/M	Initiation	+	+	+	+	+	+	+
	Maintenance	+	+	+	+	+	+	+
	Effort mobilization	+	+	+	+	+	+	+
SC	All	N/A	N/A	N/A	N/A	N/A	N/A	N/A

Note: ECFs = executive cognitive functions; MT = meta-tasking; RS = response selection; I/M = initiation/maintenance; SC = social cognition.

demonstrated in a recent meta-analysis (Calamia, Markon, & Tranel, 2013). From among the various ways in which reliabilities can be computed, internal consistency, test-retest, and alternate form reliabilities are most relevant here.

First, with respect to internal consistency, some tests of EF actually do not readily lend themselves to measuring this type of reliability because technically they do not represent a composite of multiple items. Consider, for example, the internal consistency of the trail making test. Perhaps the most appropriate way to assess this would be to measure the amount of time elapsed from one circle to the next. This could potentially be accomplished if using an electronic version of the test. However, when using the typical paper-and-pencil version, the error term associated with the experimenter's capacity to precisely time these brief periods would likely overwhelm the actual reliability of the test. Similar problem arises for Stroop color-word interference tests and, to a lesser degree, for fluency measures and tower tests, to name a few. Thus, internal consistency is often not reported for many EF tests.

When internal consistencies are reported, they typically rely on some form of split-half reliability, such as correlating the number of items completed within the first half of the time allotted for test completion and the second half of the allotted time. For example, on the D-KEFS Verbal Fluency (Delis, Kaplan, & Kramer, 2001), internal consistency is based on the correlation among the four 15-second intervals in which the examinee generates responses across the 1-minute period allotted for task completion. In other cases, if a test has more than one condition, internal consistency is assumed to be reflected in the correlation of the two (or more) conditions with each other.

Second, with respect to test-retest reliability, one needs to consider that some tests of EF do not lend themselves to valid use in a repeat assessment. This is because for some tests a repeated administration will fundamentally alter the construct that is being measured. For example, once a patient has been given the Wisconsin Card Sorting Test, he or she understands that the sorting principle will periodically change without warning. Thus, assuming normal episodic memory, a repeat administration simply requires that a patient maintain mental set while performing the task; the patient does *not* need to figure out why responses that were previously correct are suddenly incorrect, and no longer needs to apply reasoning and problem-solving strategies. Consequently, a repeat administration not only fails to assess the construct of interest but also leads to a constriction of range at the upper end, which in turn leads to lower reliability coefficients (Calamia et al., 2013). Similarly, on the various tower tests, once the patient figures out a strategy, he or she no longer has to engage in reasoning or problem-solving when given the test for a second time (Welsh & Huizinga, 2005). In other words, the patient will simply rely on what he or she has learned during prior test administration.

Another problem with test-retest reliability of EF tests has to do with the fact that the construct itself is not completely stable. For example, it is now well understood that EF represents a "depletable" resource that is quite vulnerable to dynamic changes in response to various situational factors (see the section on situational factors in Chapter 9). This means that performance on measures of EF will fluctuate depending on the patient's cognitive and emotional frame of mind at the time of testing; another way to think about this is that tests of EF are just as sensitive to the *state* of EF as they are to the EF *trait*. This is in contrast to many other neurocognitive domains, which have not been shown to exhibit quite the same degree of variability from one day (or situation) to the next and are thus generally thought to represent a fairly stable trait.

Lastly, virtually by definition, mild deficits in EF will typically present not as mildly impaired performances across all tests or all administrations but as somewhat erratic performances from one test to the next, as well as from one administration to the next. That is, weaknesses or mild impairments in EF present as occasional and rather unpredictable lapses in performance, rather than a reliable and stable decrement (A. A. Gamaldo, An, Allaire, Kitner-Triolo, & Zonderman, 2012; Pietrzak et al., 2009). This particular characteristic of EF performance, then, necessarily leads to lower test-retest reliability. In addition, reliabilities will be differentially affected by age and education, depending on how demanding a given test is. Specifically, the normative age/education band that finds the test intermediately difficult may present with performance lapses (and low test-retest reliability), but those normative bands that find the test either very easy or very difficult may perform more consistently (and exhibit higher test-retest reliability). Because different tests "catch" different normative bands at that "intermediate" range, test-retest reliabilities are related to age and education in a somewhat erratic manner. This can be readily gleaned from test manuals in which reliabilities are reported separately for different subsets of the normative sample (Delis et al., 2001). Table 8.3 illustrates a simplified version of such associations.

In sum, low test-retest reliabilities may speak less to the reliability of the measure and more to the limited stability of the construct. This is particularly suggested by the fact that the correlations of EF tasks with other measures

Table 8.3 Hypothetical implications for reliability given different age-groups and test difficulties

TEST DIFFICULTY	AGE-GROUP		
	YOUNG	MIDDLE	OLD
Easy	Reliably easy	Reliably easy	**Erratic**
Intermediate	Reliably easy	**Erratic**	Reliably difficult
Difficult	**Erratic**	Reliably difficult	Reliably difficult

administered during the same session are sometimes higher than the tests' own test-retest reliabilities. If the test-retest coefficients reflected actual reliabilities of the test, if would be a statistical paradox (or a spurious findings) for those tests to exhibit higher correlations with other measures.

There are some additional limitations to how well reliability may be determined for EF tests. In particular, as discussed earlier, all EF tests rely not only on EF processes but also on a slew of lower-order component processes. These lower-order processes account for a sizable portion of the EF test variance. For example, on the D-KEFS Trail Making, simple sequencing of letters or numbers (analogous to Trails A) accounts for approximately 25% to 35% of variance in the number-letter sequencing condition (analogous to Trails B) when combined across the entire normative sample (Delis et al., 2001). Similar figures characterize the association between the interference condition of the D-KEFS Color-Word Interference test and the word reading or color naming conditions of that test. That is, correlations between performances on tasks assessing component processes and those assessing EF tend to range from about .4 (in younger samples) to about .6 (in older samples; Delis et al., 2001). Because reliabilities on many EF tests tend to be in a similar range as their correlations with tasks measuring relevant component processes, and because reliabilities of many tasks assessing component processes tend to be higher than reliabilities of EF tests, it is actually not at all clear how much of the reliable variance in a repeated test administration is due to the reliability of the EF aspects of the task, and how much of it simply captures the reliable variance in a given component process.

As an example of this point, the test-retest reliabilities for the nine executive tests in the D-KEFS battery (Delis et al., 2001) range from .24 to .80

(mean = .57, median = .58). In contrast, test-retest reliabilities for the component process tasks range from .56 to .77 (mean = .65, median = .61). Thus, it is possible that much of the EF reliability is simply due to the component variance. Table 8.4 provides an illustration of this issue, using reported reliabilities of EF and component process tasks for the D-KEFS Trail Making. The fourth column illustrates that it is possible, for example, that the reliability of letter sequencing (i.e., a component task) could *fully* account for a retest performance on the number-letter sequencing condition (i.e., the EF task).

Given these limitations, it would be important to report reliabilities of scores *after* component processes have been accounted for (e.g., the reliability of the contrast between the letter sequencing and the number-letter sequencing conditions). Unfortunately, across various manuals of EF tests, such reliabilities are not always reported.

Reliability and Clinical Practice. Given that measures of EF are fairly notorious for having poorer reliabilities than tests designed to tap into other neurocognitive constructs (Calamia et al., 2013), clinicians need to take care not to overinterpret performances on individual EF tests. Rather, it is advisable to administer multiple measures of EF, with the understanding that there may be quite some variability among performances. It is not uncommon for someone to score in the superior range on one test and in the impaired range on another. On repeat assessment, the opposite pattern between the two tests may emerge. This is because impaired performances most likely reflect *lapses* in EF against the backdrop of otherwise normal ability and should be interpreted as a potential risk for lapses in daily life.

To deal with this issue, clinicians should interpret the variability, rather than single scores. Additionally, clinicians may also choose to compute a mean scaled (or other standard) score across all EF tasks, as such composites have been repeatedly shown to be more reliable than individuals tasks, with internal consistency coefficients sometimes surpassing .80. Such composites are particularly valuable for repeat evaluations aimed at assessment of change. Additionally, clinicians are encouraged to maintain a database of test scores from their own patient samples so that they can directly examine the reliabilities of composites in their settings and their patient populations. Table 8.5 shows some examples of known reliabilities for composite scores from published research, as well as additional previously unpublished reliabilities generated for the purpose of this chapter using available datasets.

Table 8.4 Test-retest reliabilities and intercorrelations for the D-KEFS Trail Making test for ages 8–19

	COMPONENT RELIABILITY (rr)	CORRELATION B/W COMPONENT & EF (PEARSON r)	SHARED VARIANCE B/W COMPONENT AND EF (R SQUARED)	DIFFERENCE B/W EF RELIABILITY* AND SHARED VARIANCE
Visual scanning	.50	.24	.06	.14
Number sequencing	.77	.43	.18	.02
Letter sequencing	.57	.45	.20	.00
Motor speed	.82	.23	.05	.15

Note: *Test-retest reliability for the EF task (i.e., number-letter sequencing) is .20 for this age-group (Delis et al., 2001).

Table 8.5 Internal consistency reliabilities of composites of measures of EF

POPULATION (N)	TESTS IN A COMPOSITE	RELIABILITY	REFERENCE
Male criminal offenders, aged 19–49 (N = 91)	8 D-KEFS scores:		Composite not published; data set provided by Eastvold et al. research team; sample described in Eastvold, Suchy, & Strassberg, 2011.
	Trail Making Condition 4	.36	
	Letter Fluency	.76	
	Category Fluency	.81	
	Design Fluency Condition 1	.62	
	Design Fluency Condition 2	.73	
	Design Fluency Condition 3	.22	
	Color-Word Interference	.71	
	Color-Word Interference Switch	.52	
	Mean Chronbach's Alpha	.591	
	Median Chronbach's Alpha	.665	
	Composite Chronbach's Alpha	.838	
Teens with Type 1 diabetes, aged 16–18 (N = 200)	8 D-KEFS scores:		Suchy (work in progress).
	Trail Making Condition 4	.20	
	Letter Fluency	.67	
	Category Fluency	.70	
	Design Fluency Condition 1	.66	
	Design Fluency Condition 2	.43	
	Design Fluency Condition 3	.13	
	Color-Word Interference	.90	
	Color-Word Interference Switch	.80	
	Mean Chronbach's Alpha	.561	
	Median Chronbach's Alpha	.665	
	Composite Chronbach's Alpha	.830	

Male sex offenders and community controls, aged 21–44 (N = 60)	3 scores: Stroop Color and Word Test (Golden) Ruff Figural Fluency Test Unique d. Behavioral Dyscontrol Scale	.73 .76 .87	Suchy et al., 2009
	Mean Chronbach's Alpha	**.790**	
	Median Chronbach's Alpha	**.760**	
	Composite Chronbach's Alpha	**.806**	
Community-dwelling older adults, aged 66–85 (N = 65)	4 D-KEFS scores: Trail-Making Condition 4 Letter Fluency Design Fluency all 3 conditions Tower Test	.55 .67 .50 .70	Puente, Lindbergh, & Miller, 2015
	Mean Chronbach's Alpha	**.555**	
	Median Chronbach's Alpha	**.610**	
	Composite Chronbach's Alpha	**.795**	
Healthy, community-dwelling adolescents, aged 13–16 (N = 236)	8 D-KEFS scores: Trail-Making Condition 4 Letter Fluency Category Fluency Category Fluency Switching Color-Word Interference Color-Word Interference Switch Card Sorting Tower Test	.20 .67 .70 .65 .90 .80 .58 .51	Composite not published; data set provided by Anderson et al. research team; sample described in Anderson et al., 2009

(continued)

Table 8.5 (Continued)

POPULATION (N)	TESTS IN A COMPOSITE	RELIABILITY	REFERENCE
	Mean Chronbach's Alpha	.626	
	Median Chronbach's Alpha	.660	
	Composite Chronbach's Alpha	.776	
Community-dwelling older adults, aged 60–87 (N = 50)	5 D-KEFS scores: Trail-Making Condition 4 Letter Fluency Category Switching Fluency Design Fluency all 3 conditions Color-Word Interference Switch	.55 .67 .70 .50 .57	Kraybill, Thorgusen, & Suchy, 2013
	Mean Chronbach's Alpha	.598	
	Median Chronbach's Alpha	.570	
	Composite Chronbach's Alpha	.754	
Community-dwelling older adults, aged 60–85 (N = 61)	4 D-KEFS scores: Trail-Making Condition 4 Letter Fluency Design Fluency all 3 conditions Tower Test	.55 .67 .50 .70	Puente, Lindbergh, & Miller, 2015
	Mean Chronbach's Alpha	.555	
	Median Chronbach's Alpha	.610	
	Composite Chronbach's Alpha	.753	

Community-dwelling older adults, aged 60–92 (N = 45)	4 D-KEFS scores:		Mitchell & Miller, 2008
	Trail-Making Condition 4	.55	
	Letter Fluency	.67	
	Design Fluency all 3 conditions	.50	
	Tower Test	.70	
	Mean Chronbach's Alpha	**.555**	
	Median Chronbach's Alpha	**.610**	
	Composite Chronbach's Alpha	**.750**	
Children with high-functioning autism, aged 10–17 (N = 57)	5 D-KEFS scores:		Composite not published; data set provided by Larson et al. research team; sample described in Gidley Larson & Suchy, 2014
	Design Fluency Condition 1	.66	
	Design Fluency Condition 2	.43	
	Design Fluency Condition 3	.13	
	Color-Word Interference	.90	
	Color-Word Interference Switch	.80	
	Mean Chronbach's Alpha	**.584**	
	Median Chronbach's Alpha	**.660**	
	Composite Chronbach's Alpha	**.723**	
Community-dwelling older adults, aged 58–87 (N = 72)	5 D-KEFS scores:		Kraybill & Suchy, 2011
	Trail-Making Condition 4	.55	
	Letter Fluency	.67	
	Category Switching Fluency	.70	
	Design Fluency all 3 conditions	.50	
	Color-Word Interference Switch	.57	

(*continued*)

Table 8.5 (Continued)

POPULATION (N)	TESTS IN A COMPOSITE	RELIABILITY	REFERENCE
	Mean Chronbach's Alpha	.598	
	Median Chronbach's Alpha	.570	
	Composite Chronbach's Alpha	.700	
Mean for Single Tests		.607	
Median for Single Tests		.665	
Mean for Composites		.775	
Median for Composites		.776	

Validity

Validity refers to how well a given test measures what it is purported to measure. Several types of validity are particularly relevant to us as clinicians. These are (a) criterion validity, (b) concurrent validity, and (c) construct validity.

Criterion and Ecological Validity. With respect to *criterion validity*, the key question is whether performance on a given test relates to some external (and clinically relevant) criterion. For example, is poor performance on a given test related to a particular diagnosis? Or, alternatively, is poor performance related to a particular lesion location?

Closely related to criterion validity is the concept of *ecological validity*, which typically refers to how well test performance relates to behavior in daily life. That is, can we use patients' performances on tests of EF to predict everyday outcomes, such as driving ability, job performance, the ability to perform instrumental activities of daily living, or the ability to manage one's medications? Although many studies have now demonstrated that performances on measures of EF do in fact correlate with such outcomes (Boyle, Cohen, Paul, Moser, & Gordon, 2002; Jefferson et al., 2006; Koehler et al., 2011; Kraybill & Suchy, 2011; Kraybill et al., 2013; Niewoehner et al., 2012; Perna, Loughan, & Talka, 2012; Rapp et al., 2005; Suchy, Blint, & Osmon, 1997), clinicians nevertheless feel quite uncertain about whether they can predict patients' functioning in daily life based purely on performances on measures of EF. These concerns are warranted for several reasons.

First, it is well understood that clinical assessments are conducted in a highly structured environment in which the clinician provides a variety of scaffolding. For example, if a patient is anxious, the clinician takes care to ease the patient's concerns so as to allow him or her to fully focus on test performance; if a patient is unmotivated, the clinician provides repeated encouragements. Additionally, clinicians provide a variety of prompts that help patients stay on track. For example, if a patient becomes disengaged, the clinician will prompt with "keep going," and if a patient becomes distracted, the clinician will once again reorient the patient to the test. Consequently, although the test scores may reflect the patient's ability in a well-structured, ideal environment, they do not provide a picture of how well or poorly the patient would perform if left to his or her own devices. Yet, independent functioning is by definition just that: being able to function when left to one's own devices. In fact, independent functioning needs to occur not only in the absence of scaffolding but also in the presence of various environmental distractors or stressors. For example, one needs to continue to function even if not feeling well, or even in the middle of a personal crisis such as the death of a loved one or a divorce.

A second reason for poor ecological validity when considered in the context of a given patient is the fact that, as mentioned earlier, executive problems present as erratic lapses in performance or functioning. Thus, a patient may be assessed on a good day and show no problems on test performance. Yet, such a patient may still exhibit lapses in EF at home during stressful times. In contrast, another patient may exhibit subtle weaknesses in EF across the board and thus be at risk for executive lapses in daily life, yet, depending on the amount of scaffolding and support the patient receives at home, such lapses may or may not occur. In other words, executive lapses may represent a low-frequency occurrence that is difficult to measure and difficult to predict. Yet, even a single lapse can have devastating consequences.

A third reason for poor ecological validity of executive measures has to do with the fact that our tests tap only certain subdomains of EF. In particular, our tests are fairly good at assessing executive cognitive functions, initiation and set maintenance, and inhibition (though all these subdomains are mutually confounded in typical clinical measures). In contrast, most of the typical EF tests are fairly poor for assessment of meta-tasking abilities or social cognition.

A fourth reason for poor ecological validity of executive measures is the fact that the executive demands of many situations encountered in daily life depend less on the situation itself, and more on a person's temperament or proclivities toward certain behaviors. For example, a person whose temperament is characterized by a strong tendency to seek rewards will have to rely on EF more heavily when needing to say no to rewarding stimuli (such as food) than a person whose temperament is characterized by a strong tendency to avoid punishment (such as being scolded by one's physician).

Lastly, because an important purpose of a neuropsychological evaluation is to aid with diagnosis, many evaluations focus on determining whether a patient has evidenced a decline or a change in functioning. For that reason, the test scores that we use clinically are corrected for age and, in many instances, for educational attainment and other demographic characteristics. Directly translating such scores into daily functioning is difficult, as the patient characteristics themselves explain part of the variance in functionality. Thus, when making judgments about daily functionality, perhaps we should compare our patients' scores to normative samples of *functional* individuals rather than to a sample of age- and education-matched controls. For example, a brain surgeon with a mild EF impairment relative to age- and education-matched peers may best stop operating on people's brains, but this mild impairment is likely completely inconsequential when it comes to driving ability, the ability to manage one's medications, or the ability to take care of any other instrumental activities of daily living independently.

Lest we despair, let us nevertheless remind ourselves of what our tests *can* accomplish. For example, if a patient has moderate to severe deficits, then prediction of a higher risk of failures in daily functioning is certainly warranted. However, clinicians need to be clear that we can only predict the *risk* for failures in functioning, rather than a *certainty* that serious failures will occur. Thus, if we recommend that a patient stop driving because of the risk of attentional errors, we should not feel disappointed or blame our procedures if the patient then continues to drive for another year without an incident.

Concurrent Validity. In addition to criterion and ecological validities, *concurrent validity* is also important to us as clinicians. Concurrent validity examines whether performance on one measure is closely related to, or could even be substituted with, performance on another measure. This type of validity tells us whether one test measures a similar ability or construct as another test. Although concurrent validity is often used as a means to an end, that is, to validate newly developed measures, a good understanding of different tests' concurrent validity is highly relevant in clinical practice. This is because clinicians often find themselves in situations in which a patient had already been given a particular measure by another clinician, or when a test is spoiled by an administrator error or some unavoidable environmental event such as a fire alarm or a loss of electric power. In such situations, clinicians can readily replace one test with another if they have good working knowledge of how well two tests relate to one another. Such information can often be gleaned from test manuals and, in many cases, from empirical literature. Additionally, clinicians are encouraged to maintain a database of patient test scores so they can examine correlations among tests in their own patient population.

Lastly, *construct validity* represents a higher-order type of validity that can be viewed as the cumulative knowledge gained from other types of validity testing. Construct validity refers to the degree to which a given test actually measures the *construct* that it is purported to measure. When it comes to tests of EF, it becomes readily apparent that test validation is not easily accomplished because the construct itself is actually not all that well defined or understood. Although the advances in cognitive neuroscience have allowed us to have a better understanding of the various elemental processes and subdomains of EF, the development of the typical clinical measures that we use with our patients long predates such advances. Consequently, validation of tests of EF has generally relied on two approaches: first, determining whether a test is sensitive to frontal lobe damage, and second, determining whether a new test correlates with older tests that have already been validated. These approaches, especially when used in combination, are unsatisfying and inherently circular because a validation that is based on a correlation with another test that itself was only validated based on sensitivity to frontal lobe damage does not offer much new information about the test's ability to tap the EF construct. In contrast, with increasing interest in ecological validity, demonstrating the test's relationship to daily functioning greatly contributes to the validation of the test against an external index of the EF construct.

Test and Battery Selection

There are many clinical tests that are purported to rely on EF. In their text *Neuropsychological Assessment*, Lezak and colleagues (2004) list well over 20 informal tasks, standardized tests, and comprehensive test batteries in the chapter on assessment of EF. Similarly, in the third edition of their compendium of neuropsychological tests, Strauss, Sherman, and Spreen (2006) classify 13 tests as measures of EF, with additional tests that are often considered to assess EF (e.g., trail making) listed under attention. Clearly, a detailed description of all available tests of EF not only would be beyond the scope of this chapter but also would be inherently redundant with other excellent, highly comprehensive resources that are already available elsewhere. To avoid duplicating extant information, the remainder of this chapter focuses on recommendations about how to go about selecting EF tests for your assessment battery. The following presents some frequently asked questions that clinicians pose when selecting tests for assessment of EF.

Which Tests Measure EF? As mentioned earlier, there is some disagreement about which tests should be classified as assessing EF. For example, although many clinicians consider the alphanumeric sequencing condition of the various trail making tests as measures of EF, some classify these conditions as assessing attention. Similarly, although verbal fluency is typically classified as a measure of EF, it is sometimes listed under verbal abilities. Conversely, the Digit Symbol Coding test is typically considered to measure speed of processing, and the Rey-O Complex Figure Test is typically considered to measure visual-constructional abilities, but some researchers and clinicians classify both of these tests as measures of EF. These inconsistencies are understandable, given that no one test measures only one construct. In fact, as discussed earlier in this chapter, performances on all measures of EF rely on other component processes (see Table 8.1); conversely, many tests that are typically classified as measuring nonexecutive constructs do, in reality, rely on at least some aspects of EF. Table 8.6 provides an overview of which EF subdomains are needed for performance of classic "nonexecutive" tests.

Given the nonspecificity of typical clinical tests, one may wonder how we ever manage to interpret test results. Lest we despair, it is important to consider that it is typically the impaired ability that drives test performance and, especially in cases of severe impairment, overwhelms the contributions of the remaining processes. As an example, although most factor analyses of the WAIS subtests yield four-factor solutions, factor analyses conducted with individuals over the age of 70 become overwhelmingly driven by speed of processing, such that all timed subtests fall on a single factor (Wechsler, 1997). In other words, visual-spatial abilities are obscured by the more prominent decline in speed of processing that occurs with advanced age. Thus, clinicians need to consider where the principal limitations of a given patient are and then interpret the tests accordingly; for example, if the patient's performances on all language tests are impaired, it is not appropriate to interpret verbal fluency as a measure of EF.

How Many EF Tests Do I Need to Include in My Battery? There are several reasons for administering multiple tests of EF in any given assessment session. First, as discussed earlier in this chapter, tests of EF are notoriously unreliable, not only because of the test characteristics but also because the construct itself dynamically alters due to a number of situational factors. As seen in Table 8.4, administration of multiple tests improves reliability. Second, as also discussed earlier, weaknesses in EF often present as *lapses* rather than as weaker performances across the board. Administration of multiple tests is more likely to capture such lapses. Importantly, variability in performance across several EF measures is diagnostic in its own right. Third, the nonspecificity of EF tests (i.e., their reliance on nonexecutive component processes) makes it virtually impossible to interpret a single EF test because any one test may be fatally confounded by some other neurocognitive weakness. Thus, for example, it is advisable to administer both verbal and nonverbal tests of EF, and to examine both timed and untimed aspects of performance.

Because no research thus far has made a clear statement about the ideal number of EF tests in a given battery or for a given population, it is not possible to provide a definitive answer to this question. Additionally, the lengths

Table 8.6   Executive contributions to performance on "nonexecutive" tests

PRIMARY CONSTRUCTS AND TEST EXAMPLES	EF CONTRIBUTIONS
Processing speed • Digit Symbol Coding • Symbol Search	ECFs (working memory) I/M (initiation, maintenance, effort mobilization) RS (inhibition, discrepancy detection)
Visual-spatial/constructional abilities • Rey-O Complex Figure • Block Design	ECFs (working memory, mental flexibility) I/M (initiation, maintenance, effort mobilization) RS (inhibition, discrepancy detection)
Nonverbal reasoning • WAIS-IV Matrices • Raven's Matrices	ECFs (working memory, mental flexibility, goal-directed retrieval)
Language comprehension • Token Test	ECFs (working memory)
Verbal reasoning • WAIS-IV Similarities • WAIS-IV Comprehension	ECFs (working memory, mental flexibility, goal-directed retrieval)
Verbal learning • CVLT • HVLT	ECFs (working memory, goal-directed retrieval) I/M (initiation, maintenance, effort mobilization) RS (inhibition, discrepancy detection)
Sustained attention • CPT	I/M (initiation, maintenance, effort mobilization) RS (inhibition, discrepancy detection)

Note: ECFs = executive cognitive function; I/M = initiation/maintenance; RS = response selection; CLVT = California Verbal Learning Test; HVLT = Hopkins Verbal Learning Test; CPT = Continuous Performance Test.

Table 8.7 Solutions for addressing gaps in typical clinical batteries used for assessment of EF

GAPS IN TYPICAL CLINICAL BATTERIES	SOLUTION	NOTES	REFERENCE
Social cognition	WAIS-IV Advanced Clinical Solutions Social Cognition Battery	Social Perception subtest can be used as a screener to conserve time.	Pearson, 2009
Meta-tasking	Modified Six Elements Test and Zoo Map subtests from the Behavioural Assessment of Dysexecutive Syndrome (BADS)	Only British norms are available at present. Will also be impaired if ECFs are impaired.	B. Wilson et al., 1996
Threat sensitivity and contingency updating	Iowa Gambling Task	May also be impaired if ECFs are impaired.	Bechara, 2007

of test batteries tend to differ for practical reasons, including the purpose, the setting, and the population. In light of these practical issues, the reader may consider the following: The administration of the WCST tests takes about 20 to 30 minutes, and the administration of the Trail Making, the Color-Word Interference, and the Verbal and Design Fluencies from the D-KEFS also takes about 20 to 30 minutes. Thus, if time is an issue, it may be advisable to choose several shorter tasks rather than one long test.

How Do I Make Sure My Assessment Taps into All Facets of EF? At first blush it may appear that the most convenient and logical way of selecting tests of EF would be to classify them by which EF subdomains they are related to, so as to ascertain screening of all aspects of EF and to facilitate determination of which EF subdomain is impaired. Unfortunately, this cannot be easily accomplished, as various subdomains of EF are mutually interconnected, and any given test of EF relies on multiple EF subdomains (see Table 8.2). Consequently, rather than selecting tests that *uniquely* tap into a given subdomain, clinicians are encouraged to select a battery of tests that *together* tap as many subdomains and elemental processes as possible. As seen in Table 8.2, classic measures of EF jointly accomplish this goal for the majority of subdomains and elemental processes, but some areas are chronically underrepresented. These are (a) the subdomains of meta-tasking and social cognition, and (b) the elemental processes of threat sensitivity and contingency updating. Table 8.7 provides some guidance on how to address these gaps.

Chapter Summary

There are many psychometric challenges when assessing EF, including limited reliability of EF measures, limited stability of the EF construct, and potential changes in the construct itself when the same test is administered more than once. To maximize test-rest reliability, clinicians are encouraged to consider using composites of several EF tests. When selecting tests of EF, clinicians need to take care to (a) carefully consider reliability and validity issues, (b) have means of controlling for component processes, such as contrasting the alphanumeric sequencing condition of trail making with a simple numeric sequencing condition, (c) ensure that the battery of tests they use samples as many subdomains of EF and as many elemental processes as possible, and (d) administer several tests so as to allow meaningful sampling of behavior and allow for variability across tests to emerge.

9

Interpretive Considerations

EF Umbrella Versus EF Subdomains

Thus far, much of this text has focused on delineating different subdomains of executive functioning (EF). Here, we will review the *clinical utility* of understanding the underlying elemental processes that contribute to each EF subdomain, as well as the advantages of having a firm grasp on the constellations of symptoms that make up each syndrome.

It is understood that time constraints and available assessment methods preclude clinicians from fully and thoroughly evaluating every neurocognitive process that may contribute to a given patient's complaints or functional limitations. To deal with this reality, clinicians can use their knowledge of EF subdomains as a framework when supplementing formal assessment data with relevant interview questions, as outlined in Chapter 7. For example, by understanding that the disorganized syndrome is characterized by deficient time-based and event-based prospective memory, the clinician can choose strategic interview questions that will provide important information about the patient's prospective memory, which will then contribute to the determination of whether the patient does in fact suffer from the disorganized syndrome. In turn, a thorough understanding of the disorganized syndrome will allow the clinician to extrapolate from the available test data to potential problems in daily life, facilitating provision of concrete and relevant recommendations. In addition to providing a framework that guides the assessment process and recommendations, understanding the different EF syndromes can add specificity to differential diagnosis, as is the case, for example, with the inappropriate syndrome being associated with the behavioral variant of frontotemporal lobar degeneration (bvFTD).

All that said, clinicians need to be realistic when it comes to differentiating among individual EF syndromes. As stated earlier, test scores alone are not sufficient for identifying specific EF deficits because performance on most tests relies on multiple processes and multiple EF subdomains. Additionally, in some cases, neither the patient nor the collateral source may have adequate insight to provide reliable and valid answers to interview questions that could elucidate the nature of the patient's difficulties. These issues are further compounded by the fact that pure syndromes are relatively rare, as many patients present with a combination of several syndromes or only partial features of a syndrome. Thus, the tenacity with which a clinician pursues differentiation among individual EF syndromes should depend on whether such differentiation will add specificity to a differential diagnosis or have important ramifications for daily functioning. For example, as mentioned earlier, the inappropriate syndrome can uniquely contribute to the differential diagnosis (bvFTD); thus, in cases of suspected bvFTD, the clinician should take extra care to adequately assess relevant subdomains, such as social cognition (SC). In contrast, in cases of moderate traumatic brain injury (TBI), a less coherent mixture of symptoms is likely, and diagnosis is already known. Thus, functional implications of deficits, rather than syndrome differential, may be a more realistic and important goal.

Trait Versus State in EF Assessment

Another key issue that clinicians need to carefully consider before proceeding to interpretation of their data is whether the results they have obtained reflect the patient's EF as a stable trait, or whether they reflect a fluctuating state. It is, or course, customary for clinicians to comment in their reports on whether the assessment results on the whole are a reasonably accurate reflection of the patient's abilities, or whether various proximal factors, such anxiety or fatigue, limit interpretability. It is somewhat less customary to comment on the *differential* impact various intervening variables can have on EF as compared with other neurocognitive domains. Yet, in recent years, much research has increasingly shown that EF represents the most "depletable" of all neurocognitive resources. Consequently, how well or poorly one performs on measures of EF *on a given day* depends on a slew of situational factors, such as the amount of sleep the night before, emotional distress during or even before the testing takes place, or presence of pain or physical discomfort. Unfortunately, no specific guidelines exist on how exactly to "correct" for such situational factors. Thus, the best clinicians can do at present is to simply be vigilant and to take into consideration that performances on *EF tests specifically* may have been affected. Of note, many factors, such as sedative medications, have a somewhat generalized impact on cognition. The following section reviews those factors that appear to impact EF differentially.

Lack of Sleep. A number of studies have found that greater sleep quality and sleep efficiency are associated with better performance on measures of EF among healthy young adults (Benitez & Gunstad, 2012; Guoping, Kan, Danmin, & Fuen, 2008; Plessow, Kiesel, Petzold, & Kirschbaum, 2011), preschool children (Bernier, Beauchamp, Bouvette-Turcot, Carlson, & Carrier, 2013), and healthy older adults (Sutter, Zöllig, Allemand, & Martin, 2012). Additionally, poor sleep quality has been shown to be associated with further decrements in EF in clinical populations, such as patients with HIV infection (C. E. Gamaldo et al., 2013) or Parkinson's disease (Stavitsky, Neargarder, Bogdanova, McNamara, & Cronin-Golomb, 2012). Importantly, at least some studies have found that the association between sleep and cognition is *specific* to EF and does not extend to other cognitive domains (Bernier et al., 2013; Stavitsky et al., 2012).

That said, some studies have failed to find a direct association between poor performance on EF measures and *objective* sleep quality or sleep duration, finding instead that *subjective* sleepiness predicts poor EF performance (Anderson, Storfer-Isser, Taylor, Rosen, & Redline, 2009). Additionally, at least one study has suggested that the association between sleep deprivation and EF may be explained by decrements in speed of processing (Tucker, Whitney, Belenky, Hinson, & Van Dongen, 2010); thus, more research is needed on the specific vulnerability of EF to poor sleep. However, at least one study has found that individuals with higher trait EF may be less vulnerable to the deleterious impact of sleep deprivation (Killgore, Grugle, Reichardt, Killgore, & Balkin, 2009), a finding that may potentially explain inconsistencies among study results. Regardless of the mechanism, from a clinical standpoint, poor sleep has the potential to have a deleterious impact on test performance in general and on EF in particular. Thus, it is advisable that clinicians interpret with caution test data collected from patients who complain of sleepiness or who report unusually poor sleep quality or duration during the night prior to testing.

Emotion Regulation. As already discussed in prior chapters, emotion regulation is a nonunitary construct that consists of two broad categories: regulation of how we feel (e.g., employing cognitive reappraisal) and regulation of how we act (e.g., suppressing laughter or crying, or suppressing even subtle facial manifestations of a feeling). This latter type of emotion regulation is known as *emotional* or *expressive suppression* and, due to its deleterious impact on EF, is the principal focus of this section. Incidentally, suppression is actually a misnomer because *exaggeration* of emotional expressions (e.g., smiling when not feeling like smiling) appears to have a similarly depleting impact on EF and is therefore often subsumed under the same emotion regulation category.

The deleterious effect of emotional/expressive suppression on EF has been extensively studied within the realm of social and experimental psychology. This research shows that individuals who engage in excessive emotional/expressive suppression are at risk for subsequent lapses in response selection (RS), such as engaging in aggressive acts or inappropriate sexual behaviors, impulsive spending, or breaking diets (Baumeister & Alquist, 2009; Baumeister, Bratslavsky, Muraven, & Tice, 1998; Gailliot & Baumeister, 2007; Muraven, Tice, & Baumeister, 1998). Additionally, emotional/expressive suppression is associated with decrements in the executive cognitive functions (ECFs), evidenced by an increased tendency to be persuaded by illogical arguments or make logic errors, difficulties with cognitive decision-making, and poorer performance on typical measures of EF and working memory (Baumeister & Alquist, 2009; Pocheptsova, Amir, Dhar, & Baumeister, 2009; Schmeichel, Vohs, & Baumeister, 2003; Schmeichel et al., 2008; Schmeichel & Zell, 2007). Importantly, it appears that the depletion effect is fairly specific to EF, above and beyond simple attention and speed of processing, and above and beyond the impact of depressive symptoms (Franchow & Suchy, 2015).

It has been suggested that the mutual depletion between EF and emotional/expressive suppression is simply a reflection of the fact that both constructs are theoretically (Baumeister, Schmeichel, Vohs, Kruglanski, & Higgins, 2007) and neuroanatomically related (Goldin, McRae, Ramel, & Gross, 2008). In fact, virtually by definition, successful emotional/expressive suppression requires that one be able to engage in inhibition and error monitoring, as well as have social and emotional awareness. Additionally, similar to EF, emotional/expressive suppression can be highly effortful and consumes considerable metabolic resources (Beer, John, Scabini, & Knight, 2006; Gailliot et al., 2007). Importantly, it appears that the depletion of EF is not resolved when emotional/

expressive suppression demands are terminated, but rather persists for some time afterward (Schmeichel et al., 2003; Stucke & Baumeister, 2006). In fact, we have recently demonstrated that the depletion may continue throughout the day and may impact performance on tests of EF by as much as two thirds of a standard deviation (i.e., 2 Scaled Scores; Franchow & Suchy, 2015).

The ramifications of this effect on test performance are considerable. First, this means that test performance can vary by a margin large enough so as to place patients into different descriptive categories (e.g., mildly impaired versus low average). Second, because of the lasting effects of depletion beyond the depleting situation or event, patients who have had high emotional/expressive suppression demands on the day of testing may perform more poorly regardless of the scaffolding provided by the examiner. This statement is further supported by the fact that the typical clinical supports were made available to examinees during testing in the Franchow and Suchy (2015) study, yet depletion was still evident in the results. Consequently, clinicians should carefully consider the patient's current and *recent* emotion regulation burdens and their unique impact on EF. Some examples of increased expressive suppression demands are listed in Table 9.1.

Table 9.1 Examples of situations that may lead to executive depletion due to high expressive suppression demands

EXPRESSIVE SUPPRESSION BURDEN	TYPICAL SITUATION
Suppressing tears/crying	Patient experienced a recent loss of a loved one.
Suppressing anger	Patient has had a "bad day" prior to coming for the evaluation, feeling hurt or affronted on several occasions.
Suppressing giddiness	Patient has recently received life-changing good news.
Suppressing anxiety	Patient gave a presentation in class prior to coming for the evaluation.
Enhancing smiling	Patient had a job interview prior to coming for the evaluation.

Interpretive Considerations

Pain. There is considerable evidence that both chronic and acute pain have deleterious impact on EF (Nes, Roach, & Segerstrom, 2009). Similar to research on emotion regulation, studies suggest that pain affects EF uniquely (i.e., to the exclusion of other cognitive domains; Karp et al., 2006; Scherder et al., 2008), or at least that it affects EF more strongly than other cognitive abilities (Jongsma et al., 2011). Although there is some preliminary evidence that different subdomains of EF are differentially affected by pain (Oosterman, Derksen, van Wijck, Kessels, & Veldhuijzen, 2012), more research is needed before definitive conclusions can be drawn. Importantly, even though some of the decrements in EF among patients with pain can be explained by the associated depression, sleep disruption, and use of pain medications, pain nevertheless still emerges as a significant predictor of EF above and beyond these other factors (Jongsma et al., 2011; Karp et al., 2006).

It has been suggested that one of the mechanisms behind the relationship between pain and EF deficits is related to emotion regulation, as addressed in the previous section. Specifically, there is evidence that patients rely on EF to help them control pain, thereby depleting executive resources (Glass et al., 2011; Nes et al., 2009; Silvestrini & Rainville, 2013). Additionally, patients need to regulate not only their subjective experience of pain but also their pain-related behaviors, such as grimacing or postural changes (Nes et al., 2009). Lastly, the physiologic stress associated with the experience of pain may also further contribute to cognitive changes via the deleterious impact of chronic cortisol elevations (Hinkelmann et al., 2009). This notion is supported by research that has shown that chronic pain is associated with neurodegenerative changes among older adults (Jongsma et al., 2011), and that pain has a greater deleterious impact on EF among patients with dementia (Scherder et al., 2008).

Referral Question: Diagnostic Decision-making and Estimating Premorbid EF

Once the clinician decides about the interpretability of EF results, the next most important interpretive consideration has to do with the nature of the referral question, specifically whether the question focuses primarily on diagnostic impressions or functional outcome. Of course, in many cases, both diagnosis and functioning need to be addressed.

When making diagnostic decisions, arguably the most foundational questions the clinician needs to address are whether there has been a decline in cognition from a premorbid baseline, and whether the nature and severity of such a decline are consistent with a particular diagnosis. Thus, the more accurately the clinician estimates premorbid executive functioning, the more accurate determinations about a potential decline can take place. To accomplish this, all patient characteristics that are known to systematically relate to premorbid EF need to be considered. Such relevant characteristics are reviewed in the following.

Demographics. It is well accepted that certain person-specific characteristics, such as age, gender, educational attainment, and ethnicity, relate to performances on cognitive measures, including EF (Constantinidou, Christodoulou, & Prokopiou, 2012; Dorbath, Hasselhorn, & Titz, 2013; Gladsjo et al., 1999; Martins, Maruta, Freitas, & Mares, 2013; Tripathi, Kumar, Bharath, Marimuthu, & Varghese, 2014). What this typically means in clinical neuropsychological assessment is that all scores are converted to standard scores that are adjusted for relevant demographics (usually age and educational background, and sometimes gender and ethnicity). Using such norms, the clinician determines how much a given patient's current functioning deviates from an estimated premorbid baseline. However, clinicians should interpret normative comparisons thoughtfully, taking into consideration that demographic normative adjustments offer only a gross approximation of a given patient's actual background, functioning only as convenient (and somewhat simplistic) proxies for more complex underlying constructs. For example, there are considerable regional differences in the quality of one's education, and factors such as acculturation and socioeconomic status are known to be confounded with ethnicity and race (Manly, 2005). Consequently, other factors, such as the complexity of occupational demands as described in Chapter 7, should also be considered so as to further fine-tune the normative estimates.

Personality. Aside from demographics, there are other person-specific characteristics that are known to systematically relate to EF performance and yet are not considered during the norming process. The most notable among these is personality (not to be confused with personality *disorders*, which are covered in Chapter 12). Specifically, research shows that EF represents a heritable trait, with individual differences in EF being related to specific genes, particularly those controlling the various aspects of the dopaminergic system. The integrity of the dopaminergic system in turn relates to certain stable ways of relating to the world (i.e., stable personality traits). For a review, see P. G. Williams and colleagues (2009).

Briefly, personality research has consistently found five stable dimensions of personality (De Fruyt, De Bolle, McCrae, Terracciano, & Costa, 2009; Wilberg, Karterud, Pedersen, Urnes, & Costa, 2009). These are neuroticism, extraversion, openness to experience, conscientiousness, and agreeableness. From among these, neuroticism (i.e., a tendency to experience emotional arousal and distress) and openness to experience (i.e., a tendency to be cognitively and behaviorally inquisitive, imaginative, and reflective) are most strongly related to EF.

With respect to neuroticism, there is evidence that neuroticism that is clinically elevated is associated with poorer EF (Murdock, Oddi, & Bridgett, 2013; P. G. Williams et al., 2010). However, it has also been suggested that neuroticism may be associated with cognition in a curvilinear fashion, similar to the way in which arousal relates to cognition (Suchy, 2011, p. 229; P. G. Williams et al., 2009). In other words, consistent with the Yerkes-Dodson law (Yerkes & Dodson, 1908), intermediate levels of arousal are ideal for optimal test performance; similarly, intermediate levels of neuroticism may be needed for optimal EF. This is because, in many typical situations, intermediate levels of neuroticism are likely to lead to intermediate levels of arousal. In contrast, extremely high or extremely low neuroticism tends to be associated with maladaptively high or low arousal, respectively, and thus interfering with optimal cognition.

In contrast to neuroticism, openness to experience appears to have an unequivocally linear relationship with EF, such that greater openness is related to higher intelligence as well as better EF (Franchow et al., 2013; Murdock et al., 2013; P. G. Williams et al., 2010). Importantly, although individuals with higher educational achievement also tend to be higher on openness, openness contributes to intelligence above and beyond education, particularly at lower educational levels (Franchow et al., 2013). For these reasons, it has been suggested that inclusion of personality scores in regression-based computations of T scores may improve accuracy of estimating a patient's expected or premorbid level of performance (Suchy, 2011, p. 251), though more research is needed to demonstrate the clinical utility of such an approach. Meanwhile, particularly for individuals for whom the quality of education is questionable, normatively high levels of openness to experience may represent a better estimate of premorbid EF than education alone, such that at least a slight educational adjustment upward may be warranted (Franchow et al., 2013).

Referral Question: Daily Functioning and Prediction of Functional Lapses

In contrast to diagnostic decision-making, which relies on determining whether a patient has evidenced a decline, a different interpretive process needs to be applied when making a determination about whether a patient can perform certain activities, including occupational and educational duties, or instrumental activities of daily living (IADLs). Specifically, although a patient may exhibit normal functioning given his or her demographics (and thus be deemed neuropsychologically "healthy"), such a patient may not be able to perform certain activities in daily life. For example, an 85-year-old patient with 8 years of education who performs in the average range relative to demographically adjusted norms may receive a clean bill of health as far as neurodegenerative conditions are concerned. However, this patient's cognitive resources, although "normal," may not be adequate for management of complex financial matters. Such a patient may also not have adequate resources for independent management of complex medical regimens, such as those associated with Type 2 diabetes or HIV, or for using the Internet to obtain important information, such as transportation schedules or addresses and phone numbers. Thus, clinicians need to consider whether a given patient's cognitive resources match the situational demands at hand. Relevant factors to consider are reviewed in the following.

Intrinsic Resources and Task Complexity. Research overwhelmingly suggests that EF represents a neurocognitive domain that is the most strongly associated with the ability to execute IADLs (Kraybill & Suchy, 2011; Kraybill et al., 2013; Martyr & Clare, 2012; Suchy et al., 2011). Despite this overwhelming effect, EF alone does *not* appear to be sufficient. Rather, several studies have demonstrated that general mental status (McGuire, Ford, & Ajani, 2006), as well as cognitive reserve as reflected in intellectual functioning or educational attainment (Duda, Puente, & Miller, 2014; Starr & Lonie, 2008), also contribute to the ability to perform IADLs well. In fact, although some authors have suggested that the association between cognitive reserve and functionality is mediated by EF (Puente, Lindbergh, & Miller, 2015), other research has shown that *both* IQ and EF *independently* predict functionality and/or medication self-management in several populations, including patients with TBI (Perna et al., 2012), schizophrenia (Maeda et al., 2006), and bipolar disorder (Martinez-Aran et al., 2009), as well as older adults (Hart & Bean, 2011).

There are several reasons for why cognitive reserve/mental status *together* with EF should contribute to success in daily life. First, individuals with higher IQ or higher mental status appear to employ more efficient cognitive strategies when performing tasks, and consequently require fewer EF resources (S. Graham et al., 2010; Perfetti et al., 2009). Second, greater cognitive reserve is associated with greater semantic knowledge about a variety of situations, allowing greater reliance on crystallized intelligence rather than novel problem-solving. Lastly, individuals with higher IQ appear to have greater insight into their own deficits or weaknesses; such insight, in conjunction with higher EF, likely facilitates deployment of compensation strategies, thereby facilitating and prolonging functionality (Gerretsen, Plitman, Rajji, & Graff-Guerrero, 2014; Suchy et al., 2011).

In sum, although EF is unequivocally most strongly associated with successful daily functioning, EF capacity should nevertheless be considered in the context of other intrinsic resources, such as a patient's general intelligence, educational background, and overall mental status.

In addition to cognitive reserve and mental status, task complexity also interacts with EF. This is especially true when intrinsic resources, as discussed earlier, are also taken into consideration. Specifically, performance of even simple tasks tends to require considerable EF resources for individuals who are older, cognitively compromised, or less intelligent, but performance of the very same tasks may have virtually no EF involvement among individuals who are comparatively younger, healthier, or more intelligent (Cappell, Gmeindl, & Reuter-Lorenz, 2010; Ohsugi, Ohgi, Shigemori, & Schneider, 2013). In other words, for a given daily activity, average or even below average EF may be all that is required from many young, healthy, intelligent adults. In contrast, EF may be absolutely essential for performance of even a simple activity by older adults or intellectually compromised individuals, such that above average or perhaps even superior EF may be necessary for adequate functioning. To complicate matters further, it also appears that greater task complexity can sometimes overwhelm available resources of older or less able individuals, leading to a *disengagement* of EF resources and a subsequent failure to perform or initiate task (Clément, Gauthier, & Belleville, 2013; Perfetti et al., 2009).

Given these interactions between intrinsic characteristics and task complexity, it is possible that some daily tasks that *require error-free performance* may be too complex for even normal, cognitively healthy individuals. Consistent with this notion, we have found that normal EF was associated with error-free performance of IADLs only among those community-dwelling healthy older adults who also exhibited *above average* intellectual functioning (Suchy et al., 2011). Similarly, in our preliminary examination of a sample of adolescents with Type 1 diabetes, we have found not only that IQ (along with EF) related to disease management (S. L. Turner et al., 2015), but also that those who managed to maintain healthy blood glucose levels on a sustained basis had *above average* crystallized intelligence and had mothers with advanced degrees.[1] Although such findings certainly support the adage that to err is human, in some situations even a single mistake may have dire ramifications; consequently, clinical recommendations need to carefully weigh possible outcomes.

Incidentally, although task complexity is typically thought to reflect greater working memory load or the requirement to switch among multiple tasks, it also appears to matter whether the context in which the task is performed is novel or familiar. We have found that simply introducing a novel context to an otherwise *overlearned* task increased the task's reliance on EF and resulted in slower performance (Euler, Niermeyer, & Suchy, 2015). Consequently, clinicians need to consider that even familiar IADLs may become executively more demanding for patients who move to a new home or a new apartment.

Complexity of Daily Life. Although it is perhaps obvious to most clinicians, it nevertheless warrants mentioning that the complexity of one's daily life also has an impact on the available EF resources. Daily life complexity refers to the sheer number of tasks one needs to accomplish in a day. The greater the number of tasks, the greater the need for interleaving individual tasks' subgoals with each other, or for "squeezing" simple, one-step tasks in between more complex tasks. Under such circumstances, accomplishing even a simple IADL relies on meta-tasking (MT) ability, and the possibility of simply failing to remember to perform a given IADL increases manyfold. Thus, when judging whether a patient has adequate cognitive resources to perform a given task (e.g., medication management), clinicians should consider not only the complexity of the task itself but also the complexity of the patient's life on the whole.

Temperament. Certain temperamental characteristics also will have an impact on the degree to which certain environmental distractors will interfere

---

[1] Data from NIDDKD grant number 1R01DK092939, "A self-regulation approach to diabetes adherence into emerging adulthood," used with permission from Cynthia Berg and Deborah Wiebe, MPIs.

with task completion. Depending on a given person's temperamental sensitivity to reward versus punishment, as well as individual likes and dislikes, rewards and threats in the environment will exert differential pulls and pushes that may either facilitate or interfere with task completion. In this section, the word *temperament* is used somewhat broadly, including not only general threat and reward sensitivities and the relevant physiologic outcomes but also specific physiologically based predispositions, such as attraction to alcohol, sweet foods, or sexual activity. Thus, although one person may find it executively taxing to abstain from alcohol, another person may find abstaining from alcohol executively inconsequential but be executively taxed by a requirement to avoid sweets or to refrain from engaging in unsafe sex. Unfortunately, it is not possible, at least not at present, to quantify such tendencies so as to "correct" for them in neuropsychological evaluations. Nevertheless, clinicians need to recognize that such temperamentally determined pulls and pushes exist and that they will to some extent always compromise our ability to predict the likelihood of an executive lapse in a given patient.

In addition to the temperamentally determined pulls and pushes, temperament also determines the magnitude of one's emotional response to certain stimuli. Thus, for one person an affront by a sales clerk may be "water off their back," but for another it may be a reason for emotional upset that lasts for the rest of the day. It follows that the latter person is much more at risk for becoming executively depleted due to excessive emotion regulation demands. The more depletable person then is also at a greater risk for EF lapses on a regular basis.

Pulling It All Together: Contextually Valid Executive Assessment

It is a virtual truism in the world of clinical neuropsychology that measures of EF have limited ecological validity. This has led some to reject the construct of EF altogether (Stuss & Alexander, 2000), while leading others to embark on the development of measures that would deliver more ecological assessments of patients' daily functionality. Such new tests typically aim to mimic daily life by asking patients to perform various IADLs, such as shopping or running errands in a city, using a virtual environment (Campbell et al., 2009; Jansari et al., 2014; Jovanovski, Zakzanis, Campbell, et al., 2012; Jovanovski, Zakzanis, Ruttan, et al., 2012; Klinger, Cao, Douguet, & Fuchs, 2009; Renison, Ponsford, Testa, Richardson, & Brownfield, 2012). These new advances are highly creative, technologically sophisticated, and attractive as research tools. However, it is not yet clear whether they could realistically replace more neurocognitively based measures of EF in neuropsychological evaluations, or whether they should instead target rehabilitation settings where they could be used for assessments and rehabilitation of specific IADL skills. The distinction, although subtle, is important: On the one hand, neuropsychological assessments focus on neurocognitive processes as they relate to brain health, extrapolating from that perspective to daily functioning. On the other hand, assessments of IADLs examine whether a person can perform a particular daily task, regardless of neurocognitive underpinnings—that is, not only cognitive but also perceptual or physical limitations could account for poor performance.

Aside from this distinction, virtual reality solutions alone cannot address the issues discussed earlier in this chapter, such as individual differences in patients' lifestyles (and daily life complexity) or temperamental pulls and pushes. Thus, although such assessment solutions likely have incremental validity above and beyond traditional neuropsychological tests, such incremental validity may be limited to estimates of a patient's ability *only* in situations that are highly comparable to a given virtual scenario.

Consider, for example, a 16-year-old taking a virtual driving test. Assuming sufficient practice and normal cognition, it is likely the teen will pass. However, does the result of the driving test translate into actual driving safety on the road? Likely not. There are several reasons for this. First, it is well recognized that EF of adolescents is not yet fully mature (Stuss, 1992), making them prone to executive lapses. Second, it is also now well recognized that adolescents are particularly sensitive to, and prone to impulsively pursuing, social rewards (Stautz & Cooper, 2014; Weigard, Chein, Albert, Smith, & Steinberg, 2014). Although adolescents' immature EF may well be adequate for safe driving under ideal circumstances (or to pass a virtual driving test), it has been shown that introduction of competing contingencies that are socially rewarding (e.g., other teens in the car) will increase the possibility that an EF lapse will occur (Stautz & Cooper, 2014; Weigard et al., 2014). In other words, the teen's immature EF *in combination with* his temperamental characteristics (i.e., excessive attraction to social rewards) increases the chances of a lapse and thus makes for a combination that can be, quite literally, deadly. This vulnerability of teens to lapses is so well accepted now that some states, such as California, prohibit teen drivers from being behind the wheel if other teens are present in the car.

The preceding example shows that both traditional approaches to EF assessment and the virtual driving test ultimately fail ecologically: That is, neither realistically predicts whether driving lapses are likely. This is because both tests fail to examine other patient characteristics and the patient's real-world contexts. To address these limitations of current assessment methods, the Contextually Valid Executive Assessment (ConVExA) approach is currently under development in my laboratory. This assessment model aims to improve ecological validity of EF assessment by considering the patient's EF trait capacity (in the case of the teen, his immature EF) *in the context* of his other intrinsic resources (IQ), as well as the task complexity (driving), other environmental demands (distractions in the car), temperamental vulnerabilities (attraction to social rewards), and the seriousness of the ramifications of a lapse (car accident, injury).

Although much research needs to be done to provide explicit evidence-based ConVExA guidelines for clinicians, in principle the model can be applied in its current form to supplement or fine-tune traditional assessment methods. The following is a description of work yet to be done, as well as suggestions for how to implement the model given presently available clinical and empirical resources.

Work Yet to Be Done

(1) *Tools for better estimation of premorbid EF.* Research needs to develop formulas for incorporating information about personality, job complexity, and other relevant information into normative adjustments.

(2) *Methods for more accurate conversion of EF state (yielded by formal assessment methods) to EF trait.* We have begun this work in our laboratory, showing that we can estimate the acute burden of emotion regulation on the day of testing and extrapolate from that to the necessary adjustments to EF performance (Franchow & Suchy, 2015). The instrument (Burden of State Emotion Regulation Questionnaire; BSERQ) is currently being validated, and ongoing replication research is showing promising results.

(3) *Quantifying intrinsic resources required for error-free task completion.* Research needs to systematically examine the levels of EF, in the context of particular IQ and general mental status, required for error-free performance of specific IADLs of varying complexity. As mentioned earlier, the focus on *error-free* performance is purposeful: If a patient cannot perform a particular task without

errors while being formally assessed, then clearly errors are likely to occur in daily life as well. In situations in which even a single error can have serious ramifications for the patient's safety (or safety of others), predicting the risk of a lapse represents an important clinical goal. Information about the required minimum EF levels for error-free performance can be provided to clinicians in the form of normative tables, wherein EF scores are stratified *not* according to age or education (as is typical) but rather based on IQ and mental status. Test raw scores then are converted *not* to scaled scores but to the number of errors normatively committed on a specific IADL task in a distraction-free environment.

(4) *Tools for systematic evaluation of the complexity of the patient's daily life.* Tools for systematic evaluation of the complexity of the patient's daily life need to take the form of self-reports and informant reports. Such reports can be used to empirically *quantify* the impact of daily-life complexity on the probability of lapses, above and beyond what normative tables (described under numbers 2 and 3 above) can provide.

(5) *Tools for systematic assessment of the likelihood of becoming executively depleted on a daily basis.* A tool like this needs to include the assessment of temperamental pulls and pushes, the tendency to become upset, and the frequency and severity of pain, physical discomfort, psychological stress, and sleep deprivation. Currently, some questionnaires that examine temperamental characteristics exist, but their utility for the present purpose has not been examined. That said, the BSERQ measure described under number 2 above does assess the typical daily level of depletion and may serve for this purpose, though more research is needed.

What Can You Do Now? The preceding listing of "work yet to be done" is admittedly somewhat daunting. Nevertheless, clinicians should not despair: Much can be done in a typical clinical practice that would improve the ecological validity of EF assessment. Steps that clinicians can take are detailed in the following:

(1) To the extent possible, thoroughly assess all five EF subdomains and identify syndromes and symptoms as described throughout

this text. This will facilitate diagnostic decision-making, as well as provision of relevant recommendations.

(2) Carefully consider issues such as sleep, pain, and emotion regulation burden on the day of testing that could be affecting current test performance. Keep in mind that EF is more depletable by these issues than other cognitive domains, and qualify your interpretation of the patient's cognitive profile accordingly.

(3) Carefully consider issues such as personality, prior occupational attainment, and others addressed in detail in Chapter 7 and in the present chapter when estimating premorbid level of EF. For example, a patient with long-standing high openness to experience may have been premorbidly higher on EF than norms would suggest, whereas a patient with long-standing high neuroticism may have been premorbidly lower on EF than norms would suggest.

(4) In the interview, inquire about the complexity of IADLs that are important for the patient's safety (e.g., learn about the complexity of the patient's medication regimen), and consider this complexity in the context of the patient's IQ, educational attainment, and current general mental status (aside from current EF levels). For example, higher than average EF may be needed for complex regimens, as well as for simple regimens in the context of lower than averge IQ or lower than average mental status.

(5) In the interview, inquire about the complexity of the patient's daily life (see Table 9.2). Consider that even simple IADL demands (e.g., a simple medication regimen) may require considerable EF resources if occurring in the context of a very complex daily life.

(6) In the interview, inquire about the patient's daily tendencies to become executively depleted, such as the tendency to not get enough sleep, high frequency and severity of pain or discomfort in daily life, or the tendency to become highly emotionally upset. Consider that patients with such tendencies may exhibit considerable fluctuations in EF in their daily life. Thus, low average EF may not be sufficient for *consistently* error-free performance of IADLs.

(7) Integrate the preceding information with test data. Consider, for example, that a highly complex daily life will interfere with performance of even very simple medical regimens for patients characterized by disorganized syndrome, and that temperamental

Table 9.2 Sample topics to inquire about when determining the complexity of patient's daily life

DOMAIN OF DAILY LIFE	TOPICS TO INQUIRE ABOUT
Job	• One job versus multiple jobs • Leave job behind versus bring job home with you

IADLS	• Sharing duties vs. being solely responsible for
	  ○ Shopping
	  ○ Cooking
	  ○ Cleaning/yard work/repairs and upkeep
	  ○ Bill paying
	  ○ Ordering repairs
	  ○ Management of medical regimens (and its complexity)

Caretaking (children, spouse, parents, etc.)	• Sharing duties vs. being solely responsible for
	  ○ Shopping
	  ○ Cooking
	  ○ Cleaning/yard work/repairs and upkeep
	  ○ Bill paying
	  ○ Ordering repairs
	  ○ Management of medical regimens (and its complexity)
	• Frequency (live-in situations versus once a day versusonce a week, etc.)

Recreational activities	Frequency of organizing (alone vs. with help vs. not at all) • Get-togethers, parties, etc. • Vacations, weekend getaways, etc. • Going to the movies, plays, concerts, etc.

hypersensitivity to rewards will be particularly problematic for patients with disinhibited syndrome.

Chapter Summary

There are many considerations that can improve the interpretation and clinical utility of EF assessment. First, clinicians need to consider whether it is realistic or even clinically valuable to differentiate among EF subdomains and the corresponding syndromes for any given patient and referral question.

Second, because EF is a highly depletable cognitive domain, with test results being vulnerable to biases due to sleep deprivation, pain, or excessive emotion regulation demands on the day of testing, clinicians need to be vigilant to identify potential biases and adjust obtained EF scores accordingly. Third, for diagnostic purposes, it is important to estimate premorbid EF functioning as closely as possible, including in such estimates not only demographics but also personality and other characteristics that are known to systematically relate to EF. Fourth, to estimate a patient's ability to engage in a particular IADL, clinicians need to consider intrinsic cognitive resources beyond EF, as well as the complexity of the IADL task at hand, the complexity of the patient's daily life, and the patient's temperament. The ConVExA model offers a roadmap for future research toward addressing these clinical goals, as well as suggestions that can be implemented by clinicians given the currently available clinical resources.

PART FOUR

EXECUTIVE DYSFUNCTION IN CLINICAL POPULATIONS

This part of the book provides an overview of executively compromised patient populations typically seen by clinical neuropsychologists in their practice. The part is organized according to major groupings of disorders, including neurodevelopmental, neurodegenerative, and neuropsychiatric categories, as well as disorders associated with an acquired insult or an illness. To the extent possible, disorders are linked to the various EF syndromes, with the understanding that (a) many disorders present with a combination of syndromes or even with a global EF dysfunction, and (b) for some disorders the literature in not clear regarding the specific EF symptoms. Related to the latter point, readers should understand that *absence of evidence* does not equal *evidence of absence*. That is, for many disorders, certain subdomains may have not been adequately studied; for others, pronounced deficits in a particular subdomain may obscure deficits in another subdomain (this is particularly true for meta-tasking). Readers should note that it is beyond the scope of this book to provide an exhaustive review of the literature on all disorders that could potentially present with deficits in EF. Rather, the goal here is to help clinicians develop a sense of the scope of EF dysfunction across typical patient populations. Readers are encouraged to follow the newest literature on populations of interest.

Note that the Appendix provides a tabulated overview of the literature reviewed in this part of the book.

10

Neurodevelopmental Disorders

The term *neurodevelopmental* refers to disorders or conditions that are characterized by abnormalities in the growth and development of the central nervous system. In this chapter, our discussion will be limited to disorders that involve abnormalities in brain function or structure. Importantly, the term neurodevelopmental disorders is sometimes erroneously used to refer to disorders of childhood. However, these disorders obviously affect both children and adults; an example of such a disorder is autism. In contrast, certain conditions are *not* considered neurodevelopmental when they occur in adults but have neurodevelopmental consequences when they occur in children or pre- or perinatally. For example, brain injuries secondary to an anoxic event or a cerebrovascular accident that occur prior to birth dramatically impact future development of the brain. Cerebral palsy is an example of such a neurodevelopmental disorder. Note that traumatic brain injuries in both adults and children are covered in the chapter on acquired brain injury (Chapter 13).

Attention Deficit Hyperactivity Disorder

Attention deficit hyperactivity disorder (ADHD) is a disorder that is characterized by a persistent pattern of inattentiveness, hyperactivity, or impulsivity that interferes with normal daily functioning in both social and educational/occupational domains. Typical age of onset is in early childhood, with diagnostic criteria from the fifth edition of the *Diagnostic and Statistical Manual of Mental Disorders* (DSM-5) requiring onset prior to 12 years of age (American Psychiatric Association, 2013). Symptoms must occur in more than one setting and cannot be better accounted for by other diagnoses. Three subtypes of ADHD have been described. These are (a) the predominantly inattentive presentation, (b) the predominantly hyperactive-impulsive presentation, and (c) the combined presentation.

The neuroanatomy of ADHD has been studied extensively. This research implicates abnormalities in the frontoparietal working memory network (Cortese et al., 2012), as well as the anterior cingulate gyrus (Colla et al., 2008; O'Connell et al., 2009; A. B. Smith, Taylor, Brammer, Halari, & Rubia, 2008) and the right cerebral hemisphere (Casey, Castellanos, Giedd, & Marsh, 1997; Garcia-Sanchez, Estevez-Gonzalez, Suarez-Romero, & Junque, 1997; A. B. Smith et al., 2008). Given these neuroanatomical underpinnings, it should not be surprising that a range of EF anomalies would be present in this disorder.

Meta-analytic work confirms that individuals with ADHD exhibit executive deficits that include the subdomains of executive cognitive functions (ECFs), initiation/maintenance (I/M), and response selection (RS; Lansbergen, Kenemans, & van Engeland, 2007; Willcutt, Doyle, Nigg, Faraone, & Pennington, 2005). Limitations in social cognition (SC) are also common (Da Fonseca et al., 2009; L. M. Williams et al., 2008). Cognitive weaknesses or deficits generally cannot be explained by lower intelligence or lower education, or other comorbid disorders (Willcutt et al., 2005). Additionally, some meta-analyses have focused on examination of patient performance on specific measures. Such studies have demonstrated that children with ADHD perform poorly on the Wisconsin Card Sorting Test (Romine et al., 2004), on continuous performance tests (CPT; Pauli-Pott & Becker, 2011), and on the Stroop (or color-word interference) tests (Homack & Riccio, 2004), although poor performances on these tests are *not* specific to ADHD. Given the previously described EF limitations, difficulties with emotion regulation also represent a core symptom of ADHD (Martel, 2009). Consequently, ADHD is associated with negative emotionality (Healey, Marks, & Halperin, 2011) and depression (Wolff & Ollendick, 2006), as well as increased aggression (Melnick & Hinshaw, 2000).

There has been much interest in trying to understand the differences between the inattentive and the hyperactive/impulsive subtypes of ADHD. Such research demonstrates that individuals with primarily the inattentive presentation are often characterized by a sluggish cognitive tempo (in line with I/M deficits, or the apathetic syndrome), whereas impulsive or hyperactive patients are characterized by pervasive behavioral dysregulation (in line with RS deficits, or the disinhibited syndrome; Becker & Langberg, 2014). Although ADHD symptoms in general tend to decrease somewhat in adulthood, during childhood there may be an increase in measurable EF deficits with increasing age, especially during the transition from preschool to school age (Pauli-Pott & Becker, 2011). In general, whereas inattentiveness tends to be easier to detect with typical neuropsychological measures than impulsivity (Martel, Nikolas, & Nigg, 2007), impulsivity tends to be more readily apparent via behavioral observations, particularly in children.

Autism Spectrum Disorders

According to some classification systems, autism, Asperger's syndrome, and nonverbal learning disability represent diagnostic categories in their own right; however, *DSM-5* (American Psychiatric Association, 2013) subsumes the previously separate categories into a single autism spectrum disorder (ASD) of varying presentations and severities. Regardless of the classification system, on the whole these disorders are marked by difficulties in social skills and communication, cognitive delays, and a variety of stereotyped behaviors and interests. Because of the long tradition of separate diagnostic labels for autism and Asperger's syndrome, the literature related to each of these two presentations is reviewed separately here.

Autism. The available research on EF deficits in autism is based primarily on samples of individuals with high-functioning autism, due to the difficulty of recruiting or assessing individuals with more severe autistic features. Importantly, the exact definition of high-functioning autism varies somewhat from one study to the next; consequently, many samples may be composed of both patients with high-functioning autism and those with Asperger's syndrome. Due to this heterogeneity in samples, research findings are mixed.

Despite the mixed empirical findings, it is generally believed that individuals with autism suffer from executive deficits (Ozonoff, South, & Provencal, 2007). This is particularly consistent in parent and teacher reports and is thus commonly accepted in the clinical lore (A. S. Chan et al., 2009; Gilotty, Kenworthy, Sirian, Black, & Wagner, 2002; Humphrey, Golan, Wilson, & Sopena, 2011; Rosenthal et al., 2013). With respect to parent-reported deficits, these tend to correlate with adaptive functioning (Gilotty et al., 2002), although the appropriateness of interpreting parental reports as actual deficits in EF has been challenged (Humphrey et al., 2011).

Studies that examine EF using performance-based cognitive measures (as opposed to questionnaires) report findings that span the gamut from EF performances that are comparable to those of typically developing controls to performances that are clinically impaired (Happé, Booth, Charlton, & Hughes, 2006; Kimhi, Shoam-Kugelmas, Agam Ben-Artzi, Ben-Moshe, & Bauminger-Zviely, 2014; Kleinhans, Akshoomoff, & Delis, 2005; R. J. Landa & Goldberg, 2005; S. Robinson, Goddard, Dritschel, Wisley, & Howlin, 2009; Sachse et al., 2013). Studies that have attempted to characterize *profiles* of executive dysfunction among individuals with autism have also been inconsistent. For example, Kleinhans et al. (2005) found deficits on measures of verbal fluency in the context of normal ability to perform the color-word interference test, whereas S. Robinson and colleagues (2009) found impairments on color-word interference in the context of normal verbal fluency. Overall, studies have found both impaired and intact performances on virtually all classic measures of EF.

These mixed findings raise the question of why individuals with autism appear to function abnormally in daily life while at times performing well during formal assessments. One likely explanation is that the principal deficit in autism involves *meta-tasking* (MT). As already discussed in Chapter 3, deficient MT (or the *disorganized syndrome*) is characterized by normal performances on typical cognitive measures, in the context of functional problems in daily life. This notion is supported by a recent study (D. Williams, Boucher, Lind, & Jarrold, 2013) that found deficient prospective memory among individuals with autism (incidentally, this deficit could not be explained by poor time estimation). As a reminder, prospective memory represents one of several core elemental processes that support MT (see Chapter 3 for a full review).

In addition to MT, SC is virtually by definition impaired in individuals with ASD, likely due to abnormalities in the function and structure of the amygdala, as well as processing deficiencies in the theory of mind and mirror neuron system networks (Hornak et al., 2004; Kenemans et al., 2005; Tsuchida et al., 2010). Difficulties fairly consistently include poor recognition of facial and prosodic affect, as well as impaired empathy (Hubbard & Trauner, 2007; Humphreys et al., 2007), although at least some research suggests that emotional empathy may be relatively spared as compared with cognitive empathy (Dziobek et al., 2008).

Lastly, an interesting question about EF in this population has to do with whether executive dysfunction represents a core, primary deficit, or whether executive impairment emerges later as a secondary consequence of the disorder. At least some research with young preschoolers suggests that most symptoms of executive dysfunction begin to emerge later, only after impairments in SC become apparent (Yerys, Hepburn, Pennington, & Rogers, 2007), which typically occurs by the age of 3 years (G. Dawson, Webb, & McPartland, 2005). Also relevant is the finding that SC deficits cannot be explained by limitations in general intellectual functioning or perception (G. Dawson et al., 2005). However, this interpretation needs to be considered with caution, as progressively greater executive dysfunction during maturation is a common phenomenon in a variety of cognitive disorders that first present in childhood.

Asperger's Syndrome. As mentioned earlier, in *DSM-5* (American Psychiatric Association, 2013), Asperger's syndrome is no longer a separate diagnosis. Instead, it is classified as *autism spectrum disorder without language or intellectual impairment*. However, given that the majority of past research still uses the older label, it is included here as its own diagnostic category. Studies that specifically focus on individuals with Asperger's syndrome fairly consistently identify specific difficulties with mental flexibility, as well as with other aspects of ECFs (Ambery, Russell, Perry, Morris, & Murphy, 2006; Brady et al., 2013; Glasier, 2008; Hieger, 2006; Semrud-Clikeman, Fine, & Bledsoe, 2014). The specific deficit in mental flexibility may well be related to these patients' difficulties with perspective taking, cognitive empathy, or theory of mind (ToM), all of which are commonly impaired in this population (Baez et al., 2012; Baron-Cohen & Wheelwright, 2004; Dziobek et al., 2008). Consistent with deficits on ToM tasks, SC is virtually by definition impaired (Kaetsyri, Saalasti, Tiippana, von Wendt, & Sams, 2008; Lyons & Fitzgerald, 2004; Montgomery, Stoesz, & McCrimmon, 2013), as is the ability to regulate emotions (Semrud-Clikeman, Walkowiak, Wilkinson, & Butcher, 2010).

Of note, similar to research on high-functioning autism, some studies find no differences between patients and control groups on classic measures of EF (Hill & Bird, 2006; Li, Zou, & Li, 2005; Shamay-Tsoory, Tomer, Yaniv, & Aharon-Peretz, 2002). However, more complex tasks that tax MT abilities do tend to detect impairments even in the context of otherwise normal cognitive profile (Hill & Bird, 2006). Lastly, because Asperger's syndrome is also associated with slow performance on measures of processing speed (Holdnack, Goldstein, & Drozdick, 2011), clinicians need to take care not to confound processing speed and EF on timed tests.

Chronic Tic Disorders (CTD)

According to *DSM-5* (American Psychiatric Association, 2013), tic disorders are characterized by "sudden, rapid, recurrent, non-rhythmic movements and vocalizations." Tic disorders are commonly comorbid with other conditions, including ADHD (40–50%) and obsessive-compulsive disorder (OCD; 30–40%), and, less frequently, anger and impulse control disorders, and anxiety and mood disorders (Freeman et al., 2007). Similar to research on ASD, findings of EF deficits in children with CTD have been inconsistent, such that some studies report deficits (Chang, McCracken, & Piacentini, 2007; Watkins et al., 2005) whereas others fail to identify reliable group differences (Roessner, Albrecht, Dechent, Baudewig, & Roethenberger, 2008; Verte, Geurts, Roeyers, Oosterlaan, & Sergeant, 2005). These inconsistencies are likely in part related to considerable heterogeneity among studied samples, with some studies excluding comorbidities and others allowing inclusion of comorbid conditions, thereby potentially confounding results.

When deficits in EF are found, they typically involve working memory, planning, problem-solving, and decision-making (implicating a weakness in the domain of ECFs; Channon, Pratt, & Robertson, 2003) and response inhibition (implicating a weakness in RS; Eichele et al., 2010). Importantly, results of studies that compare patients with CTD only (i.e., without comorbidities) with patients with CTD plus comorbidities suggest that EF weaknesses may be related to comorbid psychopathologies (e.g., ADHD, OCD) rather than CTD per se (Chang et al., 2007; Channon et al., 2003; Roessner et al., 2008; Watkins et al., 2005).

In sum, although the literature can be interpreted as suggesting that individuals with CTD potentially exhibit some symptoms of the disinhibited and dysexecutive syndromes, a careful examination of comorbidities may provide clearer picture. Lastly, it is important to consider that individuals with CTD expend considerable energy on tic suppression, which may have a deleterious impact on their cognition, in particular their EF (Franchow & Suchy, 2015; Himle et al., 2012).

Intellectual Disability

Intellectual disablity refers to a category of disorders that are characterized by abnormally low intellectual functioning in conjunction with deficits in adaptive behaviors (American Psychiatric Association, 2013). There are a variety of causes of intellectual disability; these include genetic and chromosomal conditions, complications during pregnancy or birth, or an illness or injury. Additionally, *familial intellectual disability* refers to low intellectual functioning that is inherited from parents and further exacerbated by limited opportunities in a child's environment. This latter type of intellectual disability is generally viewed to be simply an extension of the normal (i.e., nonpathological) range of functioning, rather than a disorder, and is not included in this review.

The majority of research on EF among individuals with intellectual disabilities includes patients with Down syndrome, Prader-Willi syndrome, fragile X syndrome, and Williams syndrome. On the whole, this research suggests that intellectually disabled individuals do exhibit a variety of weaknesses across EF subdomains (Barisnikov, Hippolyte, & Van der Linden, 2008; Borella, Carretti, & Lanfranchi, 2013; Chevalère et al., 2013; Danielsson et al., 2010; Greer, Riby, Hamiliton, & Riby, 2013; Hartman, Houwen, Scherder, & Visscher, 2010; Hippolyte, Iglesias, Van der Linden, & Barisnikov, 2010; Jauregi et al., 2007; Kasari et al., 2001; Lanfranchi, Jerman, Dal Pont, Alberti, & Vianello, 2010; Rhodes, Riby, Park, Fraser, & Campbell, 2010; Sgaramella, Carrieri, & Barone, 2012; Wishart et al., 2007), and that the severity these deficits relates to impairments in social and occupational functionality (Gligorović & Đurović, 2014).

However, EF and IQ are highly correlated among intellectually disabled individuals (Chevalère et al., 2013), suggesting that EF deficits may simply be in line with expectations given these patients' intellectual limitations. In fact, when compared with control groups matched on IQ (typically accomplished by matching participants on *mental age*), EF weaknesses fail to emerge (Walley & Donaldson, 2005), and at least one study found that verbal abilities were a better predictor of employment status than EF (Su, Chen, Wuang, Lin, & Wu, 2008). Similarly, some research suggests that deficits in SC among intellectually disabled individuals may also be explained by IQ (Garner, Callias, & Turk, 1999; Grant, Apperly, & Oliver, 2007). One possible exception is that some individuals with intellectual disability appear to exhibit working memory deficits that are more severe than would be suggested by their IQ levels, and these weaknesses are thought to represent the mechanism behind poor reasoning (Carretti, Belacchi, & Cornoldi, 2010). Nevertheless, in interpreting these findings, one needs to consider that comparisons with controls matched for mental age may not provide a realistic picture of the actual cognitive profile, as the maturation of EF does not occur in a linear fashion relative to age and IQ.

Regarding specific etiologies of intellectual disabilities, executive weaknesses that are above and beyond the more generalized intellectual disability have been fairly consistently reported among individuals with fragile X syndrome (Bennetto, Taylor, Pennington, Porter, & Hagerman, 2001; Hooper et al., 2008; Moss & Howlin, 2009). The specific EF domains that appear to be mostly affected include ECFs (particularly working memory) and RS, whereas I/M abilities appear relatively normal (S. Baker et al., 2011; Cornish, Turk, & Hagerman, 2008; Hooper et al., 2008; Kogan et al., 2009; Murphy & Mazzocco, 2009; Wilding, Cornish, & Munir, 2002). Additionally, although deficits on ToM tasks have also been reported in this population, they appear to be secondary to working memory and intellectual deficits (Grant et al., 2007). Of note, there is a considerable gender effect in fragile X, such that boys and men with the full mutation are typically mildly to severely intellectually disabled, whereas only about 25% of girls and women exhibit intellectual impairment, with the remainder showing normal, albeit low, intellectual functioning with concomitant mild learning difficulties (Bennetto et al., 2001; Cornish et al., 2008; Rinehart, Cornish, & Tonge, 2011). Adult carriers of fragile X (i.e., presumably unaffected individuals) also exhibit mild working memory weaknesses, and are at risk for the development of fragile X–associated tremor and ataxia syndrome (FXTAS) in middle age, which is described in more detail in Chapter 11 (Neurodegenerative Disorders).

Lastly, some research suggests the possibility that declines in EF represent an early marker of neurodegenerative changes in patients with Down syndrome, with both behavioral changes (i.e., disinhibition and apathy) and declines in test performances on classic EF measures being associated with incipient global cognitive decline, potentially due to Alzheimer's disease (Adams & Oliver, 2010; S. L. Ball, Holland, Watson, & Huppert, 2010).

Congenital Injuries

Cerebral Palsy. *Cerebral palsy* is an umbrella term for a host of pre-, peri-, and postnatal brain insults resulting from a wide range of causes, including hypoxia/anoxia, ischemia, hemorrhage, infections or toxic agents, trauma, and genetic factors (Mahone & Slomine, 2008). Cerebral palsy is characterized by problems with muscle control and coordination, muscle tone, and posture and balance, with the majority (approximately 75%) of cases exhibiting spastic symptoms, and the remainder showing dyskinetic or ataxic symptoms (Blondis, 2004; Warschausky, Kaufman, & Felix, 2013). Additionally, approximately one half to two thirds of individuals with cerebral palsy also have an intellectual disability or at least one specific learning disorder (Fennell & Dikel, 2001; Schenker, Coster, & Parush, 2005). Although the validity of available assessment instruments used with this population has been questioned (Yin Foo, Guppy, & Johnston, 2013), at least one study has reported excellent to fair test-retest reliability on IQ and EF measures among children with cerebral palsy (Piovesana, Ross, Whittingham, Ware, & Boyd, 2015).

Research on neuropsychological functioning (beyond IQ) of individuals with cerebral palsy is sparse. However, neuroimaging often reveals white matter changes, including leukomalacia in the periventricular regions (Fennell & Dikel, 2001), suggesting that problems in EF might exist. Additionally, it is common for parents of children with cerebral palsy to report a variety of behavioral problems, including symptoms of externalization and hyperactivity (Brossard-Racine et al., 2013); such symptoms in turn have been shown to be related to executive weaknesses in nonneurological populations (Schoemaker, Mulder, Deković, & Matthys, 2013). Thus, not surprisingly, the few studies that have examined cognition in more depth have reported deficits in EF (Bodimeade, Whittingham, Lloyd, & Boyd, 2013) and attention (Lemay, Lê, & Lamarre, 2012). Of note, there is considerable variability in symptom profiles within studied samples due to the heterogeneity of etiologies, pathophysiology, and lesion locations and severity. Consequently, at present, no clear profile of EF dysfunction in this population has been identified (Bottcher, 2010). Future research faces challenges in finding appropriate control samples to match on motor or potential cognitive/intellectual limitations, as well as appropriate assessment approaches.

Fetal Alcohol Syndrome. Fetal alcohol syndrome (FAS) is a disorder that is associated with heavy exposure to alcohol during fetal development. It is characterized by both physical and central nervous system abnormalities, including abnormalities in the corpus callosum and the frontal lobes (Niccols, 2007). Not surprisingly, FAS is associated with a range of neurocognitive impairments in intellectual functioning, learning and memory, sensory processing, moral functioning, and language development (Nuñez, Roussotte, & Sowell, 2011). At least some research suggests that EF deficits represent a prominent feature of this disorder and that these deficits cannot be explained by other cognitive deficiencies (Connor, Sampson, Bookstein, Barr, & Streissguth, 2001; K. Kerns, Don, Mateer, & Streissguth, 1997); however, similar to research on intellectual disabilities, some studies suggest that EF deficits are in fact consistent with IQ and other cognitive impairments (Korkman, Kettunen, &

Autti-Rämö, 2003; McGee, Schonfeld, Roebuck-Spencer, Riley, & Mattson, 2008).

Regarding the type of executive dysfunction, research suggests that all subdomains are affected: Individuals with FAS often exhibit the low arousal and sluggishness associated with inattentive ADHD and the apathetic syndrome, behavioral dysregulation associated with the disinhibited syndrome, reasoning and problem-solving deficits associated with the dysexecutive syndrome, and emotional and social impairments associated with the inappropriate syndrome (Connor et al., 2001; Green et al., 2009; K. Kerns et al., 1997; Korkman et al., 2003; Mattson, Schoenfeld, & Riley, 2001; McGee et al., 2008; Monnot et al., 2002; Nuñez et al., 2011).

Importantly, many individuals who experienced prenatal exposure to alcohol do not meet the diagnostic criteria for FAS, due to the lack of the typical facial features associated with the syndrome. However, such individuals still exhibit structural and functional brain abnormalities (Astley et al., 2009a, 2009b; Sowell et al., 2008), as well as cognitive impairments that are primarily executive (Mattson et al., 2010).

Preterm Birth

Children born prior to the 37th week of gestation are considered to be preterm. With advances in medical care and life-sustaining technologies, about 1% to 2% of live births in developed countries are considered "very preterm," with birth occurring prior to the 32nd week of gestation, and a small fraction of these are considered "extremely preterm," with birth occurring prior to the 26th week of gestation (Howard, Anderson, & Taylor, 2008). Although there is considerable variability in outcomes, and gestational age is further moderated by birthweight, it is generally the case that outcomes are poorer with shorter gestational age and lower birthweight. Age at assessment further moderates the findings for some, but not all, areas of functioning, with the largest deficits found at preschool age, and some normalization of performance found after the age of 11 years (Mulder, Pitchford, Hagger, & Marlow, 2009).

In general, it is agreed that approximately 50% of children born very preterm exhibit considerable executive and attentional difficulties, and often meet the diagnostic criteria for ADHD. Both inattentive and impulsive/hyperactive presentations have been reported, with poorer ability to sustain attention and an inability to inhibit prepotent responses persisting even after controlling for IQ or other factors (Mulder et al., 2009). However, although inattentive problems appear to persist as children mature, problems with inhibitory control appear to improve with age (Howard et al., 2008; Mulder et al., 2009). In addition, persistent deficits in ECFs have also been reported, including deficits in working memory and memory retrieval, and concomitant deficits on tests of planning (Jongbloed-Pereboom, Janssen, Steenbergen, & Nijhuis-van der Sanden, 2012; Mulder et al., 2009).

Spina Bifida and Hydrocephalus

Spina bifida is a disorder characterized by an incomplete closure of the spinal canal; it is often associated with other complications in the central nervous system, including hydrocephalus and Chiari malformations (Yeates, Fletcher, & Dennis, 2008; Zabel, Jacobson, & Mahone, 2013). As reviewed by Yeates and colleagues (2008), children and adults with spina bifida exhibit on average somewhat depressed intellectual functioning, with as many as 25% exhibiting frank intellectual disability. In general, visual-spatial abilities, math skills, and SC tend to be most affected (Lindsay, 1997), with possibly as many as 50% of children with spina bifida exhibiting a profile that is consistent with nonverbal learning disability (Yeates, Loss, Colvin, & Enrile, 2003). Because the most typical site for shunting takes place in the right hemisphere (Meager, Kramer, Frim, & Lacy, 2010), some authors have suggested that shunting may be partly responsible for the cognitive and social/emotional deficits among those spina bifida patients who also present with hydrocephalus (Rissman, 2011). However, limited research for this hypothesis exists. Nevertheless, it is noteworthy that, as reviewed in Chapter 4 (response selection), Chapter 5 (initation/maintenance), and Chapter 6 (social cognition), right hemisphere dysfunction can be associated with disinhibited, apathetic, and inappropriate syndromes.

Additionally, because uncontrolled hydrocephalus is often associated with permanent damage to the periventricular white matter (Del Bigio, 2010), individuals with poorly control intracranial pressure often exhibit deficits in processing speed and some aspects of EF (Iddon, Morgan, Loveday, Sahakian, & Pickard, 2004), most notably the ECFs subdomain (Meager et al., 2010). However, there are inconsistencies in research findings, such that some studies find that greater EF deficits are associated with hydrocephalus, whether occurring in the context of spina bifida or other disorders (Iddon et al., 2004), whereas others have found that spina bifida alone results in greater impairment than hydrocephalus alone (Hampton et al., 2013). An important consideration in interpreting such inconsistencies is the etiology of hydrocephalus, the degree to which hydrocephalus is controlled, the number of shunt surgeries and revisions, and the degree to which spina bifida is associated with cerebellar involvement and Chiari malformation (Meager et al., 2010).

Chapter Summary

Many neurodevelopmental conditions are characterized by EF dysfunctions. Those reviewed in this chapter include ADHD, autism spectrum disorders, chronic tic disorders, intellectual disability, congenital injuries (cerebral palsy, fetal alcohol syndrome), preterm birth, and spina bifida and hydrocephalus. Although the nature of EF deficits is fairly well characterized in some disorders (e.g., ADHD, fetal alcohol syndrome), some disagreement continues to exist about the exact nature and severity of EF deficits in the majority of neurodevelopmental disorders. The disagreement generally stems from other cognitive/intellectual confounds that complicate interpretation (e.g., intellectual disability, autism), as well as physical disability that makes assessment difficult (e.g., cerebral palsy).

11

Neurodegenerative Disorders

Dementias of Old Age

This section covers conditions and diseases that are typically associated with cognitive deterioration in the fifth decade of life or later, although the pathophysiologic manifestations of the diseases themselves may in some cases predate symptom onset by years or even decades. This section will cover executive deficits associated with dementia diagnosis, as well as deficits that become apparent during preclinical stages of cognitive decline.

Frontotemporal Lobar Degeneration. *Frontotemporal lobal degeneration* (FTD) is the second most common neurodegenerative disease of old age after Alzheimer's disease (AD) and is often seen as the poster child for dementing illnesses that are associated with executive dysfunction. It is characterized by progressive degeneration of frontal and temporal lobes, with the age of onset being earlier when compared with other dementias, typically in the fifth to early sixth decade of life. Frontotemporal lobal degeneration is associated with three different neurobehavioral presentations, known as the behavioral variant (bvFTD), progressive nonfluent aphasia (pnfaFTD), and semantic dementia (sdFTD). This classification reflects differences in the involvement of frontal versus temporal lobes and may, in some cases, reflect relative hemispheric asymmetry with which the disease progresses. Specifically, whereas the behavioral variant is typically assumed to be associated with bilateral frontal involvement, the other two variants disproportionately affect the posterior frontal lobe and the temporal lobes, either bilaterally or primarily on the left. See Snowden (2013) for a comprehensive review.

With respect to bvFTD, the neurodegenerative process typically begins in the ventral and medial aspects of the frontal lobes, affecting, among others, von Economo neurons (E.-J. Kim et al., 2012) that are important for social cognition (SC; see Chapter 6). Only then does the neurodegenerative process gradually progress to the dorsolateral prefrontal cortex and the temporal lobes. Given this course of neurodegeneration, measurable EF deficits may not be readily apparent early on in the disease process. Instead, early symptoms often present as personality changes and include apathy, disinhibition, and social inappropriateness (Borroni et al., 2012), as well as a lack of concern about meeting the expected social demands during clinical evaluations (Rankin et al., 2008). Additional symptoms that also deserve close attention are changes in sexuality (both hyper- and hyposexuality), hyperorality/overeating, stereotyped behaviors or vocalizations (De Deyn et al., 2005; LaMarre & Kramer, 2013), and sudden onset of criminal behavior. In fact, in one study, 54% of patients with bvFTD and 56% of those with sdFTD had engaged in minor criminal behavior, as compared with only 12% of those with AD (Diehl-Schmid, Perneczky, Koch, Nedopil, & Kurz, 2013). Lastly, profound deficits in self-awareness (Rosen et al., 2014) and meta-tasking (Roca et al., 2013) can be evident early on. In sum, patients present primarily with the inappropriate syndrome, accompanied by features of the apathetic and disinhibited syndromes. Of note, whereas personality changes in other types of dementia typically present as an exaggeration of a premorbid personality (Archer et al., 2007; Gould & Hyer, 2004; Magai, Cohen, Culver, Gomberg, & Malatesta, 1997), in bvFTD gross or diametric alterations in personality can occur (Lebert, Pasquier, & Petit, 1995). For this reason, early in the course of bvFTD many patients receive psychiatric diagnoses rather than neurological diagnoses, and the initial treatments and assessments involve psychiatric, rather than neurologic, medical disciplines (LaMarre & Kramer, 2013).

Importantly, because executive cognitive functions (ECFs) may not be affected early on in the disease course, a clear pattern of executive deficits on typical clinical measures may not emerge, which sometimes causes some confusion for clinicians. In fact, some research has failed to identify any differences on EF performances between patients with bvFTD and those with AD (Giovagnoli, Erbetta, Reati, & Bugiani, 2008; Roca et al., 2013). To make matters worse, some studies report comparable deficits on tests of episodic memory in both bvFTD and AD (Hornberger & Piguet, 2012; Pennington,

Hodges, & Hornberger, 2011). For this reason, it has been suggested that test scores alone are not adequate for differentiation of bvFTD and AD. Rather, diagnostic differential may be more appropriately achieved by way of qualitative analysis of performance (such as perseverative responding and increased numbers of errors due to rule-breaking and disorganization; Kramer et al., 2003; Libon et al., 2007; Thompson, Stopford, Snowden, & Neary, 2005) and information from collateral sources (such as information about inappropriate behavior and personality changes) collected via interviews or questionnaires (De Deyn et al., 2005; Milan et al., 2007). Recently, the International Behavioural Variant FTD Criteria Consortium put forth a set of consensus symptoms; from among these, behavioral disinhibition, perseverative/compulsive behaviors, problems with empathy or sympathy, and hyperorality resulted in greatest agreement among raters, whereas apathy and neuropsychological data yielded lesser agreement (LaMarre et al., 2013).

Nevertheless, some conclusions can be drawn from test data. Among the most promising approaches for differential diagnosis is a pattern analysis of performances on letter versus semantic fluency tests. In general, whereas patients with AD show mild impairment on semantic fluency, patients with bvFTD show a greater impairment on both fluency types as compared with AD, and, importantly, greater relative impairment on letter fluency as compared with semantic fluency (Rascovsky, Salmon, Hansen, Thal, & Galasko, 2007). Additionally, especially in cases with prominent apathetic symptoms, general slowing across all timed measures may be observed among patients with bvFTD. As a supplement to traditional neuropsychological measures, tests that tap SC may also prove to be more sensitive; in fact, longitudinal research suggests that isolated early-onset deficits on tasks of theory of mind (ToM) represent a risk factor for future development of FTD (Pardini et al., 2013).

Subcortical Ischemic Vascular Dementia. Vascular dementia is a neurobehavioral syndrome that encompasses heterogeneous causes and presentations. Although in all cases the general cause is vascular disease, the specific causes can include (a) multiple large cortical infarctions (i.e., multi-infarct dementia), (b) multiple subcortical lacunar infarction (i.e., lacunar state), (c) a single strategically placed infarction, or (d) small vessel disease resulting in diffuse white matter pathology (i.e., Binswanger's disease or leukoaraiosis; K. Y. Haaland & Swanda, 2008). Because the cognitive profiles and the clinical course associated with large cortical strokes clearly depend on the number and location of lesions and as such are highly specific to any given patient, some authors do not consider those to be the same entity as vascular dementia. In other words, it is common in clinical neuropsychology to assume that the term *vascular dementia* refers to small vessel disease involving diffuse pathological changes within the periventricular white matter, as well as multiple lacunar strokes. As has been done by other authors, we will refer to this entity as *subcortical ischemic vascular dementia* (SIVD; G. E. Smith & Bondi, 2013, p. 207).

Correctly diagnosing SIVD is of key importance: Although the appropriate use of antihypertensive medications has been shown to slow down or stop the progression of this dementia (Shah et al., 2009), the use of cholinesterase inhibitors and memantine (used in Alzheimer's dementia) may be associated with adverse effects, absence of cognitive improvements, and high monetary cost (D. A. Levine & Langa, 2011). That said, clinicians need to be aware of the high comorbidity (25% to 80% across studies) of Alzheimer's and vascular pathology (Jellinger, 2008), a condition that is sometimes referred to as *mixed dementia* (Langa, Foster, & Larson, 2004).

A recent meta-analysis confirmed that vascular mild cognitive impairment (MCI) is marked by poor performances on traditional measures of EF, as well as motor symptoms and behavioral dysregulation, which are typically accompanied by prominent periventricular white matter hyperintensities (Sudo et al., 2012). Similarly, a carefully conducted study of patients with SIVD showed that the most common characteristics of the disorder include deficits on measures of EF and visual-spatial functioning, with lesser impairment on measures of delayed recall, once again in the context of prominent periventricular white matter hyperintensities and hypertension (Cosentino et al., 2004). Importantly, the often-cited "stepwise" decline as a hallmark symptom of vascular dementia has not been consistently found for SIVD (G. E. Smith & Bondi, 2013, p. 208) and is more likely to be associated with multi-infarct dementia.

With respect to the differential between SIVD and AD, a recent review (G. E. Smith & Bondi, 2013, pp. 220–228) suggests that patients with AD and SIVD do not differ from each other on EF. Rather, many studies show that the hallmark double dissociation between the two disorders is that patients with SIVD perform more poorly on measures of EF than on measures of episodic memory (particularly free delayed recall), whereas patients with AD perform more poorly on measures of episodic memory than on measures of EF.

Regarding specific profiles among EF subdomains, research in this area is limited. However, functional imaging research suggests that lacunar strokes and white matter hyperintensities have a deleterious impact on metabolism primarily in the dorsolateral prefrontal cortex, which in turn correlates with performance on typical measures of EF (B. R. Reed et al., 2004). This localization suggests that ECFs may be the most affected. This is consistent with research showing that processes related to working memory are disrupted in SIVD (Lamar, Swenson, Kaplan, & Libon, 2004).

Regarding specific assessment methodology and/or profiles of EF that might help with the differential diagnosis between SIVD and AD, some research suggests specific deficit on letter fluency, or a specifically depressed Initiation/Perseveration score on the Mattis Dementia Rating Scale among patients with SIVD (Porto, Caramelli, & Nitrini, 2007). Additionally, early in the dementing process, a single deficit in EF (especially as compared with episodic memory) is suggestive of SIVD, whereas later on in the disease process, motor and gait symptoms become more prominent (M. Chan, Lim, & Sahadevan, 2008). Lastly, declines in the pace of walking are associated with declines in EF and a diagnosis of SIVD (Verghese, Wang, Lipton, Holtzer, & Xue, 2007).

Alzheimer's Dementia. As reviewed by G. E. Smith and Bondi (2008), Alzheimer's disease represents the most common type of neurodegenerative etiology, affecting primarily people 65 years of age or older, with the risk further increasing with increasing age. The cause of the disease is unknown, although several principle mechanisms have been hypothesized, including loss of cholinergic neurons, amyloid accumulation, and vascular causes. The neurophysiologic changes in the brain have been well characterized, including their locations and concomitant cognitive deficits. Given that early on the disease targets primarily the hippocampus and posterior temporal lobe, it is understandable that the hallmark deficits of Alzheimer's dementia include problems with memory retention, and language or semantic network impairments. For additional review, see G. E. Smith and Bondi (2008).

However, deficits in EF also play a prominent role. Many studies have found that individuals with Alzheimer's disease exhibit deficits in ECFs, as evidenced on tests of working memory, reasoning and problem-solving, and general cognitive flexibility (Harrison et al., 2014; G. E. Smith & Bondi, 2008). Importantly, such deficits are apparent also among individuals with MCI who progress to Alzheimer's dementia (Bisiacchi, Borella, Bergamaschi, Carretti, & Mondini, 2008; Dickerson, Sperling, Hyman, Albert, & Blacker, 2007) and are predictive of a faster rate of decline among patients with mild dementia (Parikh et al., 2014). Additionally, research has shown that a combination of weaknesses in EF and episodic memory among apparently neurologically healthy older adults together predict the progression to Alzheimer's disease several years later (Albert et al., 2011; Chen et al., 2001). These findings are likely explained by the fact that, in addition to the hippocampus and related mesial temporal structures, tertiary cortical areas represent the primary target of the disease, both anteriorly and posteriorly (Yang et al., 2012).

In addition to deficits in ECFs, there is also considerable evidence of initiation/maintenance (I/M) deficits, particularly decreased initiation. In fact, the majority of patients' caregivers report problem with decreased initiation, with 55% reporting that patients initiate only with prompting, and 42% reporting that patients do not initiate activity even though they express willingness to engage in that activity (Cook et al., 2008). In sum, the types of executive deficits that are likely to be seen in Alzheimer's disease patients both during the prodromal period and after progression to dementia involve primarily ECFs and I/M. For detailed discussion of the topic, see G. E. Smith and Bondi (2013, pp. 169–172).

Of note, much research has demonstrated the utility of semantic or category fluency tests both for the diagnosis of AD and for differentiation of AD from other neurodegenerative processes, such as SIVD and FTD. In particular, meta-analytic research shows that patients with AD tend to exhibit poorer performances on semantic fluency as compared with letter fluency (Henry, Crawford, & Phillips, 2004); in contrast, patients with FTD and SIVD tend to exhibit the opposite pattern, or show impairment on measures of both semantic and letter fluency.

Dementia With Lewy Bodies. *Dementia with Lewy bodies* (DLB) is characterized by fluctuations in cognition (especially attention and alertness), recurrent and well-formed visual hallucinations, and features of parkinsonism. Other associated futures include, among others, REM sleep disorder, severe sensitivity to neuroleptics, as well as repeated falls, loss of consciousness, and autonomic dysregulation (Tröster, 2008). Early in the disease process cognition is characterized by deficits in EF, as well as in attention and visual-spatial abilities (Boeve, 2012; Bradshaw, Saling, Anderson, Hopwood, & Brodtmann, 2006; Molano et al., 2010; Yoon, Lee, Yong, Moon, & Lee, 2014). As the disease progresses, deficits in these domains continue to be more pronounced as compared with other dementias of similar overall severity (Collerton, Burn, McKeith, & O'Brien, 2003; Crowell, Luis, Cox, & Mullan, 2007; Kao et al., 2009; Preobrazhenskaya, Mkhitaryan, & Yakhno, 2006). Memory impairment is often absent early on and only begins to emerge as the disease progresses, although even then deficits in delayed recall and delayed recognition tend to be less severe among patients with DLB as compared with AD patients (Crowell et al., 2007; Kawai et al., 2013; Kraybill et al., 2005; Levy & Chelune, 2007; McLaughlin, Chang, & Malloy, 2012). Interestingly, the severity of visual hallucinations appears to be related to the severity of EF deficits (Cagnin et al., 2013). Lastly, patients with DLB sometimes exhibit apparent deficits in verbal comprehension, and these appear to be related to deficient working memory (Gross et al., 2012).

Regarding the specific profile of EF dysfunction, most traditional EF measures such as tests of verbal fluency, working memory, trail making, and the Stroop (Crowell et al., 2007; Hanyu et al., 2009; Johns et al., 2009; Kraybill et al., 2005; Yoon et al., 2014) are reasonably sensitive to deficits in this disease, even relative to other dementias. Although the consistently identified working memory deficits suggest a specific impairment in ECFs, marked fluctuations in performance on attentional measures suggest impaired I/M, particularly set maintenance (Bradshaw et al., 2006; Walker et al., 2000). These conclusions are consistent with caregiver reports of dysexecutive symptoms and apathy (Peavy et al., 2013). Lastly, disinhibition is not considered to be a classic symptom of DLB, but both patients and caregivers list disinhibition as a symptom of concern (Kao et al., 2009; Peavy et al., 2013).

Parkinson's Disease and Other Parkinsonian Disorders. *Parkinson's disease* (PD), whose typical age of onset is after 50 years of age, is characterized by a set of fairly specific motor symptoms that begin to emerge when approximately 70% to 80% of the pigmented cells in the substantia nigra have been lost (Tröster & Fields, 2008). Importantly, some cognitive limitations are already present in approximately one third of newly diagnosed patients (Foltynie, Brayne, Robbins, & Barker, 2004), with some 25% of newly diagnosed patients showing impaired performances on three or more cognitive tests (Muslimović, Post, Speelman, & Schmand, 2005), including measures of EF and memory (Foltynie et al., 2004; Muslimović et al., 2005).

The presence of cognitive dysfunction (in addition to motor dysfunction) early on in the disease can be explained by the fact that the frontal striatal circuits involving dorsolateral, orbitofrontal, and medial frontal cortices (including anterior cingulate gyrus) have direct and indirect pathways that link the striatum with the substantia nigra. In addition, cognitive changes may relate to dopaminergic changes in the mesocortical and mesolimbic systems (rather than just the nigro-striatal system), as well as nondopaminergic neurotransmitter systems involving norepinephrine, serotonin, and acetylcholine (for review, see Tröster & Fields, 2008). Lastly, patients with PD exhibit changes in white matter integrity (Gallagher et al., 2013), and the presence of Lewy bodies continues to be discussed as a possible cause of cognitive decline in PD (Aarsland, Perry, Brown, Larsen, & Ballard, 2005).

The estimates of the rate of frank dementia in PD vary widely. Although the most common estimates range from 20% to 40%, as many as 75% of patients who survive 10 years after diagnosis present with dementia (Aarsland & Kurz, 2010). Additionally, higher rates of dementia occur in patients who are diagnosed at an older age (Wickremaratchi, Ben-Shlomo, & Morris, 2009). Interestingly, measureable early weaknesses in EF represent a risk factor for the development of dementia (Janvin, Aarsland, & Larsen, 2005), as do more prominent gate problems (particularly freezing gate) and postural instability (as opposed to tremor), which themselves tend to be associated with more pronounced EF deficits (Dirnberger & Jahanshahi, 2013). Importantly, dementia in PD can be related to additional etiologies, with the majority of cases suspected of also having DLB (McKeith, 2002).

Regarding the type of executive deficits commonly seen in patients with PD, the majority of research suggests impaired ECFs (including planning, reasoning, working memory, memory retrieval/fluency, and mental flexibility) and I/M (primarily initiation; Beato et al., 2008; Benge, Phillips-Sabol, & Phenis, 2014; A. Costa et al., 2014; Dirnberger & Jahanshahi, 2013; Dujardin et al., 2013; Pettit, McCarthy, Davenport, & Abrahams, 2013). Additionally, deficits in SC have also been reported (Dirnberger & Jahanshahi, 2013), including deficient paralinguistic communication (Dujardin et al., 2004) and self-awareness (Kudlicka, Clare, & Hindle, 2013). These EF limitations cannot be fully explained by other potentially confounding factors such as slow speed of processing or slow motor response (Pettit et al., 2013). In general, cognitive profiles are consistent with functional imaging research that shows diminished metabolism and/or dopamine receptor binding in the dorsolateral prefrontal and anterior cingulate cortices and related subcortical circuitry (Dagher, Owen, Boecker, & Brooks, 2001; Dirnberger & Jahanshahi, 2013; Ekman et al., 2012), as well as improvements in both task performance and dorsolateral metabolism with treatment (Cools, Stefanova, Barker, Robbins, & Owen, 2002).

Importantly, not all patients exhibit remittance of cognitive problems with pharmacotherapy. In some cases, treatment-related systemic increases in dopamine may result in excess dopamine in a less affected hemisphere, especially among patients with subtle motor symptoms that are asymmetric (Tomer, Aharon-Peretz, & Tsitrinbaum, 2007). Additionally, dopaminergic treatment can be associated with increases in impulsivity or risk-taking (Cools, Barker, Sahakian, & Robbins, 2003; Gschwandtner, Aston, Renaud, & Fuhr, 2001).

Progressive supranuclear palsy (PSP) presents with symptoms that are similar to PD, with vertical gaze palsy being the most classic distinguishing feature. Progressive supranuclear palsy is much less common than PD, occurring in 5 out of 100,000 people over the age of 50 (Hoppitt et al., 2011). Consequently, it is less studied then PD, and much less is known about its cognitive profile. In general, however, it is estimated that 50% to 80% of PSP patients develop dementia. Executive deficits represent a common early symptom of PSP dementia, with approximately 70% of patients evidencing poor performances on the Initiation/Perseveration subscale of the Mattis Dementia Rating Scale and on the Frontal Assessment Battery (R. G. Brown et al., 2010; Gerstenecker, Mast, Duff, Ferman, & Litvan, 2013). In this population, EF deficits appear to be associated with the atrophy of the frontal lobes (Cordato et al., 2002) and the cerebellum (Giordano et al., 2013). Although EF deficits tend to be more severe and the decline appears to be more rapid in PSP than in PD (Soliveri et al., 2000), memory retrieval problems are comparable between the two disorders (Aarsland et al., 2003). Lastly, social/emotional awareness and receptive paralinguistic communication also appear to be impaired in PSP (Ghosh, Rowe, Calder, Hodges, & Bak, 2009).

Cortical-basal degeneration is characterized by asymmetric progressive motor rigidity, dystonia, or myoclonus that is nonresponsive (or, at best, minimally responsive) to levodopa. It is frequently associated with asymmetric ideational apraxia (Soliveri, Monza, & Paridi, 1999). Deficits in EF are common and also include deficits in memory retrieval. These deficits cannot be explained by aphasia (Hohler, Ransom, Chun, Troster, & Samii, 2003), even though nonfluent aphasia is particularly common in this disorder (N. L. Graham, Bak, Patterson, & Hodges, 2003).

Multiple-system atrophy (MSA) is an umbrella term for striatonigral degeneration, olivopontocerebellar atrophy, and Shy-Drager syndrome (for a review, see Tröster & Fields, 2008). The disorder is characterized by neurodegenerative changes that involve the basal ganglia, cerebellum, pons, and medulla oblongata, although these brain regions are involved to varying degrees in the different MSA subtypes. The disorder is characterized by ataxia, autoimmune dysfunction, and parkinsonism. Patients with MSA exhibit a cognitive profile that is highly similar to that of PD, with approximately one third of patients exhibiting deficits in EF (R. G. Brown et al., 2010; Siri et al., 2013), although some research suggests that patients with MSA are somewhat more cognitively impaired than those with PD (Kao et al., 2009). Although some studies find subtle cognitive differences among the three MSA variants (Balas, Balash, Giladi, & Gurevich, 2010), others do not (Siri et al., 2013). For additional review of neurobehavioral presentations of these disorders, see Tröster and Fields (2008).

Fragile X–Associated Tremor and Ataxia. First identified in the late 1990s (R. Hagerman et al., 2001), fragile X–associated tremor and ataxia syndrome (FXTAS) is a disorder that afflicts carriers of the FMR1 premutation allele that is associated with fragile X syndrome. The disorder is characterized by a late-onset (usually starting in the fifth decade of life) intention tremor and gait ataxia, parkinsonism, and peripheral neuropathy (Brega et al., 2008; P. J. Hagerman & Hagerman, 2004; R. Hagerman et al., 2001). Although carriers on the whole tend to exhibit lower IQ scores and some weaknesses in memory, those with FXTAS also exhibit global deficits in EF (Birch, Cornish, Hocking, & Trollor, 2014; Brega et al., 2008; Brega et al., 2009; Grigsby et al., 2008; Grigsby et al., 2006). There is also some evidence that mild EF dysfunction and weaknesses in working memory predate the onset of motor symptoms (K. M. Cornish, Hocking, Moss, & Kogan, 2011).

Amyotrophic Lateral Sclerosis. Amyotrophic lateral sclerosis (ALS) is a motor neuron disease involving both upper and lower motor neurons and presenting with muscle weakness and/or atrophy and speech and/or swallowing problems. Although ALS has classically been seen as a purely motor condition, much recent research suggests that cognition is impaired in a large subset of cases, with between 30% and 50% of patients exhibiting some cognitive limitations and as many 20% to 30% exhibiting frank cognitive impairment or dementia (Consonni et al., 2013; Oh et al., 2014; Ringholz et al., 2005; Rippon et al., 2006). Executive deficits in particular appear to represent a prominent feature of cognitive dysfunction (Rajeswaran & Nalini, 2013; Rippon et al., 2006; Zalonis et al., 2012) and continue to be present even when motor symptoms (Štukovnik, Zidar, Podnar, & Repovš, 2010) and speed of processing (Pettit et al., 2013) are taken into consideration. Executive function deficits appear to be present in both sporadic and familiar etiologies (Irwin, Lippa, & Swearer, 2007) and in both spinal (limb) and bulbar subtypes (Zalonis et al., 2012). The presence of EF deficits appears to have prognostic ramifications, predicting faster disease progression, as well as future disability or death (Elamin et al., 2013; Elamin et al., 2011; Oh et al., 2014). For further review, see Irwin et al. (2007). Given the prevalence of EF deficits, some investigators have hypothesized that ALS occurs on a continuum with FTD (Goldstein & Abrahams, 2013; Irwin et al., 2007; Strong, Lomen-Hoerth, Caselli, Bigio, & Yang, 2003). In fact, as many as 15% of ALS patients meet the diagnostic criteria for FTD (Ringholz et al., 2005).

Regarding the specific profile of EF deficits, performances on measures of verbal fluency/memory retrieval and abstract reasoning and on Stroop and trail-making tests tend to be below expectations (Quinn et al., 2012; Rajeswaran & Nalini, 2013; Rippon et al., 2006; Zalonis et al., 2012). These weaknesses are associated with metabolic and structural abnormalities in the working memory networks (Libon et al., 2012; Quinn et al., 2012), implicating ECFs. Additionally, SC is also impaired (Goldstein & Abrahams, 2013), including deficits in sarcasm comprehension (Staios et al., 2013). Lastly, given the suspected association between FTD and ALS, it should not be surprising that personality changes are sometimes reported in patients who do not exhibit other cognitive limitations (as is common early in bvFTD; Waldron, Barrash, Swenson, & Tranel, 2014).

Other Neurodegenerative Disorders

Multiple Sclerosis. Multiple sclerosis (MS) is a progressive neurodegenerative disease that primarily affects young adults between the ages of 20 and 40. Multiple sclerosis involves a chronic autoimmune process marked by degeneration of the myelin sheath surrounding axons of the central nervous system. Second only to traumatic brain injury, it is a common source of disability among young and middle-aged adults. In addition to motor, sensory, and autonomic symptoms, cognitive dysfunction is estimated to occur in more than 50% of cases across all diseases subtypes and can often be detected early on in the disease process (Amato et al., 2010; Chelune, Stott, & Pinkston, 2008). In general, however, patients with secondary progressive MS are more impaired cognitively than patients with the relapsing-remitting subtype; similarly, patients with primary progressive MS tend to be more impaired than those with the relapsing-remitting subtype when controlling for disease duration (Planche, Gibelin, Cregut, Pereira, & Clavelou, 2015; Ruet, Deloire, Charré-Morin, Hamel, & Brochet, 2013).

Because of the considerable heterogeneity of lesion location and lesion burden among patients with MS, there is some variability in the specific cognitive profiles of individual patients. Regardless, the one common denominator is slowed speed of processing (Bodling, Denney, & Lynch, 2012; Chelune et al., 2008). Because adequate speed of processing is necessary for cognitive functions that rely on complex brain networks, it should not be surprising that deficits in processing speed are also typically associated with deficits in attention and in ECFs, including working memory and memory retrieval (Ferreira, 2010). In fact, as many as 80% of patients with detectable cognitive impairments exhibit deficits in ECFs, at least among the relapsing-remitting subtype (García, Plasencia, Benito, Gómez, & Marcos, 2009); in patients with pediatric-onset MS, EF deficits appear to be present in as many as 44% of cases (Till et al., 2012). Lastly, the severity of EF deficits tends to correlate with whole brain volume and lesion burden (Parmenter et al., 2007; Till et al., 2012).

Because depression is extremely common among patients with MS, research has repeatedly examined the possibility that some or all of the cognitive deficits seen in this population could be related to the deleterious impact of depression. In general, this has *not* been supported, although the lack of this association continues to be questioned (Feinstein, 2006), as some contributions of depression and anxiety to test performance have been demonstrated (Julian & Arnett, 2009). Nevertheless, patients' *complaints* of cognitive difficulties do appear to be mediated by depression (Feinstein, 2012; Randolph, Arnett, & Freske, 2004). Given that MS patients appear to have better insight regarding their own EF deficits than do their friends or relatives (M. M. Smith & Arnett, 2010), it is possible that subtle declines in EF that are not detectable by traditional EF measures may be present in some patients and may in fact contribute to depressive symptoms.

Lastly, patients with MS exhibit deficits in SC, including impaired performances on tests of ToM and the ability to understand emotional expressions (Henry et al., 2009). Some patients with MS exhibit blunted emotional reactivity, potentially impacting their ability to learn from negative consequences, which is sometimes associated with the disinhibited syndrome (Kleeberg et al., 2004).

Chapter Summary

Many neurodegenerative conditions are characterized by EF dysfunctions. Those reviewed in this chapter include frontotemporal lobar degeneration, subcortical ischemic dementia, Alzheimer's dementia, dementia with

Lewy bodies, Parkinson's disease and other parkinsonian disorders, fragile X–associated tremor and ataxia syndrome, amyotrophic lateral sclerosis, and multiple sclerosis. Due to the important contribution behavioral testing makes to diagnostic decision-making for these disorders, the nature and severity of EF dysfunction is extensively studied and fairly well characterized. However, the assessment and diagnosis of the behavioral variant of FTD continues to represent a challenge, as traditional cognitive measures do not seem to adequately capture the typical symptoms of this syndrome.

12

Neuropsychiatric Disorders

Neuropsychiatric disorders are, virtually by definition, characterized by deficient emotion regulation and social functioning. Thus, deficits in executive functioning (EF) in general and social cognition (SC) in particular are consistently found in these populations. This chapter focuses on populations whose EF deficits are of notable clinical significance and on populations that are likely to be encountered by clinical neuropsychologists in their practice. A thorough review of all neuropsychiatric disorders associated with relative weaknesses in some aspects of EF is beyond the scope of this chapter.

Schizophrenia Spectrum Disorders

Schizophrenia spectrum refers to a set of disorders that are characterized by delusions and hallucinations, as well as differing degrees of disorganized thought processes (sometimes evidenced in disorganized speech), disorganized motor functioning, and the so-called negative symptoms (e.g., apathy, social disengagement, anhedonia, poverty of speech, and flat affect; American Psychiatric Association, 2013). The most studied among these disorders is schizophrenia, which itself consists of several subtypes, including paranoid, disorganized, catatonic, and undifferentiated.

It is well recognized that schizophrenia is associated with cognitive dysfunction, and it has been argued that cognitive deficits represent a core, stable feature of schizophrenia (R. A. Reed, Harrow, Herbener, & Martin, 2002). In fact, meta-analytic research shows that cognitive deficits in schizophrenia exhibit larger effect sizes than deficiencies in brain volume, metabolism, or receptor density (Heinrichs, 2005). Cognitive profiles in schizophrenia are consistently marked by deficits in EF (including SC), attention, and memory/learning, all of which occur in the context of generally depressed IQ (Braw, Benozio, & Levkovitz, 2012; Christensen, Patrick, Stuss, Gillingham, & Zipursky, 2013; Kopald, Mirra, Egan, Weinberger, & Goldberg, 2012; Leeson et al., 2010; Oram, Geffen, Geffen, Kavanagh, & McGrath, 2005; Yun et al., 2011). Of note, similar profiles of deficits have also been demonstrated among patients with schizoaffective disorder (Amann et al., 2012). Given that cognition is generally depressed in schizophrenia, it is possible that poor performances on EF measures simply reflect deficits in the lower-order processes. Some research has examined this question, and although lower-order processes do explain some variance in EF performance in schizophrenia populations, executive deficits persist even after controlling for these processes (Neill & Rossell, 2013; Savla et al., 2011).

While onset of schizophrenia typically occurs in late adolescence or young adulthood, longitudinal research suggests that mild cognitive problems begin to emerge during the prodromal stage (Laws, Patel, & Tyson, 2008). These further worsen with the onset of psychosis, then remain relatively stable for at least 10 years after diagnosis (Bozikas & Andreou, 2011), and finally evidence further decline after the age of 65 (Rajji & Mulsant, 2008). However, patients in remission do appear to exhibit considerable normalization of their EF performances (Braw et al., 2012). Although some studies find EF weaknesses in first-degree relatives of patients with schizophrenia, the findings are somewhat inconsistent (Jameson, Nasrallah, Northern, & Welge, 2011; Kuha et al., 2007; Sánchez-Torres et al., 2013), perhaps due to the fact that unaffected siblings may exhibit a delay in EF maturation (Bhojraj et al., 2010) rather than a deficit that persists into adulthood.

The cognitive profile of schizophrenia is consistent with neuroanatomical studies that show smaller overall brain volume, ventricular enlargement, and volume reduction in medial temporal, frontal (including anterior cingulate gyrus), and parietal lobes, as well as the cerebellum and the thalamus (Baiano et al., 2007; Minzenberg, Laird, Thelen, Carter, & Glahn, 2009; Ridler et al., 2006; Rüsch et al., 2007; Rüsch et al., 2008; Segarra et al., 2008). Additionally, white matter abnormalities in the inferior frontal cortex, anterior cingulate gyrus, the caudate nucleus, insula, and the inferior parietal lobule have been associated with impulsivity among patients with schizophrenia (Hoptman et al., 2004; Hoptman et al., 2002). Relatedly, functional imaging studies show abnormal activation patterns in dorsolateral, ventrolateral, and medial prefrontal cortices during tasks relying on executive cognitive functions (ECFs) and response selection (RS; Barch & Csernansky, 2007; Kaladjian, Jeanningros, Azorin, Anton, & Mazzola-Pomietto, 2011; Minzenberg et al., 2009; Royer et al., 2009).

It is important to note that despite what appears to be a fairly consistent literature, there is considerable variability among patients with respect to their EF abilities (Raffard & Bayard, 2012). This should not be surprising given the heterogeneity of schizophrenia itself. Consequently, a number of studies have examined whether meaningful subtypes with different cognitive profiles exist (Iampietro, Giovannetti, Drabick, & Kessler, 2012; Leeson et al., 2009; Power, Dragović, & Rock, 2013; Savla et al., 2011). Although profiles across studies vary in part as a function of different cognitive batteries, on the whole greater EF impairments are associated with greater severity of negative symptoms and disorganization (Dibben, Rice, Laws, & McKenna, 2009; Donohoe, Corvin, & Robertson, 2006; Donohoe & Robertson, 2003), as well as with problematic behaviors, poorer psychosocial adjustment, and limitations in functional independence (Iampietro et al., 2012; Meiron, Hermesh, Katz, & Weizman, 2013; Power et al., 2013; Yen et al., 2009). These findings point to the practical and clinical utility of EF assessment in this population.

Regarding the specific nature of executive deficits, ECFs are virtually universally impaired, including consistent deficits on a wide range of measures of working memory (Heinrichs, 2005; Royer et al., 2009), as well as deficits in meta-tasking (MT) that tend to be present at the first onset of psychosis and remain stable despite treatment (Liu et al., 2011). Also, given the high prevalence of negative symptoms in schizophrenia that are characterized by apathy and poor motivation, it should be expected that initiation/maintenance (I/M) would be impaired in this population as well. In fact, a number of studies have demonstrated the association of negative symptoms in general and apathy in particular with performances on measures of EF, with perhaps the most consistent deficits emerging on various Stroop tasks (Donohoe et al., 2006; Faerden et al., 2009; Fervaha, Agid, Foussias, & Remington, 2014; Fervaha et al., 2013; Holmén et al., 2012). Additionally, some studies have noted impaired motivation and sensitivity to rewards (Fervaha et al., 2013), both of which represent core features of the apathetic syndrome. However, some studies show normal I/M (Egeland, 2007; Ilonen et al., 2000; Sanz, Gómez, Vargas, & Marín, 2012). Thus, it is possible that apathy in this population is secondary to deficient ECFs and impoverished ideation, rather than a primary

I/M deficit. In general, however, motivation per se in this population is grossly understudied (Barch, 2008).

In addition to apathy, impulsivity is also sometimes described in patients with schizophrenia. In such cases, it is believed that the impulsive symptoms contribute to aggression and suicide risk (Gut-Fayand et al., 2001; Iancu et al., 2010). This notion has been in part supported by research showing that white matter abnormalities in the right inferior frontal lobe are associated both with self-reported aggression and with self-reported impulsivity among men with schizophrenia (Hoptman et al., 2002). Unfortunately, limited research exists examining impulsivity behaviorally, with poor agreement regarding the impulsivity construct further confounding the picture (Ouzir, 2013). Nevertheless, in support of the notion that impulsivity is a factor in schizophrenia, research has found that patients exhibit impaired error monitoring or discrepancy detection (Aleman, Agrawal, Morgan, & David, 2006; Silver & Goodman, 2007), which is a key feature of RS (i.e., disinhibited syndrome). Lastly, SC appears to be impaired among individuals with schizophrenia independent of their other impairments in EF (Pickup, 2008).

In sum, research consistently shows that patients with schizophrenia exhibit deficits in ECFs and SC, in conjunction with a globally depressed general cognitive and intellectual status. Less consensus exists on whether deficits also include other subdomains of EF. At least one study showed deficits in MT, but deficits in RS and I/M are not clearly delineated, in part due to sparse behavioral research and inconsistency in the use of constructs and assessment instruments. Lastly, research findings are considerably limited by the heterogeneity of schizophrenia and by the failure of many studies to clearly define their populations or to compare different schizophrenia subtypes.

Bipolar Disorder

Bipolar I, bipolar II, and cyclothymic disorders represent a "bridge" between depression and schizophrenia spectrum disorders with respect to symptomatology, genetics, and family history. On the one hand, there appears to be a shared genetic association between schizophrenia and bipolar disorders, which frequently co-occur in the same family; on the other hand, bipolar disorders are virtually by definition associated with episodes of depression (American Psychiatric Association, 2013).

Three recent meta-analyses comparing patients with schizophrenia and bipolar disorder found that patients with bipolar disorder have a neurocognitive profile that is similar to that seen in schizophrenia, but with less severe impairment (Amann et al., 2012; Ancín, Cabranes, Santos, Sánchez-Morla, & Barabash, 2013; Vöhringer et al., 2013). As is the case in research on schizophrenia, EF deficits among patients with bipolar disorder are predictive of psychosocial maladjustment (Yen et al., 2009). In addition to behavioral comparisons, functional imaging research suggests that although schizophrenia and bipolar disorder are characterized by different patterns of activation during tasks that tax memory, the two disorders show similar metabolic abnormalities during performance of executively demanding tasks (Whalley et al., 2012).

In contrast to schizophrenia, impulsivity symptoms are thought to represent a core feature of mania (Giovanelli, Hoerger, Johnson, & Gruber, 2013; S. L. Johnson, Carver, Mulé, & Joormann, 2013), although many studies unfortunately examine impulsivity using only questionnaire ratings (Saddichha & Schuetz, 2014). Studies that do examine impulsivity behaviorally are rare but have corroborated the association between disinhibition and criminal behavior, antisocial personality features, substance abuse, and history of suicide attempts among patients with bipolar disorder (Swann et al., 2011).

Depression

Although older classifications of neuropsychiatric illnesses tended to group depression and mania into a single overarching category of mood disorders, *DSM-5* provides a separate classification section for manic and depressive syndromes (American Psychiatric Association, 2013). The primary disorders included in the depressive category include disruptive mood dysregulation disorder, major depressive disorder, persistent depressive disorder (previously known as dysthymia), and premenstrual dysphoric disorder; the majority of research on the association between depressive symptoms and EF is based on patients diagnosed with major depressive disorder.

Much research with both younger and older adults supports the notion that depression has a deleterious impact on cognition in general and on EF in particular (Biringer et al., 2005; Harvey et al., 2004; Mahurin et al., 2006; Murrough, Iacoviello, Neumeister, Charney, & Iosifescu, 2011; Paelecke-Habermann, Pohl, & Leplow, 2005; Stordal et al., 2004; Taconnat et al., 2010), as well as the notion that EF limitations represent a risk factor for the development and/or maintenance of depressive symptoms (Murrough et al., 2011; Trivedi & Greer, 2014).

However, research findings are far from consistent, with some studies reporting that EF deficits associated with depression are minor at most (Jungwirth et al., 2011). Inconsistent or negative findings can likely be explained in part by the heterogeneity of samples across studies, both with respect to depression subtypes and severity and with respect to demographics (Hammar & Årdal, 2009). Studies that do focus on examining EF across subtypes of depression have begun to demonstrate some of the influences of unique patient characteristics. For example, research has shown that depressed patients with higher cortisol levels (suggesting higher levels of stress) exhibit greater EF impairment than those with lower cortisol levels (Egeland et al., 2005). Similarly, there is evidence that anxiety uniquely contributes to EF deficits above and beyond depression alone (Yochim, Mueller, & Segal, 2013), and patients who present with both depression and apathy exhibit greater EF deficits than patients with either apathy or depression alone (Nakaaki et al., 2008). Thus, studies that exclude patients with certain common comorbid characteristics are bound to report smaller EF deficits than those that allow inclusion of such comorbidities. Consequently, the degree to which any given patient suffering from depression will exhibit EF deficits cannot be readily gleaned from the literature.

Research examining the impact of treatment on EF is also marked by some inconsistencies. On the one hand, some research shows that patients' EF improves with successful treatment (Biringer et al., 2005; Trivedi & Greer, 2014). In fact, despite the well-known deleterious impact of electroconvulsive therapy (ECT) on cognition, a large-scale meta-analysis has shown improvements in EF above and beyond baseline after the ECT treatment was concluded (Semkovska & McLoughlin, 2010). On the other hand, much research also shows that mild subclinical weaknesses in EF persist in many patients even after normalization of mood (Hammar & Årdal, 2009; Paelecke-Habermann et al., 2005; Trivedi & Greer, 2014), consistent with the suggestion that executive weaknesses represent a risk factor (or a biomarker) for this disorder (Vinberg, Miskowiak, & Kessing, 2013). In line with this notion, at least some research suggests that older adults with EF deficits are less likely to respond favorably to pharmacological treatment of depression (Alexopoulos et al., 2005), and older individuals with acquired EF dysfunction due to stroke (Terroni et al., 2012), small vessel disease (Taylor, Aizenstein, & Alexopoulos, 2013), or mild cognitive impairment (MCI; Polyakova et al., 2014) are at an increased risk for the development of depression.

Regarding the profile of specific EF deficits most commonly associated with depression, it is generally believed that depressed patients are most likely to present with the dysexecutive syndrome (Christopher & MacDonald, 2005; L. S. P. de Almeida et al., 2012), consistent with the reliance of emotion regulation on ECFs (see Chapter 2), and the apathetic syndrome (Hoffstaedter, Sarlon, Grefkes, & Eickhoff, 2012; Klimkeit, Tonge, Bradshaw, Melvin, & Gould, 2011; Thomas et al., 2009), consistent with decreases in reward sensitivity among depressed individuals (see Chapter 5). Additionally, because depression appears to contribute to difficulties in daily functioning above and beyond traditionally assessed EF performance (Rog et al., 2014), it is possible that depression has a deleterious impact on those aspects of EF that cannot be readily assessed in a laboratory, namely, MT. Lastly, some weaknesses in SC are also typically present, as is the case for virtually all neuropsychiatric disorders (Bozikas et al., 2006; Weniger et al., 2004).

Anxiety

Despite the refinement of the anxiety disorders category in *DSM-5*, these disorders still represent a fairly heterogeneous group, including a wide range of conditions such as separation anxiety disorder, selective mutism, specific phobias, social anxiety disorder (previously social phobia), panic disorder, agoraphobia, generalized anxiety disorder, substance/medication-induced anxiety disorder, and anxiety disorder due to other medical condition (American Psychiatric Association, 2013). The most common among these are specific phobias and social anxiety disorder, with 12-month prevalence of approximately 8% and 7%, respectively (American Psychiatric Association, 2013). This chapter focuses primarily on social phobia because this disorder not only is quite common but also is most likely to be encountered in clinical practice and most likely to interfere with functioning in the course of daily life. Of note, *DSM-5* classifies obsessive-compulsive disorder separately from anxiety disorders.

Similar to depression, anxiety disorders in general and social phobia in particular are associated with deficits in ECFs (Topçuoğlu, Fistikci, Ekinci, Gönentür, & Agouridas, 2009). Additionally, similar to depression, there is growing evidence that subtle subclinical weaknesses in EF represent a vulnerability for the development of anxiety (Wells & Matthews, 2006). Interestingly, some aspects of EF may be stronger among anxious individuals. For example, anxiety is associated with larger than typical error-related negativity per electrophysiologic recordings (Moser, Moran, Schroder, Donnellan, & Yeung, 2013), suggesting stronger than normal error monitoring or discrepancy detection. However, it is not clear whether this actually translates into better than normal RS among anxious individuals. In fact, considering the Yerkes-Dodson law (Yerkes & Dodson, 1908), individuals with high state anxiety are likely to exhibit impaired performances across the board, due to excessive levels of anxiety-related arousal.

Obsessive-Compulsive Disorders

According to *DSM-5*, obsessive-compulsive disorders (OCDs) are related to, but not subsumed under, the anxiety disorder category. Instead, based on research and clinical evidence, OCDs as a group have emerged as a category in its own right. In addition to including the OCD proper, this category also includes body dysmorphic disorder, hoarding, trichotillomania (hair pulling), and excoriation (skin picking; American Psychiatric Association, 2013). From a pathophysiologic standpoint, it is assumed that the disruption of the same neuroanatomical networks undergirds all these disorders, as animal models of OCD have typically involved hoarding and excessive grooming or licking behaviors (Feusner, Hembacher, & Phillips, 2009; Hyman, 2007).

On the whole, adult and child patients with OCD shows deficient performances on measures of EF (Aydın, Koybasi, Sert, Mete, & Oyekcin, 2014; Dittrich & Johansen, 2013; Taner, Erdogan Bakar, & Oner, 2011), as well as persistent EF weaknesses after treatment and remittance of symptoms (Bannon, Gonsalvez, Croft, & Boyce, 2006). In a review of the literature, Olley and colleagues reported that executive deficits are primarily characterized by slow performance, perseverative responding, and difficulties utilizing feedback (Olley, Malhi, & Sachdev, 2007). In addition, electrophysiologic studies have consistently found that patients with OCD exhibit an overactive error monitoring (i.e., discrepancy detection) mechanism involving the medial prefrontal cortex (Endrass et al., 2010; Mathews, Perez, Delucchi, & Mathalon, 2012; Ruchsow et al., 2005), and, counterintuitively, this excessive error monitoring is associated with performance that is characterized by a greater number of errors and attenuated response to feedback (Endrass, Koehne, Riesel, & Kathmann, 2013). It has been hypothesized that hyperactive error monitoring represents a trait marker for OCD, as it is also found in unaffected first-degree relatives of OCD patients (Riesel, Endrass, Kaufmann, & Kathmann, 2011). Together, these findings point to a deficit in RS.

Of note, some studies have found comparable performances between patients with OCD and control groups (Bédard, Joyal, Godbout, & Chantal, 2009), and others have found that deficits can be explained by neuroleptic treatment or comorbid tic disorder (Lewin et al., 2014) and/or depression (Basso, Bornstein, Carona, & Morton, 2001). Additionally, at least one study interpreted EF weaknesses as simply reflecting a *slow* performance due to abnormalities in the frontal striatal circuitry (Roth, Baribeau, Milovan, & O'Connor, 2004). Lastly, to place these deficits in perspective, patients with OCD exhibit better EF than patients with schizophrenia (Yan, Meng, & Li, 2012) or post-traumatic stress disorder (PTSD; Miraghaie, Moradi, Hasani, Rahimi, & Mirzaie, 2013).

In sum, EF deficits in OCD appear to involve a lack of balance between elemental processes that contributes to RS, namely, deficiencies in rapid updating, in the context of overactive error monitoring. It is likely that perseverative responding is a result of a deficit in contingency updating, and slow performances are likely a function of excessive error monitoring that results in excessive inhibition of responses.

Trauma- and Stressor-Related Disorders

According to *DSM-5* (American Psychiatric Association, 2013), trauma-related conditions such as post-traumatic stress disorder are related to, but no longer subsumed under, anxiety disorders. This is because of the relative heterogeneity of PTSD presentations, such that some patients exhibit fear and anxiety, whereas many others exhibit anhedonia, externalizing and aggressive behaviors, and dissociations. The disorders in this category include reactive attachment disorder, disinhibited social engagement disorder, PTSD, acute stress disorder, and adjustment disorders. In this chapter, the principal focus is on PTSD.

A number of studies have identified poorer EF among both adults and children with PTSD (Flaks et al., 2014; Koso & Hansen, 2006; Park et al., 2014), and these findings have been further buttressed by a recent meta-analysis (Polak, Witteveen, Reitsma, & Olff, 2012). However, studies show that the EF deficits in PTSD are in part mediated by depression (Olff, Polak, Witteveen, & Denys, 2014; Polak et al., 2012), and there is some evidence that EF improves after treatment and symptom remission (K. H. Walter, Palmieri, & Gunstad, 2010). Importantly, in a review of the literature, Aupperle and colleagues concluded that the EF deficits in

PTSD primarily involve ECFs mediated by dorsolateral prefrontal cortex, and that these deficits at least in part predate the development of PTSD (Aupperle, Melrose, Stein, & Paulus, 2012). This finding is consistent with the reliance of emotion regulation strategies (e.g., reframing) on ECFs (see Chapter 2).

Disruptive, Impulse, and Conduct Disorders

Disorders in this category are characterized by problems with regulation of emotions and behaviors. Importantly, as stated previously, although virtually all psychopathology is associated with emotional and behavioral dysregulation, disorders in this category are also associated with violation of the rights of others, such as aggressive acts and destruction of property. Disorders in this category include oppositional defiant disorder (ODD), intermittent explosive disorder, conduct disorder (CD), antisocial personality disorder (ASPD), and pyromania and kleptomania (American Psychiatric Association, 2013). All these disorders are characterized by EF dysfunction.

Among the primary challenges in studying EF dysfunction in this category is the extremely high rate of comorbidities. Specifically, in children and youth, the comorbidity of oppositional defiant and conduct disorders (ODD/CD) with attention deficit hyperactivity disorder (ADHD) is thought to be greater than 80% (Perera et al., 2012). In adults, the comorbidity of ASPD with substance-related disorders is also more than 80%, with additional comorbidities with anxiety disorders, ADHD, depression, and bipolar disorder ranging from 10% to 70% (Alegria et al., 2013). Although much research has attempted to dissociate the unique contributions of the different comorbidities to EF dysfunction, the results thus far are inconclusive.

Research with children and youth has supported a gamut of hypotheses: Some studies have found greater EF deficits in ADHD as compared with ODD/CD (C. Clark, Prior, & Kinsella, 2000); some have found comparable deficits in EF in both groups, with ODD/CD also exhibiting additional deficits specifically in processing of rewards (Hobson, Scott, & Rubia, 2011); others yet have proposed that EF deficits in ODD/CD emerge only under certain reward contingences (Matthys, Vanderschuren, & Schutter, 2013). Similarly complex findings emerge in research on adults. On the whole, a recent meta-analysis (Ogilvie, Stewart, Chan, & Shum, 2011) has confirmed that ASPD is associated with weaknesses in EF but has also demonstrated the importance of other participant characteristics: The largest effect sizes were associated with criminality and externalizing behaviors, whereas only small effect sizes were associated with antisocial personality alone; additionally, greater EF deficits were found among participants who were incarcerated and also had comorbid ADHD. The latter finding likely reflects the fact that individuals who engage in antisocial behavior and become incarcerated are also less organized and more impulsive than those who elude capture. In fact, approximately 40% of adult male longer-term prison inmates have been shown to have comorbid ADHD, and these individuals exhibit greater EF weaknesses than noncriminal patients with ADHD (Ginsberg, Hirvikoski, & Lindefors, 2010).

Regarding specific EF subdomains that are affected in these populations, it is generally thought that antisocial behavior, criminality, and aggression are related to weaknesses in RS (with prominent difficulties in contingency updating and an inability to benefit from feedback), as well as prominent deficits in SC (Blair, 2001). In sum, when dealing with clients who have a history of antisocial, criminal, or aggressive behavior, clinicians can expect symptoms of disinhibited and inappropriate syndromes. It is probably not a worthwhile exercise to attempt to dissociate the exact etiology of such symptoms in the context of other comorbidities.

Personality Disorders

In *DSM-5*, personality disorder (PD) is defined as "an enduring pattern of inner experience and behavior that deviates markedly from the expectations of the individual's culture, is pervasive and inflexible, has an onset in adolescence or early adulthood, is stable over time, and leads to a distress or impairment" (American Psychiatric Association, 2013, p. 645). It is important to note that PDs are distinct from "personality" and do not necessarily map onto the currently accepted personality dimensions. Although normal personality dimensions have been shown to be associated with individual differences in EF (P. G. Williams et al., 2010; P. G. Williams et al., 2009), this chapter focuses on personality *disorders* only. The association of individual differences in EF and personality is reviewed briefly in Chapter 9.

Although there is some evidence that PDs in general are associated with poor working memory (Coolidge et al., 2009), the PD populations that have received the most attention from researchers are persons with borderline personality disorder (BPD), antisocial personality disorder (ASPD), and schizoid personality disorder (SPD). Specifically, features of primarily dysexecutive and disinhibited syndromes are evident with both BPD (Gvirts et al., 2012; V. Ø. Haaland et al., 2009; Hagenhoff et al., 2013; Lazzaretti et al., 2012; Mitropoulou et al., 2005) and ASPD (De Brito, Viding, Kumari, Blackwood, & Hodgins, 2013; Prehn et al., 2013; Roszyk, Izdebska, & Peichert, 2013), whereas fairly circumscribed symptoms of dysexective syndrome appear to be present in SPD (Hazlett et al., 2014; McClure et al., 2007; Mitropoulou et al., 2005; Vu et al., 2013). Importantly, although it is not clear whether these EF weaknesses reach the magnitude of clinical significance in some individuals, there is clear evidence that any given individual with PD may certainly perform well within normal limits (Angrilli, Sartori, & Donzella, 2013). Lastly, although patients with SPD as a group exhibit patterns of performance that are similar to those seen in schizophrenia, the magnitude of any anomalies is much smaller (Matsui, Sumiyoshi, Kato, Yoneyama, & Kurachi, 2004).

Chapter Summary

Neuropsychiatric disorders are virtually by definition associated with dysfunctional EF; thus, an exhaustive review of relevant disorders would be beyond the scope of this chapter. This chapter reviewed those disorders thought to be associated with prominent EF deficits (i.e., schizophrenia spectrum disorders and bipolar disorder), or those most typically seen in a neuropsychological practice (i.e., depression, anxiety, obsessive-compulsive disorders, trauma- and stressor-related disorders, disruptive/impulse/conduct disorders, and personality disorders). For many disorders, specificity of EF deficits in research findings is unclear, due to the high prevalence of other neuropsychiatric comorbidities, as well as comorbidity with neurodevelopmental disorders (e.g., attention deficit hyperactivity disorder). In contrast, schizophrenia is consistently and unequivocally associated with cognitive dysfunction, and impaired cognition is sometimes viewed as a key feature of this disorder.

13

Acquired Brain Insults and Medical Conditions

Traumatic Brain Injury

Traumatic brain injury (TBI) refers to damage to the brain caused by external mechanical forces. Two main classes of injuries are typically reported: (a) moderate to severe injury, characterized by extended loss of consciousness and post-traumatic amnesia (typically more than 30 minutes and more than 24 hours, respectively, though some small variations among accepted criteria exist), as well as clear neuroimaging evidence of an injury involving brain tissue; and (b) mild injury, characterized by briefer periods of loss of consciousness or post-traumatic amnesia and typically an absence of neuroimaging finding. Injuries that are associated with brief loss of consciousness or brief posttraumatic amnesia in the context of notable neuroimaging findings (e.g., contusions, edema, hemorrhage) are typically classified as *complicated mild*. For a review, see Mittenberg and Roberts (2008) and Roebuck-Spencer Sherer (2008).

There are several reasons that TBI is associated with deficits in EF. First, the most common site for contusions are frontal and temporal poles, ventral frontal regions, and, to a lesser extent, inferior aspects of the cerebellum (Gennarelli & Graham, 2005). In addition, TBI is associated with axonal shearing (Gennarelli & Graham, 2005), which results in disruption of the connections between the frontal lobes and subcortical structures, as well as coup-contre coup injuries typically involving lateral frontal and parietal lobes. As reviewed in Chapters 2 through 6, all these regions are intimately involved in a variety of EF subdomains and elemental processes. Thus, not surprisingly, it has been recommended that measures of EF that tap into executive cognitive functions (ECFs), response selection (RS), and initiation/maintenance (I/M) always be included when tracking the recovery and outcome of patients with TBI (Bagiella et al., 2010).

Although patients with a history of moderate to severe TBI often exhibit deficits on traditional measures of EF (Donovan et al., 2011; Kennedy et al., 2008; Millis et al., 2001; Ownsworth & McKenna, 2004; Sherer, Nick, Millis, & Novack, 2003), those deficits often underestimate the degree to which patients are impaired socially and occupationally (D. R. Dawson, Levine, Schwartz, & Stuss, 2000; B. Levine, Dawson, Boutet, Schwartz, & Stuss, 2000). In particular, patients suffer from irritability and poor emotion regulation, may express threats of violence, and exhibit personality changes that are highly distressing both to patients and to their loved ones (Arciniegas & Wortzel, 2014). These problems are further compounded by poor self-awareness and limited insight about deficits (Orfei, Robinson, Bria, Caltagirone, & Spalleta, 2008; Prigatano, 2005). Regarding specific profiles of EF deficits, patients with moderate to severe TBI span the gamut of EF syndromes (Lippert-Grüner, Kuchta, Hellmich, & Klug, 2006), with apathetic and disinhibited syndromes being particularly prevalent (Ciurli, Formisano, Bivona, Cantagallo, & Angelelli, 2011). Additionally, the inappropriate syndrome is reported in approximately one quarter of patients (Olver, Ponsford, & Curran, 1996), with approximately 9% exhibiting inappropriate sexual behaviors (Simpson, Sabaz, & Daher, 2013). Although the elemental processes that constitute executive cognitive functions (ECFs) and meta-tasking (MT) are also likely affected, symptoms of the dysexecutive and disorganized syndromes are in likelihood obscured by impaired I/M and RS.

Regarding mild TBI, an overwhelming majority of cases are symptom-free within 1 to 3 months (Schretlen & Shapiro, 2003); consequently, mild TBI does not represent a typical example of a disorder associated with EF deficits. However, individuals with a history of multiple mild TBIs, especially if occurring in close temporal proximity to each other, do sometimes present with EF dysfunction (Belanger, Spiegel, & Vanderploeg, 2010; Karr, Areshenkoff, & Garcia-Barrera, 2014), which may appear to be out of proportion to the severity grading of their most recent injury. Similarly, patients with *complicated* mild TBI (which is characterized by positive neuroimaging findings in the context of a loss of consciousness and post-traumatic amnesia comparable to uncomplicated TBI) may also present with mild EF difficulties that persist beyond the typical 3-moth recovery period (Kwok, Lee, Leung, & Poon, 2008), with higher premorbid cognitive reserve potentially representing a protective factor (Fay et al., 2010). Additionally, it is important to consider the possibility that some patients with mild injuries may exhibit no clear deficits on measures of EF, yet exhibit symptoms of the disorganized syndrome in their daily life. The degree to which such deficits represent a bona fide consequence of mild TBI versus premorbid cognitive or psychological limitations continues to be a source of controversy (Ruff, 2005) and is beyond the scope of this chapter.

Cerebral Vascular Accident

Cerebral vascular accidents (CVAs) entail a range of etiologies and presentations, all involving either an obstruction or a rupture within cerebral vasculature. Because small vessel disease is covered in Chapter 11 (neurodegenerative disorders), the present section focuses on large vessel disease only. Of note, neurocognitive sequelae of a stroke are dependent on many factors, including the size and location of the stroke, the age and premorbid level of functioning of the patient, and the patient's premorbid cognitive style and profile of strengths and weaknesses. Similarly, the exact localization of function is to some extent unique to each patient, as are the exact vascular distribution and the efficiency of the circle of Willis (Chuang et al., 2011; De Silva, Silva, Amaratunga, Gunasekera, & Jayesekera, 2011; Silva Neto, Brandão Câmara, & Valença, 2012; Wright et al., 2013); thus, an identical stroke may result in somewhat different neurocognitive sequelae in different patients. However, some degree of general EF dysfunction is highly common in stroke survivors, affecting approximately 50% of patients, regardless of lesion location (Pulsipher, Stricker, Sadek, & Haaland, 2013).

That said, deficits in EF are associated with strokes involving somewhat predictable distributions of the cerebral vascular system. Specifically, strokes involving anterior branches of the anterior cerebral artery are likely to affect ventral and medial convexities of the frontal lobes, possibly resulting in the disinhibited syndrome, the apathetic syndrome, the disorganized syndrome, or some combination of the three. In contrast, strokes involving the anterior branches of the middle cerebral artery are likely to affect the dorsolateral prefrontal cortex, resulting in the dysexecutive syndrome or possibly the disorganized syndrome. However, left hemisphere strokes are often associated with aphasia, which may mask EF problems. Additionally, strokes involving some portions of the parietal lobe or the cerebellum can also present with the dysexecutive syndrome, and strokes involving the right cerebral hemisphere can present with a range of executive deficits, due to the preferential roles of the right hemisphere in inhibition, attentional vigilance, emotional processing, monitoring, and gestalt processing. Lastly, involvement of the basal ganglia can present with a range of deficits, depending on which frontal-striatal circuit is involved.

Anterior Communicating Artery Aneurysm. Hemorrhages resulting from a rupture of the anterior communicating artery aneurysm (ACoAA) often present with severe cognitive impairment that is characterized by globally deficient EF and memory, with the EF deficits often further exacerbating memory problems and vice versa (A. Chan et al., 2002; Palmer & McDonald, 2000; Papagno et al., 2003; Simard, Rouleau, Brosseau, Laframboise, & Bojanowsky, 2003; Stablum, Umiltà, Mogentale, Carlan, & Guerrini, 2000). Importantly, the dual impairment in both memory and EF often leads to spontaneous confabulations, one of the hallmark presentations of ACoAA (DeLuca & Diamond, 1995; M. S. Turner, Cipolotti, & Shallice, 2010). Aside from confabulations, the exact nature of deficits varies depending on lesion location and the degree to which vasospasms exacerbate the damage caused by the hemorrhage; deficient RS and SC tend to be most prominent (Martinaud et al., 2009). Lastly, EF deficits can also be present among patients with posterior communicating artery aneurysm and middle cerebral artery aneurysm rupture and repair (Manning, Pierot, & Dufour, 2005; Papagno et al., 2003).

Oxygen Deprivation

Due to the high demands of the brain for oxygen, cognitive deficits begin to emerge with decreases in arterial oxygen prior to any damage to the brain tissue. As reviewed by Hopkins and Bigler (2008), when arterial oxygen pressure decreases to 75%, deficits in EF become evident; an additional decrease to 65% results in memory deficits, and a further decrease to 50% typically leads to unconsciousness; declines to 30 to 40% could result in death. The duration of oxygen deprivation also matters, with longer duration of ischemia leading to greater tissue damage, such that 15 minutes of global ischemia results in eventual damage to approximately 95% of the brain tissue (Busl & Greer, 2010). The neural injury itself occurs with some delay following an anoxic event, ranging from 24 hours to days or even weeks, depending on the brain region involved (Busl & Greer, 2010; Kuroiwa & Okeda, 1994; Porter, Hopkins, Weaver, Bigler, & Blatter, 2002; Shprecher & Mehta, 2010). This is because neuronal death results from a cascade of metabolic processes, including, among others, calcium influx, excitotoxicity, oxidative injury, and apoptosis (Kuroiwa & Okeda, 1994; Schurr, 2002).

Importantly, not all brain regions are equally vulnerable to declines in oxygenation: The so-called watershed-areas (i.e., areas at the end of the vascular distribution), as well as certain regions with high metabolic demands or regions with high density of excitatory amino acids (e.g., the basal ganglia and the hippocampus), are the most vulnerable. Amnesia represents perhaps the most salient cognitive deficit following anoxia due to its reliance on the hippocampus, but some of the other highly vulnerable regions are fundamentally important for normal EF; these include the dorsolateral prefrontal watershed areas, the basal ganglia and the thalamus, the Purkinje cells of the cerebellum, and the white matter (Gale et al., 1999; Hopkins & Woon, 2006; Porter et al., 2002). Consequently, in addition to memory impairment, deficits in EF represent common sequelae, occurring in as many as 46% of patients (Caine & Watson, 2000). For additional review, see Hopkins and Bigler (2008).

Although research suggests that the duration and severity of anoxia or hypoxia determine the severity of cognitive deficits (Roehrs, Merrion, Pedrosi, & Stepanski, 1995), there is also some evidence that different etiologies may be associated with different outcomes (F. C. Wilson, Harpur, Watson, & Morrow, 2003). Additionally, disorders that are associated with intermittent hypoxemia, such as chronic obstructive pulmonary disease (COPD) or sleep apnea, may present with cognitive deficits that are similar to those seen in more severe anoxic events but can be reversible or fluctuate; this is because deficits do not necessarily emerge only as a result of neuronal death but also due to potentially reversible effects, such as transient changes in the blood-brain barrier and synaptic plasticity (Gale & Hopkins, 2004; D. C. Lim & Pack, 2014).

Acute Anoxic Events. Typical examples of acute anoxic events that can lead to chronic and irreversible EF deficits include carbon monoxide poisoning, cardiac arrest, near drowning, choking, or hanging/strangling. Although, as mentioned earlier, the duration and severity of oxygen deprivation play an important role in patient outcomes, so do other situational factors. For example, is it now increasingly recognized that hypothermia has a protective role during and subsequent to ischemia (Wu & Grotta, 2013; Yenari & Han, 2012) and may increase the amount of time that the brain can survive without oxygen, as evidenced by cases of near drowning in ice water (J. D. Ball, Budrionis, & Trott, 1987; Hopkins, 2008; S. K. Hughes et al., 2002; Samuelson, Nekludov, & Levander, 2008). Additionally, treatment with hyperbaric oxygen may improve outcomes for some patients with carbon monoxide poisoning (L. K. Weaver et al., 2002). Consequently, clinical features other than the duration of oxygen deprivation may represent better predictors of long-term outcome; these include coma and post-traumatic amnesia duration and severity (Alexander, Lafleche, Schnyer, Lim, & Verfaellie, 2011; Ku, Yang, Lee, Lee, & Chou, 2010; Middelkamp et al., 2007), as well as results of initial diffusion tensor imaging (Hou et al., 2013).

Regardless, outcomes are variable. Only about 50% of cases of carbon monoxide poisoning are associated with EF dysfunction (Hopkins & Woon, 2006; Rahmani et al., 2006), and in cases of cardiac arrest, EF deficits can range from minimal to severe, potentially spanning the gamut of EF syndromes, including dysexecutive, disinhibited, and apathetic (Armengol, 2000; Baggett, Kelly, Korenman, & Ryan, 2003; C. Lim, Alexander, LaFleche, Schnyer, & Verfaellie, 2004; Peskine, Rosso, Picq, Caron, & Pradat-Diehl, 2010; Prohl, Bodenburg, & Rustenbach, 2009). Importantly, anoxic events in young children may initially appear to have excellent outcomes (J. D. Ball et al., 1987), yet long-term neuropsychological follow-ups may evidence emergence of cognitive deficit including EF dysfunction (Hopkins, 2008; Samuelson et al., 2008). Given the variability in outcome, along with emergence of bona fide deficits with time, clinicians need to be vigilant to EF dysfunction regardless of the reported characteristics of a given event.

Chronic Intermittent Hypoxemia. Obstructive sleep apnea is a disorder characterized by repeated episodes of obstruction of the upper airway while sleeping, resulting in decreases in oxygen saturation (i.e., hypoxemia), as well as repeated arousal from sleep. Patients with sleep apnea often experience excessive daytime sleepiness, fatigue, mood disturbance, and cognitive difficulties (El-Ad & Lavie, 2005). Cognitive weaknesses involve a range of domains, most typically including vigilance and attention, speed of processing, and memory, with EF representing an area of the greatest impairment (Saunamäki & Jehkonen, 2007; Waters & Bucks, 2011).

The most typical treatment for sleep apnea involves the use of continuous positive airway pressure (CPAP) therapy. Many studies have demonstrated that the use of CPAP improves daytime sleepiness, alertness, and mood, but there is considerable evidence that deficits in EF persist even with treatment (Lau, Eskes, Morrison, Rajda, & Spurr, 2010; Saunamäki & Jehkonen, 2007). Importantly, EF deficits cannot be explained by fatigue, mood disturbance, or daytime sleepiness. In fact, research has shown that although poor sleep quality is associated with declines in processing speed and increases in psychiatric symptoms (Waters & Bucks, 2011), deficits in EF appear to be related to the severity of hypoxemia (Naismith, Winter, Gotsopoulos, Hickie, & Cistulli, 2004). This finding is consistent with neuroimaging research showing that persistent cognitive deficits can be explained by permanent changes in the brain, including frontal cortical areas, anterior cingulate gyrus, and the hippocampus (Beebe & Gozal, 2002; El-Ad & Lavie, 2005; Ferini-Strambi, Marelli, Galbiati, & Castronovo, 2013). Importantly, despite residual deficits after treatment, some improvements with treatment are nevertheless evident and thus should not be dismissed. For example, the use of CPAP with older adults, including those diagnosed with neurodegenerative conditions such as Alzheimer's disease, has been shown to be accompanied by improvement in cognition (T. E. Weaver & Chasens, 2007). For additional review, see Tsai (2010).

In contrast to the extensive literature on sleep apnea, literature linking deficits in EF to COPD is somewhat scarce. However, a recent international review of studies dating back to 1957 has concluded that patients with COPD are in fact characterized by weaknesses in attention, EF, and processing speed (Areza-Fegyveres, Kairalla, Carvalho, & Nitrini, 2010).

Central Nervous System Infections

HIV. HIV infection is frequently associated with significant CNS involvement, with fully three quarters of patients exhibiting brain pathology on autopsy despite antiretroviral treatment, reflecting both the direct infiltration with HIV and the impact of other opportunistic infections (Vago et al., 2002). Infiltration of the brain with HIV is often evident early on in the disease process, and the severity of pathology increases with increases in viral loads, with as many as 45% of patients exhibiting HIV-associated neurocognitive disorders (HANDs; S. M. de Almeida, 2013). Additionally, approximately 20% of patients present with HIV-associated dementia (HAD; Manji, Jager, & Winston, 2013). Because the primary targets of HIV are the white matter and the basal ganglia (R. Paul, Cohen, Navia, & Tashima, 2002), the cognitive profile is similar to that seen in patients with subcortical dementias, particularly subcortical ischemic vascular dementia (see Chapter 11). Consequently, speed of processing, motor speed and motor control, and EF are typically affected, though other cognitive domains can be involved as well (Hardy & Hinkin, 2002; Woods, Moore, Weber, & Grant, 2009). Among the most important issues with this population is the fact that declines in EF are associated with declines in medication adherence (Lovejoy & Suhr, 2009), with clearly serious ramifications for long-term health and survival.

Epilepsy

Epilepsy is a complex disorder that is associated with a variety of etiologies; a variety of presentations, severity, and seizure frequency; and the involvement of different brain regions. Specifically, epilepsy can result from brain lesions or brain injuries (including stroke, TBI, infections, or brain tumors) or can have an idiopathic origin. Additionally, seizure activity can involve a fairly circumscribed area of the brain, or it can spread to an entire hemisphere or even generalize to the entire brain. For additional review of the topic, see G. P. Lee and Clason (2008).

Regarding cognitive limitations among individuals with seizure disorder, these are related, on the one hand, to the brain abnormalities that are the source of the seizure disorder, and, on the other hand, to the deleterious impact that seizures themselves have on the brain. Seizures that are of longer duration appear to be particularly damaging in this regard (Dlugos et al., 2013; McCusker, Kennedy, Anderson, Hicks, & Hanrahan, 2002; Tanabe, Hara, Shimakawa, Fukui, & Tamai, 2011). Age of onset is also an important factor, with onset in infancy or childhood representing a risk factor for poor cognitive outcome (Braakman et al., 2011; Luton, Burns, & Defilippis, 2010), likely due to interference with normal myelinazation, which in turn results in EF deficits regardless of the seizure focus (Hermann et al., 2010). However, it is important to consider that the impact of a childhood injury on future cognitive outcome is nonlinearly associated with age of onset due to increased vulnerability during certain critical periods (Jacobs, Harvey, & Anderson, 2007). Additionally, the type and dosage of medication and the patient's ability to tolerate the medication (R. C. Martin et al., 2005; Mula & Trimble, 2009), as well as a history of neurosurgery (Althausen et al., 2013; Lippé et al., 2010), all impact cognition to varying degrees. All these factors together contribute to the neurocognitive profile of patients with epilepsy. Lastly, it is important to consider that in adult-onset epilepsy the underlying condition causing seizures is more likely to be related to the pattern of cognitive impairment than the epilepsy itself.

Regarding the association between seizure focus and cognition, the literature is mixed. On the one hand, temporal lobe epilepsy is fairly reliably associated primarily with deficits in memory and language functions; on the other hand, differentiating frontal and temporal lobe epilepsy based on cognitive profile has been challenging. In research conducted with children, both frontal and temporal lobe epilepsy appear to be associated with deficits in EF (Longo, Kerr, & Smith, 2013), perhaps due to the disruption of white matter maturation noted earlier (Hermann et al., 2010); in contrast, research conducted with adults shows impaired memory functions in both frontal and temporal cases, with neither group showing marked EF deficits (Cahn-Weiner, Wittenberg, & McDonald, 2009).

Regarding specifically the association between frontal lobe epilepsy and EF, the literature is also inconsistent: Although some studies have found a reliable relationship between frontal lobe epilepsy and EF weaknesses (C. R. McDonald, Delis, Norman, Tecoma, & Iragui-Madoz, 2005), others find an inconsistent association at best (Longo et al., 2013; Risse, 2006). One explanation for these inconsistencies has been offered by the Cleveland Clinic group, showing that depressive symptoms prior to frontal lobe surgery predict EF postsurgically (Dulay, Busch, Chapin, Jehi, & Najm, 2013). Thus, although a subset of patients with seizure focus in the frontal lobes exhibit EF deficits, it is not the case that EF deficits on testing should be expected when localizing seizure focus to the frontal lobes.

Radiation and Chemotherapy

There is considerable evidence that chemotherapy has a deleterious impact on brain function (as reflected in impaired cognition), as well as on brain structure. The majority of this research involves patients with breast cancer. Cognitive deficits typically involve processing speed, memory, and EF, both in standard dose systemic chemotherapy (Wefel, Saleeba, Buzdar, & Meyers, 2010) and in high-dose adjuvant chemotherapy (de Ruiter et al., 2011). In fact, some research shows that more than two thirds of patients exhibit impaired performances on cognitive measures after completion of treatment (Kesler, Kent, & O'Hara, 2011; Wefel et al., 2010). However, the specificity of these findings to chemotherapy is not yet clear, with at least some research showing that similarly impaired performances result both from chemotherapy and from radiation treatment (Phillips et al., 2012). Additionally, some cognitive deficits may be related to the disease itself or to disease-associated stress and psychopathology. In fact, among men with testicular cancer treated with chemotherapy, cognitive deficits were identified both before and after treatment (Wefel et al., 2011); similarly, among women with breast cancer, cognitive deficits can be found in 21 to 30% of cases prior to treatment (Janelsins, Kesler, Ahles, & Morrow, 2014; Wefel et al., 2010). Consequently, some authors call for careful interpretation of findings thus far, as well as careful study of the primary effects of certain types of cancer on the brain (Kesler et al., 2011; W. L. Nelson & Suls, 2013).

Although the etiology of these deficits is still a matter of some debate, the behavioral findings are consistent with neuroimaging research that has shown white matter changes in patients *prior* to treatment, as well as possible compensatory activation increases in the frontoparietal working memory network (Simó, Rifà-Ros, Rodriguez-Fornells, & Bruna, 2013). Importantly, additional changes appear to emerge *after* treatment, including changes in functional connectivity in the frontoparietal working memory network (Dumas et al., 2013), and additional white matter and gray matter (primarily frontal) volume reduction and declines in frontal activation (B. C. McDonald, Conroy, Smith, West, & Saykin, 2013; Simó et al., 2013). In sum, given these imaging findings, deficits in ECFs should be expected.

In addition to adults with breast and testicular cancers, children with acute lymphoblastic leukemia have also been studied. In this population, both whole-brain radiotherapy and prophylactic chemotherapy have been shown to be related to declines in working memory and ECFs (Annett et al., 2015; de Oliveira Gomes, Leite, Garcia, Maranhão, & Hazin, 2012), and the severity of these deficits has been shown to be related to treatment intensity (Jain, Brouwers, Okcu, Cirino, & Krull, 2009).

Substance-Related and Addictive Disorders

The core characteristic of substance use disorders is the persistent and repeated use of substances despite evidence of substance-related problems in interpersonal and occupational/educational functioning. Pathological gambling is also included in this category (American Psychiatric Association, 2013). The literature on the impact of substances on cognition in general is extremely complex. The factors that need to be considered include (a) the type of the substance; (b) age of onset, frequency of use, duration of use, and cumulative dose effect; and (c) abstinence duration (Morrow, Robards, Saxton, & Metheny, 2008). Additionally, the literature is confounded by a number of factors, including socioeconomic status, general intelligence, history of abuse and neglect, and history of TBI, liver diseases, and other comorbid complications. For this reason, it is beyond the scope of this chapter to fully review this complex literature. Nevertheless, the mention of deficits in EF is virtually ubiquitous in research on substance abuse. For a review, see Yücel and colleagues (2007). It is also worth noting that much research suggests that some weaknesses in EF are premorbid and potentially represent a heritable vulnerability, rather than purely a consequence of abuse (Corral, Holguín, & Cadaveira, 2003; Kumbhani, 2008).

Regarding the specific EF subdomains, SC is often affected, including deficient paralinguistic communication and social awareness (Foisy et al., 2005; Kornreich et al., 2001; Monnot et al., 2002; Monnot et al., 2001; Philippot et al., 1999; Uekermann et al., 2005). Additionally, RS is often compromised, including poor sensitivity to threat in the context of strong sensitivity to rewards (Genovese & Wallace, 2007), as well as deficient inhibition and discrepancy detection (Wu & Grotta, 2013; Yenari & Han, 2012).

Chapter Summary

The chapter reviewed acquired brain insults and medical conditions thought to be associated with dysfunctional EF. These include traumatic brain injury (in particular moderate to severe), cerebral vascular accident (including large vessel disease and anterior communicating artery aneurysm), oxygen deprivation (both chronic intermittent hypoxia and acute anoxic events), central nervous system infections, epilepsy, the impact of radiation or chemotherapy, and substance-related and addictive disorders. In general, the exact nature of the EF deficits in many of these disorders depends on various disease characteristics, such as lesion size and location, or the disease severity, etiology, and age of onset.

Appendix

Overview of executive deficits typically associated with neuropsychological patient populations

DISORDER/ POPULATION	SYNDROME					
	DYSEXECUTIVE	DISORGANIZED	DISINHIBITED	APATHETIC	INAPPROPRIATE
ADHD	+		+ Hyperactive or combined subtype	+ Inattentive or combined subtype	+
Alzheimer's dementia	+			+	
Anoxia/hypoxia	+		+	+	
Anxiety	+		? Excessive discrepancy detection		
Asperger's syndrome	+ Mainly mental flexibility				+
Amyotrophic lateral sclerosis	+				+
Autism		+			+

(*continued*)

Overview of executive deficits typically associated with patient neuropsychological patient populations

DISORDER/POPULATION	SYNDROME					
	DYSEXECUTIVE	DISORGANIZED	DISINHIBITED	APATHETIC	INAPPROPRIATE	
Bipolar disorder	+	+	+ Represents a core feature	+	+	
Chronic tic disorders	+ Possibly explained by comorbidities		+ Possibly explained by comorbidities			
Cerebral palsy	?	?	?	?	?	
Cerebral vascular accident	+ Depends on CVA location	+ Depends on CVA location	+ Depends on CVA location	+ Depends on CVA location	+ Depends on CVA location	
Cortical-basal degeneration	+					
Dementia with Lewy bodies	+		?	+		
Depression	+	?		+	+ Mild	
Disruptive, impulsive, and conduct disorders			+		+	

Epilepsy	? Variable; greater deficits in child onset	? Variable; greater deficits in child onset	? Variable; greater deficits in child onset	? Variable; greater deficits in child onset	? Variable; greater deficits in child onset	? Variable; greater deficits in child onset	? Variable; greater deficits in child onset
Fetal alcohol syndrome	+		+	+	+	+	+
Fragile X syndrome	+		+			+	+
Fragile X–associated tremor and ataxia	+	+	+	+	+		+
Frontotemporal lobar degeneration behavioral variant	Only in advanced stages	+	+	+	+		+ Typically first symptom
HIV infection	+						
Intellectual disability	?	?	?	?	?		?
Multiple sclerosis	+				+	+	+
Multiple system atrophy	+			+	+		+ Mild

(continued)

Overview of executive deficits typically associated with patient neuropsychological patient populations

DISORDER/ POPULATION	SYNDROME					
	DYSEXECUTIVE	DISORGANIZED	DISINHIBITED	APATHETIC	INAPPROPRIATE	
Obsessive-compulsive disorders			+ Excessive discrepancy detection in context of deficient contingency updating			
Obstructive sleep apnea	+		+	+		
Parkinson's disease	+			+	+ Mild	
Post-traumatic stress disorder	+					
Preterm birth	+		+	+		
Progressive supranuclear palsy	+			+	+ Mild	
Radiation and chemotherapy	? Variable; some evidence of deficits prior to treatment	? Variable; some evidence of deficits prior to treatment	? Variable; some evidence of deficits prior to treatment	? Variable; some evidence of deficits prior to treatment	? Variable; some evidence of deficits prior to treatment	

Schizophrenia	+		+ Risk for aggression and suicide		+
Spina bifida/ hydrocephalus	+			+	+ Possibly related to right hemisphere shunt placements
Subcortical ischemic vascular dementia	+				
Substance abuse			+		+
Traumatic brain injury (moderate to severe)	+	Likely obscured by other EF deficits	+	Likely obscured by other EF deficits	+

Note: + = research has reported the syndrome in this population; ? = literature exists but is highly inconsistent and/or questioned due to methodological limitations.

References

Aarsland, D., & Kurz, M. W. (2010). The epidemiology of dementia associated with Parkinson disease. *Journal of the Neurological Sciences*, 289(1–2), 18–22.

Aarsland, D., Litvan, I., Salmon, D., Galasko, D., Wentzel-Larsen, T., & Larsen, J. P. (2003). Performance on the dementia rating scale in Parkinson's disease with dementia and dementia with Lewy bodies: Comparison with progressive supranuclear palsy and Alzheimer's disease. *Journal of Neurology, Neurosurgery and Psychiatry*, 74(9), 1215–1220.

Aarsland, D., Perry, R., Brown, A., Larsen, J. P., & Ballard, C. (2005). Neuropathology of dementia in Parkinson's disease: A prospective, community-based study. *Annals of Neurology*, 58(5), 773–776.

Abbate-Daga, G., Delsedime, N., Nicotra, B., Giovannone, C., Marzola, E., Amianto, F., & Fassino, S. (2013). Psychosomatic syndromes and anorexia nervosa. *BMC Psychiatry*, 13(14), http://www.biomedcentral.com/1471-244X/13/14.

Abler, B., Hofer, C., & Viviani, R. (2008). Habitual emotion regulation strategies and baseline brain perfusion. *Neuroreport: For Rapid Communication of Neuroscience Research*, 19(1), 21–24.

Adam, R., Leff, A., Sinha, N., Turner, C., Bays, P., Draganski, B., & Husain, M. (2013). Dopamine reverses reward insensitivity in apathy following globus pallidus lesions. *Cortex: A Journal Devoted to the Study of the Nervous System and Behavior*, 49(5), 1292–1303.

Adams, D., & Oliver, C. (2010). The relationship between acquired impairments of executive function and behaviour change in adults with Down syndrome. *Journal of Intellectual Disability Research*, 54(5), 393–405. doi: 10.1111/j.1365-2788.2010.01271.x

Addington, J., & Addington, D. (1998). Facial affect recognition and information processing in schizophrenia and bipolar disorder. *Schizophrenia Research*, 32(3), 171–181.

Addis, D. R., Sacchetti, D. C., Ally, B. A., Budson, A. E., & Schacter, D. L. (2009). Episodic simulation of future events is impaired in mild Alzheimer's disease. *Neuropsychologia*, 47(12), 2660–2671.

Addis, D. R., & Schacter, D. L. (2013). Future-oriented simulations: The role of episodic memory. *Journal of Applied Research in Memory and Cognition, 2*(4), 248–250.

Adolphs, R., Gosselin, F., Buchanan, T. W., Tranel, D., Schyns, P., & Damasio, A. R. (2005). A mechanism for impaired fear recognition after amygdala damage. *Nature, 433*(7021), 68–72.

Adrover-Roig, D., Sesé, A., Barceló, F., & Palmer, A. (2012). A latent variable approach to executive control in healthy ageing. *Brain and Cognition, 78*(3), 284–299.

Albert, M. S., DeKosky, S. T., Dickson, D., Dubois, B., Feldman, H. H., Fox, N. C., . . . Phelps, C. H. (2011). The diagnosis of mild cognitive impairment due to Alzheimer's disease: Recommendations from the National Institute on Aging–Alzheimer's Association workgroups on diagnostic guidelines for Alzheimer's disease. *Alzheimer's and Dementia, 7*(3), 270–279.

Alegria, A. A., Blanco, C., Petry, N. M., Skodol, A. E., Liu, S.-M., Grant, B., & Hasin, D. (2013). Sex differences in antisocial personality disorder: Results from the National Epidemiological Survey on Alcohol and Related Conditions. *Personality Disorders: Theory, Research, and Treatment, 4*(3), 214–222.

Aleman, A., Agrawal, N., Morgan, K. D., & David, A. S. (2006). Insight in psychosis and neuropsychological function: Meta-analysis. *British Journal of Psychiatry, 189*(3), 204–212.

Alexander, M. P. (2001). Chronic akinetic mutism after mesencephalic-diencephalic infarction: Remediated with dopaminergic medications. *Neurorehabilitation and Neural Repair, 15*(2), 151–156.

Alexander, M. P., Lafleche, G., Schnyer, D., Lim, C., & Verfaellie, M. (2011). Cognitive and functional outcome after out of hospital cardiac arrest. *Journal of the International Neuropsychological Society, 17*(2), 364–368.

Alexopoulos, G. S., Kiosses, D. N., Heo, M., Murphy, C. F., Shanmugham, B., & Gunning-Dixon, F. (2005). Executive dysfunction and the course of geriatric depression. *Biological Psychiatry, 58*(3), 204–210.

Alford, L. B. (1943). The mental state associated with cerebral lesions. *Psychosomatic Medicine, 5*, 15–19.

Allain, P., Etcharry-Bouyx, F., & Verny, C. (2013). Executive functions in clinical and preclinical Alzheimer's disease. *Revue Neurologique, 169*(10), 695–708.

Allain, P., Nicoleau, S., Pinon, K., Etcharry-Bouyx, F., Barré, J., Berrut, G., . . . Le Gall, D. (2005). Executive functioning in normal aging: A study of action planning using the Zoo Map Test. *Brain and Cognition, 57*(1), 4–7.

Allman, J. M., Tetreault, N. A., Hakeem, A. Y., Manaye, K. F., Semendeferi, K., Erwin, J. M., . . . Hof, P. R. (2010). The von Economo neurons in frontoinsular and anterior cingulate cortex in great apes and humans. *Brain Structure and Function, 214*(5–6), 495–517.

Allman, J. M., Watson, K. K., Tetreault, N. A., & Hakeem, A. Y. (2005). Intuition and autism: A possible role for von Economo neurons. *Trends in Cognitive Sciences, 9*(8), 367–373.

Althausen, A., Gleissner, U., Hoppe, C., Sassen, R., Buddewig, S., von Lehe, M., . . . Helmstaedter, C. (2013). Long-term outcome of hemispheric surgery at different ages in 61 epilepsy patients. *Journal of Neurology, Neurosurgery and Psychiatry, 84*(5), 529–536.

Al-Zahrani, S. A. (2003). Narrative discourse production of right hemisphere damaged (RHD) individuals under isolated, focused and divided-attention conditions. 63, ProQuest Information & Learning, US. Retrieved from http://search.ebscohost.com/login.aspx?direct=true&db=psyh&AN=2003-95008-055&site=ehost-live Available from EBSCOhost psyh database.

Amann, B., Gomar, J. J., Ortiz-Gil, J., McKenna, P., Sans-Sansa, B., Sarró, S., . . . Pomarol-Clotet, E. (2012). Executive dysfunction and memory impairment in schizoaffective disorder: A comparison with bipolar disorder, schizophrenia and healthy controls. *Psychological Medicine, 42*(10), 2127–2135.

Amanzio, M., Vase, L., Leotta, D., Miceli, R., Palermo, S., & Geminiani, G. (2013). Impaired awareness of deficits in Alzheimer's disease: The role of everyday executive dysfunction. *Journal of the International Neuropsychological Society, 19*(1), 63–72. doi: 10.1017/s1355617712000896

Amato, M. P., Portaccio, E., Goretti, B., Zipoli, V., Hakiki, B., Giannini, M., . . . Razzolini, L. (2010). Cognitive impairment in early stages of multiple sclerosis. *Neurological Sciences, 31*(Suppl. 2), S211–S214.

Ambery, F. Z., Russell, A. J., Perry, K., Morris, R., & Murphy, D. G. M. (2006). Neuropsychological functioning in adults with Asperger syndrome. *Autism, 10*(6), 551–564. doi: 10.1177/1362361306068507

American Psychiatric Association. (2013). *Diagnostic and statistical manual of mental disorders* (5th ed.) Arlington, VA: American Psychiatric Publishing.

Ancín, I., Cabranes, J. A., Santos, J. L., Sánchez-Morla, E., & Barabash, A. (2013). Executive deficits: A continuum schizophrenia–bipolar disorder or specific to schizophrenia? *Journal of Psychiatric Research, 47*(11), 1564–1571.

Anderson, B., Storfer-Isser, A., Taylor, H. G., Rosen, C. L., & Redline, S. (2009). Associations of executive function with sleepiness and sleep duration in adolescents. *Pediatrics, 123*(4), e701–e707.

Andreotti, C., Thigpen, J. E., Dunn, M. J., Watson, K., Potts, J., Reising, M. M., . . . Compas, B. E. (2013). Cognitive reappraisal and secondary control coping: Associations with working memory, positive and negative affect, and symptoms of anxiety/depression. *Anxiety, Stress and Coping: An International Journal, 26*(1), 20–35.

Angrilli, A., Sartori, G., & Donzella, G. (2013). Cognitive, emotional and social markers of serial murdering. *Clinical Neuropsychologist, 27*(3), 485–494. doi: 10.1080/13854046.2013.771215

Annett, R. D., Hile, S., Bedrick, E., Kunin-Batson, A. S., Krull, K. R., Embry, L., . . . Noll, R. B. (2015). Neuropsychological functioning of children treated for acute lymphoblastic leukemia: Impact of whole brain radiation therapy. *Psycho-Oncology, 24*(2), 181–189.

Anokhin, A. P., Golosheykin, S., & Heath, A. C. (2008). Heritability of frontal brain function related to action monitoring. *Psychophysiology, 45*(4), 524–534.

Anokhin, A. P., Heath, A. C., & Ralano, A. (2003). Genetic influences on frontal brain function: WCST performance in twins. *NeuroReport: For Rapid Communication of Neuroscience Research, 14*(15), 1975–1978.

Archer, N., Brown, R. G., Reeves, S. J., Boothby, H., Nicholas, H., Foy, C., . . . Lovestone, S. (2007). Premorbid personality and behavioral and psychological symptoms in probable Alzheimer disease. *American Journal of Geriatric Psychiatry, 15*(3), 202–213.

Arciniegas, D. B., & Wortzel, H. S. (2014). Emotional and behavioral dyscontrol after traumatic brain injury. *Psychiatric Clinics of North America, 37*(1), 31–53.

Areza-Fegyveres, R., Kairalla, R. A., Carvalho, C. R. R., & Nitrini, R. (2010). Cognition and chronic hypoxia in pulmonary diseases. *Dementia and Neuropsychologia, 4*(1), 14–22.

Armengol, C. G. (2000). Acute oxygen deprivation: Neuropsychological profiles and implications for rehabilitation. *Brain Injury, 14*(3), 237–250.

Arnold, L. E., Ganocy, S. J., Mount, K., Youngstrom, E. A., Frazier, T., Fristad, M., . . . Marsh, L. (2014). Three-year latent class trajectories of attention-deficit/hyperactivity disorder (ADHD) symptoms in a clinical sample not selected for ADHD. *Journal of the American Academy of Child and Adolescent Psychiatry, 53*(7), 745–760.

Aro, T., Laakso, M.-L., Määttä, S., Tolvanen, A., & Poikkeus, A.-M. (2014). Associations between toddler-age communication and kindergarten-age self-regulatory skills. *Journal of Speech, Language, and Hearing Research, 57*(4), 1405–1417.

Aron, A. R., Robbins, T. W., & Poldrack, R. A. (2004). Inhibition and the right inferior frontal cortex. *Trends in Cognitive Sciences, 8*(4), 170–177. doi: 10.1016/j.tics.2004.02.010

Aron, A. R., Robbins, T. W., & Poldrack, R. A. (2014). Inhibition and the right inferior frontal cortex: One decade on. *Trends in Cognitive Sciences, 18*(4), 177–185.

Astley, S. J., Aylward, E. H., Olson, H. C., Kerns, K., Brooks, A., Coggins, T. E., ... Richards, T. (2009a). Functional magnetic resonance imaging outcomes from a comprehensive magnetic resonance study of children with fetal alcohol spectrum disorders. *Journal of Neurodevelopmental Disorders, 1*(1), 61–80. doi: 10.1007/s11689-009-9004-0

Astley, S. J., Aylward, E. H., Olson, H. C., Kerns, K., Brooks, A., Coggins, T. E., ... Richards, T. (2009b). Magnetic resonance imaging outcomes from a comprehensive magnetic resonance study of children with fetal alcohol spectrum disorders. *Alcoholism: Clinical and Experimental Research, 33*(10), 1671–1689. doi: 10.1111/j.1530-0277.2009.01004.x

Atkinson, A. P., & Adolphs, R. (2005). Visual emotion perception: Mechanisms and processes. In L. F. Barrett, P. M. Niedenthal, & P. Winkielman (Eds.), *Emotion and consciousness* (pp. 150–182). New York, NY: Guilford Press.

Aupperle, R. L., Melrose, A. J., Stein, M. B., & Paulus, M. P. (2012). Executive function and PTSD: Disengaging from trauma. *Neuropharmacology, 62*(2), 686–694.

Aydın, P. C., Koybasi, G. P., Sert, E., Mete, L., & Oyekcin, D. G. (2014). Executive functions and memory in autogenous and reactive subtype of obsessive-compulsive disorder patients. *Comprehensive Psychiatry,55*(4), 904–911.

Bach, L. J., Happé, F., Fleminger, S., & Powell, J. (2000). Theory of mind: Independence of executive function and the role of the frontal cortex in acquired brain injury. *Cognitive Neuropsychiatry, 5*(3), 175–192.

Badaruddin, D. H., Andrews, G. L., Bölte, S., Schilmoeller, K. J., Schilmoeller, G., Paul, L. K., & Brown, W. S. (2007). Social and behavioral problems of children with agenesis of the corpus callosum. *Child Psychiatry and Human Development, 38*(4), 287–302.

Baddeley, A. D. (1998). The central executive: A concept and some misconceptions. *Journal of the International Neuropsychological Society, 4*(5), 523–526.

Baddeley, A. D., Chincotta, D., & Adlam, A. (2001). Working memory and the control of action: Evidence from task switching. *Journal of Experimental Psychology: General, 130*(4), 641–657.

Baddeley, A. D., & Della Sala, S. (1998). Working memory and executive control. In A. C. Roberts, T. W. Robbins, & L. Weiskrantz (Eds.), *The prefrontal cortex: Executive and cognitive functions* (pp. 9–21). New York, NY: Oxford University Press.

Baddeley, A. D., & Jarrold, C. (2007). Working memory and Down syndrome. *Journal of Intellectual Disability Research, 51*(12), 925–931.

Baez, S., Rattazzi, A., Gonzalez-Gadea, M. L., Torralva, T., Vigliecca, N. S., Decety, J., . . . Ibanez, A. (2012). Integrating intention and context: Assessing social cognition in adults with Asperger syndrome. *Frontiers in Human Neuroscience, 6*. doi: 10.3389/fnhum.2012.00302

Baggett, M. R., Kelly, M. P., Korenman, L. M., & Ryan, L. M. (2003). Neuropsychological deficits of a U.S. Army pilot following an anoxic event as a function of cardiac arrest. *Military Medicine, 168*(9), 769–771.

Bagiella, E., Novack, T. A., Ansel, B., Diaz-Arrastia, R., Dikmen, S., Hart, T., & Temkin, N. (2010). Measuring outcome in traumatic brain injury treatment trials: Recommendations from the Traumatic Brain Injury Clinical Trials Network. *Journal of Head Trauma Rehabilitation, 25*(5), 375–382. doi: 10.1097/HTR.0b013e3181d27fe3

Baiano, M., David, A., Versace, A., Churchill, R., Balestrieri, M., & Brambilla, P. (2007). Anterior cingulate volumes in schizophrenia: A systematic review and a meta-analysis of MRI studies. *Schizophrenia Research, 93*(1–3), 1–12.

Baird, A. D., Scheffer, I. E., & Wilson, S. J. (2011). Mirror neuron system involvement in empathy: A critical look at the evidence. *Social Neuroscience, 6*(4), 327–335.

Baker, S., Hooper, S., Skinner, M., Hatton, D., Schaaf, J., Ornstein, P., & Bailey, D. (2011). Working memory subsystems and task complexity in young boys with fragile X syndrome. *Journal of Intellectual Disability Research, 55*(1), 19–29. doi: 10.1111/j.1365-2788.2010.01343.x

Baker, S. T. (2009). Developing theory of mind and executive functions from three- to five-years-old: Cross-sectional group and longitudinal single-case approaches. 69, ProQuest Information & Learning, US. Retrieved from http://search.ebscohost.com/login.aspx?direct=true&db=psyh&AN=2009-99020-176&site=ehost-live Available from EBSCOhost psyh database.

Balas, M., Balash, Y., Giladi, N., & Gurevich, T. (2010). Cognition in multiple system atrophy: Neuropsychological profile and interaction with mood. *Journal of Neural Transmission, 117*(3), 369–375.

Ball, J. D., Budrionis, M. M., & Trott, K. L. (1987). Neuropsychological effects of cold water near-drowning in an identical twin. *International Journal of Clinical Neuropsychology, 9*(2), 71–73.

Ball, S. L., Holland, A. J., Watson, P. C., & Huppert, F. A. (2010). Theoretical exploration of the neural bases of behavioural disinhibition, apathy and executive dysfunction in preclinical Alzheimer's disease in people with Down's syndrome: Potential involvement of multiple frontal-subcortical neuronal circuits. *Journal of Intellectual Disability Research*, 54(4), 320–336. doi: 10.1111/j.1365-2788.2010.01261.x

Bannon, S., Gonsalvez, C. J., Croft, R. J., & Boyce, P. M. (2006). Executive functions in obsessive-compulsive disorder: State or trait deficits? *Australian and New Zealand Journal of Psychiatry*, 40(11–12), 1031–1038.

Barch, D. M. (2008). Emotion, motivation, and reward processing in schizophrenia spectrum disorders: What we know and where we need to go. *Schizophrenia Bulletin*, 34(5), 816–818.

Barch, D. M., & Csernansky, J. G. (2007). Abnormal parietal cortex activation during working memory in schizophrenia: Verbal phonological coding disturbances versus domain-general executive dysfunction. *American Journal of Psychiatry*, 164(7), 1090–1098.

Barisnikov, K., Hippolyte, L., & Van der Linden, M. (2008). Face processing and facial emotion recognition in adults with Down syndrome. *American Journal on Mental Retardation*, 113(4), 292–306.

Barkley, R. A. (2014). Sluggish cognitive tempo (concentration deficit disorder?): Current status, future directions, and a plea to change the name. *Journal of Abnormal Child Psychology*, 42(1), 117–125.

Baron-Cohen, S., & Wheelwright, S. (2004). The empathy quotient: An investigation of adults with Asperger syndrome or high functioning autism, and normal sex differences. *Journal of Autism and Developmental Disorders*, 34(2), 163–175.

Barrett, N. A., Large, M. M., Smith, G. L., Karayanidis, F., Michie, P. T., Kavanagh, D. J., . . . O'Sullivan, B. T. (2003). Human brain regions required for the dividing and switching of attention between two features of a single object. *Cognitive Brain Research*, 17(1), 1–13.

Bartolo, A., Benuzzi, F., Nocetti, L., Baraldi, P., & Nichelli, P. (2006). Humor comprehension and appreciation: An fMRI study. *Journal of Cognitive Neuroscience*, 18(11), 1789–1798.

Basso, M. R., Bornstein, R. A., Carona, F., & Morton, R. (2001). Depression accounts for executive function deficits in obsessive-compulsive disorder. *Neuropsychiatry, Neuropsychology, and Behavioral Neurology*, 14(4), 241–245.

Bauermeister, J. J., Barkley, R. A., Bauermeister, J. A., Martínez, J. V., & McBurnett, K. (2012). Validity of the sluggish cognitive tempo, inattention, and hyperactivity symptom dimensions: Neuropsychological and psychosocial correlates. *Journal of Abnormal Child Psychology, 40*(5), 683–697.

Baumeister, R. F., & Alquist, J. L. (2009). Is there a downside to good self-control? *Self and Identity, 8*(2–3), 115–130.

Baumeister, R. F., Bratslavsky, E., Muraven, M., & Tice, D. M. (1998). Ego depletion: Is the active self a limited resource? *Journal of Personality and Social Psychology, 74*(5), 1252–1265.

Baumeister, R. F., Schmeichel, B. J., Vohs, K. D., Kruglanski, A. W., & Higgins, E. T. (2007). Self-regulation and the executive function: The self as controlling agent. In A. W. Kruglanski & E. T. Higgins (Eds.), *Social psychology: Handbook of basic principles* (2nd ed., pp. 516–539). New York, NY: Guilford Press.

Beato, R., Levy, R., Pillon, B., Vidal, C., du Montcel, S. T., Deweer, B., . . . Cardoso, F. (2008). Working memory in Parkinson disease patients: Clinical features and response to levodopa. *Arquivos de Neuro-Psiquiatria, 66*(2-A), 147–151.

Beaucousin, V., Lacheret, A., Turbelin, M.-R., Morel, M., Mazoyer, B., & Tzourio-Mazoyer, N. (2007). FMRI study of emotional speech comprehension. *Cerebral Cortex, 17*(2), 339–352.

Bechara, A. (2007). *Iowa Gambling Task professional manual.* Lutz, FL: Psychological Assessment Resources.

Bechara, A., & Damasio, A. R. (2005). The somatic marker hypothesis: A neural theory of economic decision. *Games and Economic Behavior, 52*(2), 336–372.

Bechara, A., Damasio, A. R., Damasio, H., & Anderson, S. W. (1994). Insensitivity to future consequences following damage to human prefrontal cortex. *Cognition, 50*(1), 7–15.

Bechara, A., Damasio, H., & Damasio, A. (2000). Emotion, decision making and the orbitofrontal cortex. *Cerebral Cortex, 10*, 295–307. doi: papers://B9ADBC58-3831-4D93-BEE7-6A784A58423D/Paper/p93

Bechara, A., Damasio, H., Tranel, D., & Damasio, A. R. (1997). Deciding advantageously before knowing the advantageous strategy. *Science, 275*(5304), 1293–1294.

Bechara, A., Damasio, H., Tranel, D., & Damasio, A. R. (2005). The Iowa Gambling Task and the somatic marker hypothesis: Some questions and answers. *Trends in Cognitive Sciences, 9*(4), 159–162.

Bechara, A., Tranel, D., Damasio, H., & Adolphs, R. (1995). Double dissociation of conditioning and declarative knowledge relative to the amygdala and hippocampus in humans. *Science, 269*(5227), 1115–1118.

Becker, S. P., Fite, P. J., Garner, A. A., Greening, L., Stoppelbein, L., & Luebbe, A. M. (2013). Reward and punishment sensitivity are differentially associated with ADHD and sluggish cognitive tempo symptoms in children. *Journal of Research in Personality*, 47(6), 719–727.

Becker, S. P., & Langberg, J. M. (2014). Attention-deficit/hyperactivity disorder and sluggish cognitive tempo dimensions in relation to executive functioning in adolescents with ADHD. *Child Psychiatry and Human Development*, 45(1), 1–11. doi: 10.1007/s10578-013-0372-z

Bédard, M.-J., Joyal, C. C., Godbout, L., & Chantal, S. (2009). Executive functions and the obsessive-compulsive disorder: On the importance of subclinical symptoms and other concomitant factors. *Archives of Clinical Neuropsychology*, 24(6), 585–598.

Beebe, D. W., & Gozal, D. (2002). Obstructive sleep apnea and the prefrontal cortex: Towards a comprehensive model linking nocturnal upper airway obstruction to daytime cognitive and behavioral deficits. *Journal of Sleep Research*, 11(1), 1–16.

Beer, J. S., John, O. P., Scabini, D., & Knight, R. T. (2006). Orbitofrontal cortex and social behavior: Integrating self-monitoring and emotion-cognition interactions. *Journal of Cognitive Neuroscience*, 18, 871–879. doi: papers://B9ADBC58-3831-4D93-BEE7-6A784A58423D/Paper/p6093

Belanger, H. G., Spiegel, E., & Vanderploeg, R. D. (2010). Neuropsychological performance following a history of multiple self-reported concussions: A meta-analysis. *Journal of the International Neuropsychological Society*, 16(2), 262–267.

Benatti, B., Dell'Osso, B., Arici, C., Hollander, E., & Altamura, A. C. (2014). Characterizing impulsivity profile in patients with obsessive-compulsive disorder. *International Journal of Psychiatry in Clinical Practice*, 18(3), 156–160.

Benge, J., Phillips-Sabol, J., & Phenis, R. (2014). The neuropsychological assessment battery categories test as a measure of executive dysfunction in patients with Parkinson's disease and essential tremor: An exploratory study. *Clinical Neuropsychologist*, 28(6), 1008–1018. doi: 10.1080/13854046.2014.950985

Benitez, A., & Gunstad, J. (2012). Poor sleep quality diminishes cognitive functioning independent of depression and anxiety in healthy young adults. *Clinical Neuropsychologist*, 26(2), 214–223.

Bennetto, L., Taylor, A. K., Pennington, B. F., Porter, D., & Hagerman, R. J. (2001). Profile of cognitive functioning in women with the fragile X mutation. *Neuropsychology*, 15(2), 290–299. doi: 10.1037/0894-4105.15.2.290

Berghorst, L. H., Bogdan, R., Frank, M. J., & Pizzagalli, D. A. (2013). Acute stress selectively reduces reward sensitivity. *Frontiers in Human Neuroscience*, 7(133), doi: 10.3389/fnhum.2013.00133.

Berlin, H. A., Rolls, E. T., & Iversen, S. D. (2005). Borderline personality disorder, impulsivity, and the orbitofrontal cortex. *American Journal of Psychiatry*, 162(12), 2360–2373.

Bernad, M. d. M., Servera, M., Grases, G., Collado, S., & Burns, G. L. (2014). A cross-sectional and longitudinal investigation of the external correlates of sluggish cognitive tempo and ADHD-inattention symptoms dimensions. *Journal of Abnormal Child Psychology*, 42(7), 1225–1236.

Bernier, A., Beauchamp, M. H., Bouvette-Turcot, A. A., Carlson, S. M., & Carrier, J. (2013). Sleep and cognition in preschool years: Specific links to executive functioning. *Child Development*, 84(5), 1542–1553.

Berntson, G. G., Bechara, A., Damasio, H., Tranel, D., & Cacioppo, J. T. (2007). Amygdala contribution to selective dimensions of emotion. *Social Cognitive and Affective Neuroscience*, 2(2), 123–129.

Berridge, K. C., & Kringelbach, M. L. (2008). Affective neuroscience of pleasure: Reward in humans and animals. *Psychopharmacology*, 199(3), 457–480.

Berryhill, M. E., & Olson, I. R. (2008). Is the posterior parietal lobe involved in working memory retrieval? Evidence from patients with bilateral parietal lobe damage. *Neuropsychologia*, 46(7), 1775–1786.

Bhojraj, T. S., Diwadkar, V. A., Sweeney, J. A., Prasad, K. M., Eack, S. M., Montrose, D. M., & Keshavan, M. S. (2010). Longitudinal alterations of executive function in non-psychotic adolescents at familial risk for schizophrenia. *Progress in Neuro-Psychopharmacology and Biological Psychiatry*, 34(3), 469–474.

Bigler, E. D. (2001). The lesion(s) in traumatic brain injury: Implications for clinical neuropsychology. *Archives of Clinical Neuropsychology*, 16(2), 95–131.

Birch, R. C., Cornish, K. M., Hocking, D. R., & Trollor, J. N. (2014). Understanding the neuropsychiatric phenotype of fragile x–associated tremor ataxia syndrome: A systematic review. *Neuropsychology Review*, 24(4), 491–513.

Biringer, E., Lundervold, A., Stordal, K., Mykletun, A., Egeland, J., Bottlender, R., & Lund, A. (2005). Executive function improvement upon remission of recurrent unipolar depression. *European Archives of Psychiatry and Clinical Neuroscience*, 255(6), 373–380.

Bisiacchi, P. S., Borella, E., Bergamaschi, S., Carretti, B., & Mondini, S. (2008). Interplay between memory and executive functions in normal and pathological aging. *Journal of Clinical and Experimental Neuropsychology, 30*(6), 723–733.

Blair, R. J. R. (2001). Neurocognitive models of aggression, the antisocial personality disorders, and psychopathy. *Journal of Neurology, Neurosurgery and Psychiatry, 71*(6), 727–731.

Blonder, L. X., Heilman, K. M., Ketterson, T., Rosenbek, J., Raymer, A., Crosson, B., . . . Gonzalez-Rothi, L. (2005). Affective facial and lexical expression in aprosodic versus aphasic stroke patients. *Journal of the International Neuropsychological Society, 11*(6), 677–685.

Blondis, T. A. (2004). Neurodevelopmental motor disorders: Cerebral palsy and neuromuscular diseases. In D. Dewey & D. E. Tupper (Eds.), *Developmental motor disorders: A neuropsychological perspective* (pp. 113–136). New York, NY: Guilford Press.

Blume, A. W., Marlatt, G. A., & Schmaling, K. B. (2000). Executive cognitive function and heavy drinking behavior among college students. *Psychology of Addictive Behaviors, 14*(3), 299–302. doi: 10.1037/0893-164x.14.3.299

Boakes, J., Chapman, E., Houghton, S., & West, J. (2008). Facial affect interpretation in boys with attention deficit/hyperactivity disorder. *Child Neuropsychology, 14*(1), 82–96.

Bodimeade, H. L., Whittingham, K., Lloyd, O., & Boyd, R. N. (2013). Executive function in children and adolescents with unilateral cerebral palsy. *Developmental Medicine and Child Neurology, 55*(10), 926–933.

Bodling, A. M., Denney, D. R., & Lynch, S. G. (2012). Individual variability in speed of information processing: An index of cognitive impairment in multiple sclerosis. *Neuropsychology, 26*(3), 357–367.

Boeve, B. F. (2012). Mild cognitive impairment associated with underlying Alzheimer's disease versus Lewy body disease. *Parkinsonism and Related Disorders, 18*(Suppl. 1), S41–S44.

Bogdanova, Y., & Cronin-Golomb, A. (2013). Alexithymia and apathy in Parkinson's disease: Neurocognitive correlates. *Behavioural Neurology, 27*(4), 535–545.

Borella, E., Carretti, B., & Lanfranchi, S. (2013). Inhibitory mechanisms in Down syndrome: Is there a specific or general deficit? *Research in Developmental Disabilities, 34*(1), 65–71. doi: 10.1016/j.ridd.2012.07.017

Borod, J. C., Bloom, R. L., Brickman, A. M., Nakhutina, L., & Curko, E. A. (2002). Emotional processing deficits in individuals with unilateral brain damage. *Applied Neuropsychology, 9*(1), 23–36.

Borroni, B., Grassi, M., Premi, E., Gazzina, S., Alberici, A., Cosseddu, M., . . . Padovani, A. (2012). Neuroanatomical correlates of behavioural phenotypes in behavioural variant of frontotemporal dementia. *Behavioural Brain Research*, 235(2), 124–129.

Boschloo, L., Vogelzangs, N., van den Brink, W., Smit, J. H., Beekman, A. T. F., & Penninx, B. W. J. H. (2013). The role of negative emotionality and impulsivity in depressive/anxiety disorders and alcohol dependence. *Psychological Medicine*, 43(6), 1241–1253.

Bottcher, L. (2010). Children with spastic cerebral palsy, their cognitive functioning, and social participation: A review. *Child Neuropsychology*, 16(3), 209–228.

Boyle, P. A., Cohen, R. A., Paul, R., Moser, D., & Gordon, N. (2002). Cognitive and motor impairments predict functional declines in patients with vascular dementia. *International Journal of Geriatric Psychiatry*, 17(2), 164–169.

Bozikas, V. P., & Andreou, C. (2011). Longitudinal studies of cognition in first episode psychosis: A systematic review of the literature. *Australian and New Zealand Journal of Psychiatry*, 45(2), 93–108.

Bozikas, V. P., Tonia, T., Fokas, K., Karavatos, A., & Kosmidis, M. H. (2006). Impaired emotion processing in remitted patients with bipolar disorder. *Journal of Affective Disorders*, 91(1), 53–56.

Braakman, H. M. H., Vaessen, M. J., Hofman, P. A. M., Debeij-van Hall, M. H. J. A., Backes, W. H., Vles, J. S. H., & Aldenkamp, A. P. (2011). Cognitive and behavioral complications of frontal lobe epilepsy in children: A review of the literature. *Epilepsia*, 52(5), 849–856.

Bradshaw, J. M., Saling, M., Anderson, V., Hopwood, M., & Brodtmann, A. (2006). Higher cortical deficits influence attentional processing in dementia with Lewy bodies, relative to patients with dementia of the Alzheimer's type and controls. *Journal of Neurology, Neurosurgery and Psychiatry*, 77(10), 1129–1135.

Brady, D. I., Schwean, V. L., Saklofske, D. H., McCrimmon, A. W., Montgomery, J. M., & Thorne, K. J. (2013). Conceptual and perceptual set-shifting executive abilities in young adults with Asperger's syndrome. *Research in Autism Spectrum Disorders*, 7(12), 1631–1637. doi: 10.1016/j.rasd.2013.09.009

Brand, M., Grabenhorst, F., Starcke, K., Vandekerckhove, M. M. P., & Markowitsch, H. J. (2007). Role of the amygdala in decisions under ambiguity and decisions under risk: Evidence from patients with Urbach-Wiethe disease. *Neuropsychologia*, 45(6), 1305–1317.

Braw, Y., Benozio, A., & Levkovitz, Y. (2012). Executive functioning during full and partial remission (positive and negative symptomatic remission) of schizophrenia. *Schizophrenia Research*, 142(1–3), 122–128.

Brega, A. G., Goodrich, G., Bennett, R. E., Hessl, D., Engle, K., Leehey, M. A., . . . Grigsby, J. (2008). The primary cognitive deficit among males with fragile X–associated tremor/ataxia syndrome (FXTAS) is a dysexecutive syndrome. *Journal of Clinical and Experimental Neuropsychology, 30*(8), 853–869.

Brega, A. G., Reynolds, A., Bennett, R. E., Leehey, M. A., Bounds, L. S., Cogswell, J. B., . . . Grigsby, J. (2009). Functional status of men with the fragile X premutation, with and without the tremor/ataxia syndrome (FXTAS). *International Journal of Geriatric Psychiatry, 24*(10), 1101–1109.

Brossard-Racine, M., Waknin, J., Shikako-Thomas, K., Shevell, M., Poulin, C., Lach, L., . . . Majnemer, A. (2013). Behavioral difficulties in adolescents with cerebral palsy. *Journal of Child Neurology, 28*(1), 27–33.

Brown, A. D., Addis, D. R., Romano, T. A., Marmar, C. R., Bryant, R. A., Hirst, W., & Schacter, D. L. (2014). Episodic and semantic components of autobiographical memories and imagined future events in post-traumatic stress disorder. *Memory, 22*(6), 595–604.

Brown, R. G., Lacomblez, L., Landwehrmeyer, B. G., Bak, T., Uttner, I., Dubois, B., . . . Leigh, N. P. (2010). Cognitive impairment in patients with multiple system atrophy and progressive supranuclear palsy. *Brain: A Journal of Neurology, 133*(8), 2382–2393.

Brown, R. J., Bouska, J. F., Frow, A., Kirkby, A., Baker, G. A., Kemp, S., . . . Reuber, M. (2013). Emotional dysregulation, alexithymia, and attachment in psychogenic nonepileptic seizures. *Epilepsy and Behavior, 29*(1), 178–183.

Brown, S. W., Collier, S. A., & Night, J. C. (2013). Timing and executive resources: Dual-task interference patterns between temporal production and shifting, updating, and inhibition tasks. *Journal of Experimental Psychology: Human Perception and Performance, 39*(4), 947–963. doi: 10.1037/a0030484

Brüne, M., Schöbel, A., Karau, R., Benali, A., Faustmann, P. M., Juckel, G., & Petrasch-Parwez, E. (2010). Von Economo neuron density in the anterior cingulate cortex is reduced in early onset schizophrenia. *Acta Neuropathologica, 119*(6), 771–778.

Brydges, C. R., Fox, A. M., Reid, C. L., & Anderson, M. (2014). Predictive validity of the N2 and P3 ERP components to executive functioning in children: A latent-variable analysis. *Frontiers in Human Neuroscience, 8*(80), doi: 10.3389/fnhum.2014.00080.

Brydges, C. R., Reid, C. L., Fox, A. M., & Anderson, M. (2012). A unitary executive function predicts intelligence in children. *Intelligence, 40*(5), 458–469.

Burgess, G. C., Depue, B. E., Ruzic, L., Willcutt, E. G., Du, Y. P., & Banich, M. T. (2010). Attentional control activation relates to working memory in attention-deficit/hyperactivity disorder. *Biological Psychiatry*, 67(7), 632–640.

Burgess, P. W., Dumontheil, I., Gilbert, S. J., Okuda, J., Schölvinck, M. L., & Simons, J. S. (2008). On the role of rostral prefrontal cortex (area 10) in prospective memory. In M. Kliegel, M. A. McDaniel, & G. O. Einstein (Eds.), *Prospective memory: Cognitive, neuroscience, developmental, and applied perspectives* (pp. 235–260). New York, NY: Taylor and Francis Group.

Burgess, P. W., Gilbert, S. J., & Dumontheil, I. (2008). Function and localization within rostral prefrontal cortex (area 10). In J. Driver, P. Haggard, & T. Shallice (Eds.), *Mental processes in the human brain* (pp. 203–223). New York, NY: Oxford University Press.

Burgess, P. W., Gonen-Yaacovi, G., & Volle, E. (2011). Functional neuroimaging studies of prospective memory: What have we learnt so far? *Neuropsychologia*, 49(8), 2246–2257.

Burgess, P. W., Veitch, E., de Lacy Costello, A., & Shallice, T. (2000). The cognitive and neuroanatomical correlates of multitasking. *Neuropsychologia*, 38(6), 848–863.

Burke, C. J., Brünger, C., Kahnt, T., Park, S. Q., & Tobler, P. N. (2013). Neural integration of risk and effort costs by the frontal pole: Only upon request. *Journal of Neuroscience*, 33(4), 1706–1713.

Burns, G. L., Servera, M., del Mar Bernad, M., Carrillo, J. M., & Cardo, E. (2013). Distinctions between sluggish cognitive tempo, ADHD-IN, and depression symptom dimensions in Spanish first-grade children. *Journal of Clinical Child and Adolescent Psychology*, 42(6), 796–808.

Busl, K. M., & Greer, D. M. (2010). Hypoxic-ischemic brain injury: Pathophysiology, neuropathology and mechanisms. *NeuroRehabilitation*, 26(1), 5–13.

Butti, C., Santos, M., Uppal, N., & Hof, P. R. (2013). Von Economo neurons: Clinical and evolutionary perspectives. *Cortex: A Journal Devoted to the Study of the Nervous System and Behavior*, 49(1), 312–326.

Cabeza, R., & Nyberg, L. (2000). Imaging cognition II: An empirical review of 275 PET and fMRI studies. *Journal of Cognitive Neuroscience*, 12(1), 1–47.

Cagnin, A., Gnoato, F., Jelcic, N., Favaretto, S., Zarantonello, G., Ermani, M., & Dam, M. (2013). Clinical and cognitive correlates of visual hallucinations in dementia with Lewy bodies. *Journal of Neurology, Neurosurgery and Psychiatry*, 84(5), 505–510.

Cahn-Weiner, D. A., Wittenberg, D., & McDonald, C. (2009). Everyday cognition in temporal lobe and frontal lobe epilepsy. *Epileptic Disorders*, *11*(3), 222–227.

Cai, W., & Leung, H.-C. (2009). Cortical activity during manual response inhibition guided by color and orientation cues. *Brain Research*, *1261*, 20–28. doi: 10.1016/j.brainres.2008.12.073

Caine, D., & Watson, J. D. G. (2000). Neuropsychological and neuropathological sequelae of cerebral anoxia: A critical review. *Journal of the International Neuropsychological Society*, *6*(1), 86–99.

Calamia, M., Markon, K., & Tranel, D. (2013). The robust reliability of neuropsychological measures: Meta-analyses of test-retest correlations. *Clinical Neuropsychologist*, *27*(7), 1077–1105. doi: 10.1080/13854046.2013.809795

Cameron, O. G., & Minoshima, S. (2002). Regional brain activation due to pharmacologically induced adrenergic interoceptive stimulation in humans. *Psychosomatic Medicine*, *64*(6), 851–861.

Campbell, Z., Zakzanis, K. K., Jovanovski, D., Joordens, S., Mraz, R., & Graham, S. J. (2009). Utilizing virtual reality to improve the ecological validity of clinical neuropsychology: An fMRI case study elucidating the neural basis of planning by comparing the Tower of London with a three-dimensional navigation task. *Applied Neuropsychology*, *16*(4), 295–306. doi: 10.1080/09084280903297891

Cappell, K. A., Gmeindl, L., & Reuter-Lorenz, P. A. (2010). Age differences in prefontal recruitment during verbal working memory maintenance depend on memory load. *Cortex: A Journal Devoted to the Study of the Nervous System and Behavior*, *46*(4), 462–473. doi: 10.1016/j.cortex.2009.11.009

Carlson, S. M., Moses, L. J., & Breton, C. (2002). How specific is the relation between executive function and theory of mind? Contributions of inhibitory control and working memory. *Infant and Child Development*, *11*(2), 73–92.

Carlson, S. M., & Wang, T. S. (2007). Inhibitory control and emotion regulation in preschool children. *Cognitive Development*, *22*(4), 489–510.

Carr, L., Iacoboni, M., Dubeau, M. C., Mazziotta, J. C., & Lenzi, G. L. (2003). Neural mechanisms of empathy in humans: A relay from neural systems for imitations to limbic areas. *Proceedings of the National Academy of Sciences*, *100*, 5497–5502.

Carretti, B., Belacchi, C., & Cornoldi, C. (2010). Difficulties in working memory updating in individuals with intellectual disability. *Journal of Intellectual Disability Research*, *54*(4), 337–345. doi: 10.1111/j.1365-2788.2010.01267.x

Carrington, S. J., & Bailey, A. J. (2009). Are there theory of mind regions in the brain? A review of the neuroimaging literature. *Human Brain Mapping, 30*(8), 2313–2335.

Casey, B. J., Castellanos, F. X., Giedd, J. N., & Marsh, W. L. (1997). Implication of right frontostriatal circuitry in response inhibition and attention-deficit/hyperactivity disorder. *Journal of the American Academy of Child and Adolescent Psychiatry, 36*(3), 374–383.

Cauda, F., Torta, D. M. E., Sacco, K., D'Agata, F., Geda, E., Duca, S., . . . Vercelli, A. (2013). Functional anatomy of cortical areas characterized by von Economo neurons. *Brain Structure and Function, 218*(1), 1–20.

Cavanna, A. E., Bertero, L., Cavanna, S., Servo, S., Strigaro, G., & Monaco, F. (2009). Persistent akinetic mutism after bilateral paramedian thalamic infarction. *Journal of Neuropsychiatry and Clinical Neurosciences, 21*(3), 351.

Cendes, F., Andermann, F., Gloor, P., Evans, A., Jones-Gotman, M., Watson, C., . . . Lopez-Cendes, I. (1993). MRI volumetric measurement of amygdala and hippocampus in temporal lobe epilepsy. *Neurology, 43*, 719–725.

Chamberlain, S. R., & Sahakian, B. J. (2007). The neuropsychiatry of impulsivity. *Current Opinion in Psychiatry, 20*(3), 255–261.

Chamorro-Premuzic, T., & Furnham, A. (2008). Personality, intelligence and approaches to learning as predictors of academic performance. *Personality and Individual Differences, 44*(7), 1596–1603.

Chan, A., Ho, S., & Poon, W. S. (2002). Neuropsychological sequelae of patients treated with microsurgical clipping or endovascular embolization for anterior communicating artery aneurysm. *European Neurology, 47*(1), 37–44.

Chan, A. S., Cheung, M.-c., Han, Y. M. Y., Sze, S. L., Leung, W. W., Man, H. S., & To, C. Y. (2009). Executive function deficits and neural discordance in children with autism spectrum disorders. *Clinical Neurophysiology, 120*(6), 1107–1115. doi: 10.1016/j.clinph.2009.04.002

Chan, M., Lim, W. S., & Sahadevan, S. (2008). Stage-independent and stage-specific phenotypic differences between vascular dementia and Alzheimer's disease. *Dementia and Geriatric Cognitive Disorders, 26*(6), 513–521.

Chan, R. C. K., Guo, M., Zou, X., Li, D., Hu, Z., & Yang, B. (2006). Multitasking performance of Chinese children with ADHD. *Journal of the International Neuropsychological Society, 12*(4), 575–579.

Chan, Y.-C., Chou, T.-L., Chen, H.-C., Yeh, Y.-C., Lavallee, J. P., Liang, K.-C., & Chang, K.-E. (2013). Towards a neural circuit model of verbal humor processing: An fMRI study of the neural substrates of incongruity detection and resolution. *Neuroimage, 66,* 169–176.

Chang, S. W., McCracken, J. T., & Piacentini, J. C. (2007). Neurocognitive correlates of child obsessive compulsive disorder and Tourette syndrome. *Journal of Clinical and Experimental Neuropsychology, 29*(7), 724–733.

Channon, S., Pratt, P., & Robertson, M. M. (2003). Executive function, memory, and learning in Tourette's syndrome. *Neuropsychology, 17*(2), 247–254.

Chapman, B., Duberstein, P., & Lyness, J. M. (2007). Personality traits, education, and health-related quality of life among older adult primary care patients. *Journals of Gerontology: Series B: Psychological Sciences and Social Sciences* 62B(6), P343–P352.

Charlton, R. A., Barrick, T. R., Lawes, I. N. C., Markus, H. S., & Morris, R. G. (2010). White matter pathways associated with working memory in normal aging. *Cortex: A Journal Devoted to the Study of the Nervous System and Behavior, 46*(4), 474–489.

Chein, J. M., Moore, A. B., & Conway, A. R. A. (2011). Domain-general mechanisms of complex working memory span. *Neuroimage, 54*(1), 550–559.

Chelune, G. J., Stott, H., & Pinkston, J. (2008). Multiple sclerosis. In J. E. Morgan & J. H. Ricker (Eds.), *Textbook of clinical neuropsychology* (pp. 599–615). New York, NY: Psychology Press.

Chen, P., Ratcliff, G., Belle, S. H., Cauley, J. A., DeKosky, S. T., & Ganguli, M. (2001). Patterns of cognitive decline in presymptomatic Alzheimer disease. *Archives of General Psychiatry, 58*(9), 853–858.

Chevalère, J., Postal, V., Jauregui, J., Copet, P., Laurier, V., & Thuilleaux, D. (2013). Assessment of executive functions in Prader-Willi syndrome and relationship with intellectual level. *Journal of Applied Research in Intellectual Disabilities, 26*(4), 309–318.

Chikazoe, J. (2010). Localizing performance of go/no-go tasks to prefrontal cortical subregions. *Current Opinion in Psychiatry, 23*(3), 267–272.

Cho, Y. T., Fromm, S., Guyer, A. E., Detloff, A., Pine, D. S., Fudge, J. L., & Ernst, M. (2013). Nucleus accumbens, thalamus and insula connectivity during incentive anticipation in typical adults and adolescents. *Neuroimage, 66,* 508–521.

Chow, T. W., Binns, M. A., Cummings, J. L., Lam, I., Black, S. E., Miller, B. L., . . . van Reekum, R. (2009). Apathy symptom profile and behavioral associations in frontotemporal dementia vs dementia of Alzheimer type. *Archives of Neurology, 66*(7), 888–893.

Christensen, B. K., Patrick, R. E., Stuss, D. T., Gillingham, S., & Zipursky, R. B. (2013). CE verbal episodic memory impairment in schizophrenia: A comparison with frontal lobe lesion patients. *Clinical Neuropsychologist, 27*(4), 647–666. doi: 10.1080/13854046.2013.780640

Christopher, G., & MacDonald, J. (2005). The impact of clinical depression on working memory. *Cognitive Neuropsychiatry, 10*(5), 379–399.

Chuang, Y. M., Chang, Y. J., Chang, C. H., Huang, K. L., Chang, T. Y., Wu, T. C., . . . Lee, T. H. (2011). Correlation between the flow pattern of the circle of Willis and segmental perfusion asymmetry after carotid artery revascularization. *European Journal of Neurology, 18*(9), 1132–1138.

Cicerone, K., Levin, H., Malec, J., Stuss, D., & Whyte, J. (2006). Cognitive rehabilitation interventions for executive function: Moving from bench to bedside in patients with traumatic brain injury. *Journal of Cognitive Neuroscience, 18*(7), 1212–1222. doi: 10.1162/jocn.2006.18.7.1212

Ciurli, P., Formisano, R., Bivona, U., Cantagallo, A., & Angelelli, P. (2011). Neuropsychiatric disorders in persons with severe traumatic brain injury: Prevalence, phenomenology, and relationship with demographic, clinical, and functional features. *Journal of Head Trauma Rehabilitation, 26*(2), 116–126.

Clark, C., Prior, M., & Kinsella, G. J. (2000). Do executive function deficits differentiate between adolescents with ADHD and oppositional defiant/conduct disorder? A neuropsychological study using the Six Elements Test and Hayling Sentence Completion Test. *Journal of Abnormal Child Psychology, 28*(5), 403–414.

Clark, L., Manes, F., Antoun, N., Sahakian, B. J., & Robbins, T. W. (2003). The contributions of lesion laterality and lesion volume to decision-making impairment following frontal lobe damage. *Neuropsychologia, 41*(11), 1474–1483.

Clément, F., Gauthier, S., & Belleville, S. (2013). Executive functions in mild cognitive impairment: Emergence and breakdown of neural plasticity. *Cortex: A Journal Devoted to the Study of the Nervous System and Behavior, 49*(5), 1268–1279. doi: 10.1016/j.cortex.2012.06.004

Clifford, J. S., Boufal, M. M., & Kurtz, J. E. (2004). Personality traits and critical thinking: Skills in college students' empirical tests of a two-factor theory. *Assessment, 11*(2), 169–176.

Cohen, J. R., Berkman, E. T., & Lieberman, M. D. (2013). Intentional and incidental self-control in ventrolateral prefrontal cortex. In D. T. Stuss & R. T. Knight (Eds.), *Principles of frontal lobe function* (2nd ed., pp. 417–440). New York, NY: Oxford University Press.

Colla, M., Ende, G., Alm, B., Deuschle, M., Heuser, I., & Kronenberg, G. (2008). Cognitive MR spectroscopy of anterior cingulate cortex in ADHD: Elevated choline signal correlates with slowed hit reaction times. *Journal of Psychiatric Research, 42*(7), 587–595.

Collerton, D., Burn, D., McKeith, I., & O'Brien, J. (2003). Systematic review and meta-analysis show that dementia with Lewy bodies is a visual-perceptual and attentional-executive dementia. *Dementia and Geriatric Cognitive Disorders, 16*(4), 229–237.

Cona, G., Arcara, G., Amodio, P., Schiff, S., & Bisiacchi, P. S. (2013). Does executive control really play a crucial role in explaining age-related cognitive and neural differences? *Neuropsychology, 27*(3), 378–389.

Connelly, M., & Denney, D. R. (2007). Regulation of emotions during experimental stress in alexithymia. *Journal of Psychosomatic Research, 62*(6), 649–656.

Connor, P. D., Sampson, P. D., Bookstein, F. L., Barr, H. M., & Streissguth, A. P. (2001). Direct and indirect effects of prenatal alcohol damage on executive function. *Developmental Neuropsychology, 18*(3), 331–354.

Consonni, M., Iannaccone, S., Cerami, C., Frasson, P., Lacerenza, M., Lunetta, C., . . . Cappa, S. F. (2013). The cognitive and behavioural profile of amyotrophic lateral sclerosis: Application of the consensus criteria. *Behavioural Neurology, 27*(2), 143–153.

Constantinidou, F., Christodoulou, M., & Prokopiou, J. (2012). The effects of age and education on executive functioning and oral naming performance in Greek Cypriot adults: The neurocognitive study for the aging. *Folia Phoniatrica et Logopaedica, 64*(4), 187–198. doi: 10.1159/000340015

Cook, C., Fay, S., & Rockwood, K. (2008). Decreased initiation of usual activities in people with mild-to-moderate Alzheimer's disease: A descriptive analysis from the VISTA clinical trial. *International Psychogeriatrics, 20*(5), 952–963.

Coolidge, F. L., Segal, D. L., & Applequist, K. (2009). Working memory deficits in personality disorder traits: A preliminary investigation in a nonclinical sample. *Journal of Research in Personality, 43*(3), 355–361.

Cools, R., Barker, R. A., Sahakian, B. J., & Robbins, T. W. (2003). L-dopa medication remediates cognitive inflexibility, but increases impulsivity in patients with Parkinson's disease. *Neuropsychologia, 41*(11), 1431–1441.

Cools, R., Stefanova, E., Barker, R. A., Robbins, T. W., & Owen, A. M. (2002). Dopaminergic modulation of high-level cognition in Parkinson's disease: The role of the prefrontal cortex revealed by PET. *Brain: A Journal of Neurology, 125*(3), 584–594.

Cordato, N. J., Pantelis, C., Halliday, G. M., Velakoulis, D., Wood, S. J., Stuart, G. W., . . . Morris, J. G. L. (2002). Frontal atrophy correlates with behavioural changes in progressive supranuclear palsy. *Brain: A Journal of Neurology*, 125(4), 789–800.

Cornish, K. M., Hocking, D. R., Moss, S. A., & Kogan, C. S. (2011). Selective executive markers of at-risk profiles associated with the fragile X permutation. *Neurology*, 77(7), 618–622.

Cornish, K. M., Turk, J., & Hagerman, R. (2008). The fragile X continuum: New advances and perspectives. *Journal of Intellectual Disability Research*, 52(6), 469–482. doi: 10.1111/j.1365-2788.2008.01056.x

Corral, M., Holguín, S. R., & Cadaveira, F. (2003). Neuropsychological characteristics of young children from high-density alcoholism families: A three-year follow-up. *Journal of Studies on Alcohol*, 64(2), 195–199.

Cortese, S., Kelly, C., Chabernaud, C., Proal, E., Di Martino, A., Milham, M. P., & Castellanos, F. X. (2012). Toward systems neuroscience of ADHD: A meta-analysis of 55 fMRI studies. *American Journal of Psychiatry*, 169(10), 1038–1055. doi: 10.1176/appi.ajp.2012.11101521

Cosentino, S. A., Jefferson, A. L., Carey, M., Price, C. C., Davis-Garrett, K., Swenson, R., & Libon, D. J. (2004). The clinical diagnosis of vascular dementia: A comparison among four classification systems and a proposal for a new paradigm. *Clinical Neuropsychologist*, 18(1), 6–21.

Cossart, R., Aronov, D., & Yuste, R. (2003). Attractor dynamics of network UP states in the neocortex. *Nature*, 423(6937), 283–288.

Costa, A., Caltagirone, C., & Carlesimo, G. A. (2011). Prospective memory impairment in mild cognitive impairment: An analytical review. *Neuropsychology Review*, 21(4), 390–404.

Costa, A., Carlesimo, G. A., & Caltagirone, C. (2012). Prospective memory functioning: A new area of investigation in the clinical neuropsychology and rehabilitation of Parkinson's disease and mild cognitive impairment. Review of evidence. *Neurological Sciences*, 33(5), 965–972.

Costa, A., Monaco, M., Zabberoni, S., Peppe, A., Perri, R., Fadda, L., . . . Carlesimo, G. A. (2014). Free and cued recall memory in Parkinson's disease associated with amnestic mild cognitive impairment. *PLoS ONE*, 9(1).

Costa, P. T., & McCrae, R. R. (1992). *Manual for the Revised NEO Personality Inventory (NEO-PI-R) and the NEO Five-Factor Inventory (NEO-PI)*. Odessa, FL: Psychological Assessment Resources.

Costafreda, S. G., Fu, C. H. Y., Lee, L., Everitt, B., Brammer, M. J., & David, A. S. (2006). A systematic review and quantitative appraisal of fMRI studies of verbal fluency: Role of the left inferior frontal gyrus. *Human Brain Mapping*, 27(10), 799–810.

Cox, S. M. L., Andrade, A., & Johnsrude, I. S. (2005). Learning to like: A role for human orbitofrontal cortex in conditioned reward. *Journal of Neuroscience*, 25(10), 2733–2740.

Craig, A. D. (2009). How do you feel—now? The anterior insula and human awareness. *Nature Reviews Neuroscience*, 10(1), 59–70.

Craik, F. I. M., & Bialystok, E. (2006). Planning and task management in older adults: Cooking breakfast. *Memory and Cognition*, 34(6), 1236–1249.

Critchley, H. D. (2009). Psychophysiology of neural, cognitive and affective integration: fMRI and autonomic indicants. *International Journal of Psychophysiology*, 73(2), 88–94. doi: papers://B9ADBC58-3831-4D93-BEE7-6A784A58423D/Paper/p2431

Critchley, H. D., Wiens, S., Rotshtein, P., Ohman, A., & Dolan, R. J. (2004). Neural systems supporting interoceptive awareness. *Nature Neuroscience*, 7(2), 189–195.

Crone, E. A., Wendelken, C., Donohue, S. E., & Bunge, S. A. (2006). Neural evidence for dissociable components of task-switching. *Cerebral Cortex*, 16(4), 475–486.

Crowell, T. A., Luis, C. A., Cox, D. E., & Mullan, M. (2007). Neuropsychological comparison of Alzheimer's disease and dementia with lewy bodies. *Dementia and Geriatric Cognitive Disorders*, 23(2), 120–125.

Cummings, J. L., & Miller, B. L. (2007). Conceptual and clinical aspects of the frontal lobes. In B. L. Miller & J. L. Cummings (Eds.), *The human frontal lobes: Functions and disorders* (2nd ed., pp. 12–21). New York, NY: Guilford Press.

Cusack, R., Mitchell, D. J., & Duncan, J. (2010). Discrete object representation, attention switching, and task difficulty in the parietal lobe. *Journal of Cognitive Neuroscience*, 22(1), 32–47.

Czernecki, V., Pillon, B., Houeto, J. L., Pochon, J. B., Levy, R., & Dubois, B. (2002). Motivation, reward, and Parkinson's disease: Influences of dopatherapy. *Neuropsychologia*, 40(13), 2257–2267.

Da Fonseca, D., Seguier, V., Santos, A., Poinso, F., & Deruelle, C. (2009). Emotion understanding in children with ADHD. *Child Psychiatry and Human Development*, 40(1), 111–121.

Dagher, A., Owen, A. M., Boecker, H., & Brooks, D. J. (2001). The role of the striatum and hippocampus in planning: A PET activation study in Parkinson's disease. *Brain: A Journal of Neurology*, 124(5), 1020–1032.

Danielsson, H., Henry, L., Rönnberg, J., & Nilsson, L.-G. (2010). Executive functions in individuals with intellectual disability. *Research in Developmental Disabilities, 31*(6), 1299–1304. doi: 10.1016/j.ridd.2010.07.012

Davis, K. D., Pope, G. E., Crawley, A. P., & Mikulis, D. J. (2004). Perceptual illusion of "paradoxical heat" engages the insular cortex. *Journal of Neurophysiology, 92*(2), 1248–1251.

Dawson, D. R., Levine, B., Schwartz, M., & Stuss, D. T. (2000). Quality of life following traumatic brain injury: A prospective study. *Brain and Cognition, 44*(1), 35–39.

Dawson, G., Webb, S. J., & McPartland, J. (2005). Understanding the nature of face processing impairment in autism: Insights from behavioral and electrophysiological studies. *Developmental Neuropsychology, 27*(3), 403–424.

de Almeida, L. S. P., Jansen, K., Köhler, C. A., Pinheiro, R. T., da Silva, R. A., & Bonini, J. S. (2012). Working and short-term memories are impaired in postpartum depression. *Journal of Affective Disorders, 136*(3), 1238–1242.

de Almeida, S. M. (2013). Cognitive impairment and major depressive disorder in HIV infection and cerebrospinal fluid biomarkers. *Arquivos de Neuro-Psiquiatria, 71*(9-B), 689–692.

De Brito, S. A., Viding, E., Kumari, V., Blackwood, N., & Hodgins, S. (2013). Cool and hot executive function impairments in violent offenders with antisocial personality disorder with and without psychopathy. *PLoS ONE, 8*(6).

De Bruin, W. B., Del Missier, F., & Levin, I. P. (2012). Individual differences in decision-making competence. *Journal of Behavioral Decision Making, 25*(4), 329–330.

De Deyn, P. P., Engelborghs, S., Saerens, J., Goeman, J., Mariën, P., Maertens, K., . . . Pickut, B. A. (2005). The Middelheim Frontality Score: A behavioural assessment scale that discriminates frontotemporal dementia from Alzheimer's disease. *International Journal of Geriatric Psychiatry, 20*(1), 70–79.

De Fruyt, F., De Bolle, M., McCrae, R. R., Terracciano, A., & Costa, P. T., Jr. (2009). Assessing the universal structure of personality in early adolescence: The NEO-PI-R and NEO-PI-3 in 24 cultures. *Assessment, 16*(3), 301–311.

de Gelder, B., Vroomen, J., Pourtois, G., & Weiskrantz, L. (1999). Non-conscious recognition of affect in the absence of striate cortex. *Neuroreport: For Rapid Communication of Neuroscience Research, 10*(18), 3759–3763.

de Gelder, B., Vroomen, J., Pourtois, G., & Weiskrantz, L. (2000). Affective blindsight: Are we blindly led by emotions? Response to Heywood and Kentridge (2000). *Trends in Cognitive Sciences, 4*(4), 126–127.

Del Bigio, M. R. (2010). Neuropathology and structural changes in hydrocephalus. *Developmental Disabilities Research Reviews, 16*(1), 16–22.

Del Missier, F., Mäntylä, T., & De Bruin, W. B. (2012). Decision-making competence, executive functioning, and general cognitive abilities. *Journal of Behavioral Decision Making, 25*(4), 331–351.

Delis, D. C., Kaplan, E., & Kramer, J. (2001). *Delis-Kaplan Executive Function System: Examiner's manual.* San Antonio, TX: Psychological Corporation.

Delis, D. C., Jacobson, M., Bondi, M. W., Hamilton, J. M., & Salmon, D. P. (2003). The myth of testing construct validity using factor analysis or correlations with normal or mixed clinical populations: Lessons from memory assessment. *Journal of the International Neuropsychological Society, 9*(6), 936–946.

DeLuca, J., & Diamond, B. J. (1995). Aneurysm of the anterior communicating artery: A review of neuroanatomical and neuropsychological sequelae. *Journal of Clinical and Experimental Neuropsychology, 17*(1), 100–121. doi: 10.1080/13803399508406586

de Oliveira Gomes, E. R., Leite, D. S., Garcia, D. F., Maranhão, S., & Hazin, I. (2012). Neuropsychological profile of patients with acute lymphoblastic leukemia. *Psychology and Neuroscience, 5*(2), 175–182.

de Ruiter, M. B., Reneman, L., Boogerd, W., Veltman, D. J., Van Dam, F. S. A. M., Nederveen, A. J., . . . Schagen, S. B. (2011). Cerebral hyporesponsiveness and cognitive impairment 10 years after chemotherapy for breast cancer. *Human Brain Mapping, 32*(8), 1206–1219.

De Silva, K. R. D., Silva, R., Amaratunga, D., Gunasekera, W. S. L., & Jayesekera, R. W. (2011). Types of the cerebral arterial circle (circle of Willis) in a Sri Lankan Population. *BMC Neurology, 11*(5).

Desmond, J. E. (2001). Cerebellar involvement in cognitive function: Evidence from neuroimaging. *International Review of Psychiatry, 13*(4), 283–294.

Desmurget, M. (2013). Searching for the neural correlates of conscious intention. *Journal of Cognitive Neuroscience, 25*(6), 830–833.

DeYoung, C. G. (2015). Openness/intellect: A dimension of personality reflecting cognitive exploration. In M. Mikulincer, P. R. Shaver, M. L. Cooper, & R. J. Larsen (Eds.), *APA handbook of personality and social psychology: Vol. 4. Personality processes and individual differences* (pp. 369–399). Washington, DC: American Psychological Association.

Dibben, C. R. M., Rice, C., Laws, K., & McKenna, P. J. (2009). Is executive impairment associated with schizophrenic syndromes? A meta-analysis. *Psychological Medicine, 39*(3), 381–392.

Dickerson, B. C., Sperling, R. A., Hyman, B. T., Albert, M. S., & Blacker, D. (2007). Clinical prediction of Alzheimer disease dementia across the spectrum of mild cognitive impairment. *Archives of General Psychiatry, 64*(12), 1443–1450.

Diehl-Schmid, J., Perneczky, R., Koch, J., Nedopil, N., & Kurz, A. (2013). Guilty by suspicion? Criminal behavior in frontotemporal lobar degeneration. *Cognitive and Behavioral Neurology, 26*(2), 73–77.

Dietrich, S., Hertrich, I., Alter, K., Ischebeck, A., & Ackermann, H. (2008). Understanding the emotional expression of verbal interjections: A functional MRI study. *Neuroreport: For Rapid Communication of Neuroscience Research, 19*(18), 1751–1755.

DiGirolamo, G. J., Kramer, A. F., Barad, V., Cepeda, N. J., Weissman, D. H., Milham, M. P., . . . McAuley, E. (2001). General and task-specific frontal lobe recruitment in older adults during executive processes: A fMRI investigation of task-switching. *NeuroReport: For Rapid Communication of Neuroscience Research, 12*(9), 2065–2071.

Dillon, D. G., Holmes, A. J., Jahn, A. L., Bogdan, R., Wald, L. L., & Pizzagalli, D. A. (2008). Dissociation of neural regions associated with anticipatory versus consummatory phases of incentive processing. *Psychophysiology, 45*(1), 36–49.

Dirnberger, G., & Jahanshahi, M. (2013). Executive dysfunction in Parkinson's disease: A review. *Journal of Neuropsychology, 7*(2), 193–224.

Dittrich, W. H., & Johansen, T. (2013). Cognitive deficits of executive functions and decision-<?font ?>making in obsessive<?font aid:cstyle="crs_ITC Berkeley Oldstyle Std"?>-compulsive disorder. *Scandinavian Journal of Psychology, 54*(5), 393–400.

Dlugos, D., Shinnar, S., Cnaan, A., Hu, F., Moshé, S., Mizrahi, E., . . . Glauser, T. (2013). Pretreatment EEG in childhood absence epilepsy: Associations with attention and treatment outcome. *Neurology, 81*(2), 150–156.

Dolan, M., & Fullam, R. (2006). Face affect recognition deficits in personality-disordered offenders: Association with psychopathy. *Psychological Medicine, 36*(11), 1563–1569.

Donohoe, G., Corvin, A., & Robertson, I. H. (2006). Evidence that specific executive functions predict symptom variance among schizophrenia patients with a predominantly negative symptom profile. *Cognitive Neuropsychiatry, 11*(1), 13–32.

Donohoe, G., & Robertson, I. H. (2003). Can specific deficits in executive functioning explain the negative symptoms of schizophrenia? A review. *Neurocase, 9*(2), 97–108.

Donovan, N. J., Heaton, S. C., Kimberg, C. I., Wen, P.-S., Waid-Ebbs, J. K., Coster, W., . . . Velozo, C. A. (2011). Conceptualizing functional cognition in traumatic brain injury rehabilitation. *Brain Injury*, 25(4), 348–364.

Dorbath, L., Hasselhorn, M., & Titz, C. (2013). Effects of education on executive functioning and its trainability. *Educational Gerontology*, 39(5), 314–325. doi: 10.1080/03601277.2012.700820

Dosenbach, N. U. F., Fair, D. A., Miezin, F. M., Cohen, A. L., Wenger, K. K., Dosenbach, R. A. T., . . . Petersen, S. E. (2007). Distinct brain networks for adaptive and stable task control in humans. *Proceedings of the National Academy of Sciences of the United States of America*, 104(26), 11073–11078.

Dougherty, D. M., Mathias, C. W., Marsh, D. M., Moeller, F. G., & Swann, A. C. (2004). Suicidal behaviors and drug abuse: Impulsivity and its assessment. *Drug and Alcohol Dependence*, 76(Suppl. 7), S93–S105.

Dovis, S., Van der Oord, S., Wiers, R. W., & Prins, P. J. M. (2013). What part of working memory is not working in ADHD? Short-term memory, the central executive and effects of reinforcement. *Journal of Abnormal Child Psychology*, 41(6), 901–917.

Downey, J. (1923). *The Will-Temperament and its testing*. New York: World Book.

Duda, B., Puente, A. N., & Miller, L. S. (2014). Cognitive reserve moderates relation between global cognition and functional status in older adults. *Journal of Clinical and Experimental Neuropsychology*, 36(4), 368–378. doi: 10.1080/13803395.2014.892916

Duffy, J. D., Campbell, J. J., III, Salloway, S. P., & Malloy, P. F. (2001). Regional prefrontal syndromes: A theoretical and clinical overview. In S. P. Salloway, P. F. Malloy, & J. D. Duffy (Eds.), *The frontal lobes and neuropsychiatric illness* (pp. 113–123). Arlington, VA: American Psychiatric Publishing.

Dujardin, K., Blairy, S., Defebvre, L., Duhem, S., Noël, Y., Hess, U., & Desteé, A. (2004). Deficits in decoding emotional facial expressions in Parkinson's disease. *Neuropsychologia*, 42(2), 239–250.

Dujardin, K., Tard, C., Duhamel, A., Delval, A., Moreau, C., Devos, D., & Defebvre, L. (2013). The pattern of attentional deficits in Parkinson's disease. *Parkinsonism and Related Disorders*, 19(3), 300–305.

Dulay, M. F., Busch, R. M., Chapin, J. S., Jehi, L., & Najm, I. (2013). Executive functioning and depressed mood before and after unilateral frontal lobe resection for intractable epilepsy. *Neuropsychologia*, 51(7), 1370–1376.

Dumas, J. A., Makarewicz, J., Schaubhut, G. J., Devins, R., Albert, K., Dittus, K., & Newhouse, P. A. (2013). Chemotherapy altered brain functional connectivity in women with breast cancer: A pilot study. *Brain Imaging and Behavior, 7*(4), 524–532.

Dunbar, R. I. M. (1998). The social brain hypothesis. *Evolutionary Anthropology, 6*(5), 178–190.

Dyer, K. F. W., Bell, R., McCann, J., & Rauch, R. (2006). Aggression after traumatic brain injury: Analysing socially desirable responses and the nature of aggressive traits. *Brain Injury, 20*(11), 1163–1173.

Dyrud, J. E., & Donnelly, C. (1969). Executive functions of the ego: Clinical and procedural relevance. *Archives of General Psychiatry, 20*(3), 257–261.

Dziobek, I., Rogers, K., Fleck, S., Bahnemann, M., Heekeren, H. R., Wolf, O. T., & Convit, A. (2008). Dissociation of cognitive and emotional empathy in adults with Asperger syndrome using the Multifaceted Empathy Test (MET). *Journal of Autism and Developmental Disorders, 38*(3), 464–473.

Eastvold, A., Suchy, Y., & Strassberg, D. (2011). Executive function profiles of pedophilic and nonpedophilic child molesters. *Journal of the International Neuropsychological Society, 17*(2), 295–307.

Edin, F., Klingberg, T., Johansson, P., McNab, F., Tegner, J., & Compte, A. (2009). Mechanism for top-down control of working memory capacity. *Proceedings of the National Academy of Sciences of the United States of America, 106*(16), 6802–6807.

Egeland, J. (2007). Differentiating attention deficit in adult ADHD and schizophrenia. *Archives of Clinical Neuropsychology, 22*(6), 763–771.

Egeland, J., Lund, A., Landrø, N. I., Rund, B. R., Sundet, K., Asbjørnsen, A., . . . Stordal, K. I. (2005). Cortisol level predicts executive and memory function in depression, symptom level predicts psychomotor speed. *Acta Psychiatrica Scandinavica, 112*(6), 434–441.

Eichele, H., Eichele, T., Hammar, A., Freyberger, H. J., Hugdahl, K., & Plessen, K. J. (2010). Go/nogo performance in boys with Tourette syndrome. *Neuropsychology, 16*(2), 162–168.

Ekman, U., Eriksson, J., Forsgren, L., Mo, S. J., Riklund, K., & Nyberg, L. (2012). Functional brain activity and presynaptic dopamine uptake in patients with Parkinson's disease and mild cognitive impairment: A cross-sectional study. *Lancet Neurology, 11*(8), 679–687.

El-Ad, B., & Lavie, P. (2005). Effect of sleep apnea on cognition and mood. *International Review of Psychiatry, 17*(4), 277–282.

Elamin, M., Bede, P., Byrne, S., Jordan, N., Gallagher, L., Wynne, B., . . . Hardiman, O. (2013). Cognitive changes predict functional decline in ALS: A population-based longitudinal study. *Neurology, 80*(17), 1590–1597.

Elamin, M., Phukan, J., Bede, P., Jordan, N., Byrne, S., Pender, N., & Hardiman, O. (2011). Executive dysfunction is a negative prognostic indicator in patients with ALS without dementia. *Neurology, 76*(14), 1263–1269.

Endrass, T., Koehne, S., Riesel, A., & Kathmann, N. (2013). Neural correlates of feedback processing in obsessive-compulsive disorder. *Journal of Abnormal Psychology, 122*(2), 387–396.

Endrass, T., Schuermann, B., Kaufmann, C., Spielberg, R., Kniesche, R., & Kathmann, N. (2010). Performance monitoring and error significance in patients with obsessive-compulsive disorder. *Biological Psychology, 84*(2), 257–263.

Eslinger, P. J., & Damasio, A. R. (1985). Severe disturbance of higher cognition after bilateral frontal lobe ablation: Patient EVR. *Neurology, 35*(12), 1731–1741.

Euler, M., Niermeyer, M., & Suchy, Y. (2015). Neurocognitive and neurophysiological correlates of motor planning during familiar and novel contexts. *Neuropsychology*, doi.org/10.1037/neu0000219.

Faerden, A., Vaskinn, A., Finset, A., Agartz, I., Barrett, E. A., Friis, S., . . . Melle, I. (2009). Apathy is associated with executive functioning in first episode psychosis. *BMC Psychiatry, 9*(1), doi: 10.1186/1471-244X-9-1.

Fahie, C. M., & Symons, D. K. (2003). Executive functioning and theory of mind in children clinically referred for attention and behavior problems. *Journal of Applied Developmental Psychology, 24*(1), 51–73.

Farsides, T., & Woodfield, R. (2003). Individual differences and undergraduate academic success: The roles of personality, intelligence, and application. *Personality and Individual Differences, 34*(7), 1225–1243.

Fassbender, C., Foxe, J. J., & Garavan, H. (2006). Mapping the functional anatomy of task preparation: Priming task-appropriate brain networks. *Human Brain Mapping, 27*(10), 819–827.

Fassbender, C., Murphy, K., Foxe, J. J., Wylie, G. R., Javitt, D. C., Robertson, I. H., & Garavan, H. (2004). A topography of executive functions and their interactions revealed by functional magnetic resonance imaging. *Cognitive Brain Research, 20*(2), 132–143.

Faure, A., Reynolds, S. M., Richard, J. M., & Berridge, K. C. (2008). Mesolimbic dopamine in desire and dread: Enabling motivation to be generated by localized glutamate disruptions in nucleus accumbens. *Journal of Neuroscience, 28*(28), 7184–7192.

Fay, T. B., Yeates, K. O., Taylor, H. G., Bangert, B., Dietrich, A., Nuss, K., . . . Wright, M. (2010). Cognitive reserve as a moderator of postconcussive symptoms in children with complicated and uncomplicated mild traumatic brain injury. *Journal of the International Neuropsychological Society, 16*(1), 94–105. doi: 10.1017/s1355617709991007

Feinstein, A. (2006). Mood disorders in multiple sclerosis and the effects on cognition. *Journal of the Neurological Sciences, 245*(1–2), 63–66.

Feinstein, A. (2012). Multiple sclerosis and cognitive dysfunction: How accurate are patients' self-assessments? *European Journal of Neurology, 19*(4), 535–536.

Fellows, L. K., & Farah, M. J. (2003). Ventromedial frontal cortex mediates affective shifting in humans: Evidence from a reversal learning paradigm. *Brain: A Journal of Neurology, 126*(8), 1830–1837. doi: 10.1093/brain/awg180

Fellows, L. K., & Farah, M. J. (2005). Different underlying impairments in decision-making following ventromedial and dorsolateral frontal lobe damage in humans. *Cerebral Cortex, 15*(1), 58–63.

Fennell, E. B., & Dikel, T. N. (2001). Cognitive and neuropsychological functioning in children with cerebral palsy. *Journal of Child Neurology, 16*(1), 58–63.

Ferini-Strambi, L., Marelli, S., Galbiati, A., & Castronovo, C. (2013). Effects of continuous positive airway pressure on cognitition and neuroimaging data in sleep apnea. *International Journal of Psychophysiology, 89*(2), 203–212.

Fernandez-Duque, D., & Black, S. E. (2005). Impaired recognition of negative facial emotions in patients with frontotemporal dementia. *Neuropsychologia, 43*(11), 1673–1687.

Ferreira, M. L. B. (2010). Cognitive deficits in muliple sclerosis: A systematic review. *Arquivos de Neuro-Psiquiatria, 68*(4), 632–641.

Fervaha, G., Agid, O., Foussias, G., & Remington, G. (2014). Effect of intrinsic motivation on cognitive performance in schizophrenia: A pilot study. *Schizophrenia Research, 152*(1), 317–318.

Fervaha, G., Graff-Guerrero, A., Zakzanis, K. K., Foussias, G., Agid, O., & Remington, G. (2013). Incentive motivation deficits in schizophrenia reflect effort computation impairments during cost-benefit decision-making. *Journal of Psychiatric Research, 47*(11), 1590–1596.

Feusner, J. D., Hembacher, E., & Phillips, K. A. (2009). The mouse who couldn't stop washing: Pathologic grooming in animals and humans. *CNS Spectrums, 14*(9), 503–513.

Fischman, M. W., & Foltin, R. W. (1992). Self-administration of cocaine by humans: A laboratory perspective. In CIBA Foundation Symposium (Author), *Cocaine: Scientific and social dimensions* (pp. 165–173). Oxford, England. Wiley.

Flaks, M. K., Malta, S. M., Almeida, P. P., Bueno, O. F. A., Pupo, M. C., Andreoli, S. B., . . . Bressan, R. A. (2014). Attentional and executive functions are differentially affected by post-traumatic stress disorder and trauma. *Journal of Psychiatric Research*, 48(1), 32–39.

Fling, B. W., Cohen, R. G., Mancini, M., Nutt, J. G., Fair, D. A., & Horak, F. B. (2013). Asymmetric pedunculopontine network connectivity in parkinsonian patients with freezing of gait. *Brain: A Journal of Neurology*, 136(8), 2405–2418. doi: 10.1093/brain/awt172

Foisy, M.-L., Philippot, P., Verbanck, P., Pelc, I., Van Der Straten, G., & Kornreich, C. (2005). Emotional facial expression decoding impairment in persons dependent on multiple substances: Impact of a history of alcohol dependence. *Journal of Studies on Alcohol*, 66(5), 673–681.

Foltynie, T., Brayne, C. E. G., Robbins, T. W., & Barker, R. A. (2004). The cognitive ability of an incident cohort of Parkinson's patients in the UK: The CamPaIGN study. *Brain: A Journal of Neurology*, 127(3), 550–560.

Fossella, J. A., Sommer, T., Fan, J., Pfaff, D., & Posner, M. I. (2003). Synaptogenesis and heritable aspects of executive attention. *Mental Retardation and Developmental Disabilities Research Reviews*, 9(3), 178–183.

Franchow, E. I., & Suchy, Y. (2015). Naturally-occurring expressive suppression in daily life depletes executive functioning. *Emotion*, 15(1), 78–89.

Franchow, E. I., Suchy, Y., Thorgusen, S. R., & Williams, P. G. (2013). More than education: Openness to experience contributes to cognitive reserve in older adulthood. *Journal of Aging Science*, 1(109). doi: 10.4172/2329-8847.1000109

Fredrikson, M., Furmark, T., Olsson, M. T., Fischer, H., Andersson, J., & Långström, B. (1998). Functional neuroanatomical correlates of electrodermal activity: A positron emission tomographic study. *Psychophysiology*, 35(2), 179–185.

Freeman, R. D., Fast, D. K., Burd, L., Kerbeshian, J., Robertson, M. M., & Sandor, P. (2007). An international perspective on Tourette syndrome: Selected findings from 3500 individuals in 22 countries. *Developmental Medicine and Child Neurology*, 42(7), 436–447.

Friedman, N. P., Miyake, A., Corley, R. P., Young, S. E., DeFries, J. C., & Hewitt, J. K. (2006). Not all executive functions are related to intelligence. *Psychological Science*, 17(2), 172–179.

Frisch, S., Förstl, S., Legler, A., Schöpe, S., & Goebel, H. (2012). The interleaving of actions in everyday life multitasking demands. *Journal of Neuropsychology*, 6(2), 257–269.

Fuchs, R. A., Ramirez, D. R., & Bell, G. H. (2008). Nucleus accumbens shell and core involvement in drug context–induced reinstatement of cocaine seeking in rats. *Psychopharmacology, 200*(4), 545–556.

Gaesser, B., Spreng, R. N., McLelland, V. C., Addis, D. R., & Schacter, D. L. (2013). Imagining the future: Evidence for a hippocampal contribution to constructive processing. *Hippocampus, 23*(12), 1150–1161.

Gailliot, M. T., & Baumeister, R. F. (2007). Self-regulation and sexual restraint: Dispositionally and temporarily poor self-regulatory abilities contribute to failures at restraining sexual behavior. *Personality and Social Psychology Bulletin, 33*(2), 173–186. doi: 10.1177/0146167206293472

Gailliot, M. T., Baumeister, R. F., DeWall, C. N., Maner, J. K., Plant, E. A., Tice, D. M., . . . Schmeichel, B. J. (2007). Self-control relies on glucose as a limited energy source: Willpower is more than a metaphor. *Journal of Personality and Social Psychology, 92*(2), 325–336.

Gale, S. D., & Hopkins, R. O. (2004). Effects of hypoxia on the brain: Neuroimaging and neuropsychological findings following carbon monoxide poisoning and obstructive sleep apnea. *Journal of the International Neuropsychological Society, 10*(1), 60–71.

Gale, S. D., Hopkins, R. O., Weaver, L. K., Bigler, E. D., Booth, E. J., & Blatter, D. D. (1999). MRI, quantitative MRI, SPECT and neuropsychological findings following carbon monoxide poisoning. *Brain Injury, 13*(4), 229–243.

Gallagher, C., Bell, B., Bendlin, B., Palotti, M., Okonkwo, O., Sodhi, A., . . . Alexander, A. (2013). White matter microstructural integrity and executive function in Parkinson's disease. *Journal of the International Neuropsychological Society, 19*(3), 349–354.

Gamaldo, A. A., An, Y., Allaire, J. C., Kitner-Triolo, M. H., & Zonderman, A. B. (2012). Variability in performance: Identifying early signs of future cognitive impairment. *Neuropsychology, 26*(4), 534–540.

Gamaldo, C. E., Gamaldo, A., Creighton, J., Salas, R. E., Selnes, O. A., David, P. M., . . . Smith, M. T. (2013). Evaluating sleep and cognition in HIV. *Journal of Acquired Immune Deficiency Syndromes, 63*(5), 609–616.

García, M. C., Plasencia, P. M., Benito, Y. A., Gómez, J. J. B., & Marcos, A. R. (2009). Executive function and memory in patients with relapsing-remitting multiple sclerosis. *Psicothema, 21*(3), 416–420.

Garcia-Sanchez, C., Estevez-Gonzalez, A., Suarez-Romero, E., & Junque, C. (1997). Right hemisphere dysfunction in subjects with attention-deficit disorder with and without hyperactivity. *Journal of Child Neurology, 12*(2), 107–115.

Gardner, E., Vik, P., & Dasher, N. (2013). Strategy use on the Ruff Figural Fluency Test. *Clinical Neuropsychologist, 27*(3), 470–484. doi: 10.1080/13854046.2013.771216

Garner, C., Callias, M., & Turk, J. (1999). Executive function and theory of mind performance of boys with fragile-X syndrome. *Journal of Intellectual Disability Research, 43*(6), 466–474. doi: 10.1046/j.1365-2788.1999.00207.x

Garon, N., Bryson, S. E., & Smith, I. M. (2008). Executive function in preschoolers: A review using an integrative framework. *Psychological Bulletin, 134*(1), 31–60.

Gazzaley, A., D'Esposito, M., Miller, B. L., & Cummings, J. L. (2007). Unifying prefrontal cortex function: Executive control, neural networks, and top-down modulation. In B. L. Miller & J. C. Cummings (Eds.), *The human frontal lobes: Functions and disorders* (2nd ed., pp. 187–206). New York, NY: Guilford Press.

Geburek, A. J., Rist, F., Gediga, G., Stroux, D., & Pedersen, A. (2013). Electrophysiological indices of error monitoring in juvenile and adult attention deficit hyperactivity disorder (ADHD)—A meta-analytic appraisal. *International Journal of Psychophysiology, 87*(3), 349–362.

Gendolla, G. H. E. (2012). Implicit affect primes effort: A theory and research on cardiovascular response. *International Journal of Psychophysiology, 86*(2), 123–135.

Gennarelli, T. A., & Graham, D. I. (2005). Neuropathology. In J. M. Silver, T. W. McAllister, & S. C. Yudofsky (Eds.), *Textbook of traumatic brain injury* (pp. 27–50). Arlington, VA: American Psychiatric Publishing.

Genovese, J. E. C., & Wallace, D. (2007). Reward sensitivity and substance abuse in middle school and high school students. *Journal of Genetic Psychology, 168*(4), 465–469.

George, M. S., Kellner, C. H., Bernstein, H., & Goust, J. M. (1994). A magnetic resonance imaging investigation into mood disorders in multiple sclerosis: A pilot study. *Journal of Nervous and Mental Disease, 182*(7), 410–412.

Gerlach, K. D., Spreng, R. N., Gilmore, A. W., & Schacter, D. L. (2011). Solving future problems: Default network and executive activity associated with goal-directed mental simulations. *NeuroImage, 55*(4), 1816–1824.

Gerretsen, P., Plitman, E., Rajji, T. K., & Graff-Guerrero, A. (2014). The effects of aging on insight into illness in schizophrenia: A review. *International Journal of Geriatric Psychiatry, 29*(11), 1145–1161. doi: 10.1002/gps.4154

Gerstenecker, A., Mast, B., Duff, K., Ferman, T. J., & Litvan, I. (2013). Executive dysfunction is the primary cognitive impairment in progressive supranuclear palsy. *Archives of Clinical Neuropsychology, 28*(2), 104–113.

Geuze, E., Vermetten, E., & Bremner, J. D. (2005). MR-based in vivo hippocampal volumetrics: 2. Findings in neuropsychiatric disorders. *Molecular Psychiatry, 10*(2), 160–184.

Ghosh, B. C. P., Rowe, J. B., Calder, A. J., Hodges, J. R., & Bak, T. H. (2009). Emotion recognition in progressive supranuclear palsy. *Journal of Neurology, Neurosurgery and Psychiatry, 80*(10), 1143–1145.

Gidley Larson, J. C., & Suchy, Y. (2014). Does language guide behavior in children with autism? *Journal of Autism and Developmental Disorders, 44*(9), 2147–2161.

Gilotty, L., Kenworthy, L., Sirian, L., Black, D. O., & Wagner, A. E. (2002). Adaptive skills and executive function in autism spectrum disorders. *Child Neuropsychology, 8*(4), 241–248. doi: 10.1076/chin.8.4.241.13504

Ginot, E. (2009). The empathic power of enactments: The link between neuropsychological processes and an expanded definition of empathy. *Psychoanalytic Psychology, 26*(3), 290–309.

Ginsberg, Y., Hirvikoski, T., & Lindefors, N. (2010). Attention deficit hyperactivity disorder (ADHD) among longer-term prison inmates is a prevalent, persistent and disabling disorder. *BMC Psychiatry, 10*(112), doi: 10.1186/1471-244X-10-112.

Giordano, A., Tessitore, A., Corbo, D., Cirillo, G., de Micco, R., Russo, A., . . . Tedeschi, G. (2013). Clinical and cognitive correlates of regional gray matter atrophy in progressive supranuclear palsy. *Parkinsonism and Related Disorders, 19*(6), 590–594.

Giovagnoli, A. R., Erbetta, A., Reati, F., & Bugiani, O. (2008). Differential neuropsychological patterns of frontal variant frontotemporal dementia and Alzheimer's disease in a study of diagnostic concordance. *Neuropsychologia, 46*(5), 1495–1504.

Giovanelli, A., Hoerger, M., Johnson, S. L., & Gruber, J. (2013). Impulsive responses to positive mood and reward are related to mania risk. *Cognition and Emotion, 27*(6), 1091–1104.

Gladsjo, J. A., Schuman, C. C., Evans, J. D., Peavy, G. M., Miller, S. W., & Heaton, R. K. (1999). Norms for letter and category fluency: Demographic corrections for age, education, and ethnicity. *Assessment, 6*(2), 147–178. doi: 10.1177/107319119900600204

Glasier, P. C. (2008). The clinical and ecological utility of executive function assessment in children with attention-deficit/hyperactivity disorder or Asperger's syndrome. 68, ProQuest Information & Learning, US. Retrieved from http://search.ebscohost.com/login.aspx?direct=true&db=psyh&AN=2008-99020-258&site=ehost-live Available from EBSCOhost psyh database.

Glass, J. M., Williams, D. A., Fernandez-Sanchez, M.-L., Kairys, A., Barjola, P., Heitzeg, M. M., . . . Schmidt-Wilcke, T. (2011). Executive function in chronic pain patients and healthy controls: Different cortical activation during response inhibition in fibromyalgia. *Journal of Pain, 12*(12), 1219–1229.

Gligorović, M., & Đurović, N. B. (2014). Inhibitory control and adaptive behaviour in children with mild intellectual disability. *Journal of Intellectual Disability Research, 58*(3), 233–242. doi: 10.1111/jir.12000

Gloor, P., & Aggleton, J. P. (1992). Role of the amygdala in temporal lobe epilepsy. In J. P. Aggleton (Ed.), *The amygdala: Neurobiological aspects of emotion, memory, and mental dysfunction* (pp. 505–538). New York, NY: Wiley-Liss.

Gold, B. T., Powell, D. K., Xuan, L., Jicha, G. A., & Smith, C. D. (2010). Age-related slowing of task switching is associated with decreased integrity of frontoparietal white matter. *Neurobiology of Aging, 31*(3), 512–522.

Goldberg, E. (1986). Varieties of perseveration: A comparison of two taxonomies. *Journal of Clinical and Experimental Neuropsychology, 8*(6), 710–726.

Goldberg, E., Bilder, R. M., Hughes, J. E., & Antin, S. P. (1989). A reticulo-frontal disconnection syndrome. *Cortex: A Journal Devoted to the Study of the Nervous System and Behavior, 25*(4), 687–695.

Goldin, P. R., McRae, K., Ramel, W., & Gross, J. J. (2008). The neural bases of emotion regulation: Reappraisal and suppression of negative emotion. *Biological Psychiatry, 63*(6), 577–586.

Goldman-Rakic, P. S., Leung, H.-C., Stuss, D. T., & Knight, R. T. (2002). Functional architecture of the dorsolateral prefrontal cortex in monkeys and humans. In D. T. Stuss & R. T. Knight (Eds.), *Principles of frontal lobe function* (pp. 85–95). New York, NY: Oxford University Press.

Goldstein, L. H., & Abrahams, S. (2013). Changes in cognition and behaviour in amyotrophic lateral sclerosis: Nature of impairment and implications for assessment. *Lancet Neurology, 12*(4), 368–380.

Goldstein, L. H., Bernard, S., Fenwick, P. B., & Burgess, P. W. (1993). Unilateral frontal lobectomy can produce strategy application disorder. *Journal of Neurology, Neurosurgery and Psychiatry, 56*(3), 274–276. doi: 10.1136/jnnp.56.3.274

Gould, S. L., & Hyer, L. A. (2004). Dementia and behavioral disturbance: Does premorbid personality really matter? *Psychological Reports, 95*(3, Pt. 2), 1072–1078.

Grabenhorst, F., Rolls, E. T., Margot, C., da Silva, M. A. A. P., & Velazco, M. I. (2007). How pleasant and unpleasant stimuli combine in different brain regions: Odor mixtures. *Journal of Neuroscience, 27*(49), 13532–13540.

Grafman, J. (1988). Interesting data in search of a theory. *PsycCRITIQUES*, *33*(11), 956–957.

Graham, N. L., Bak, T., Patterson, K., & Hodges, J. R. (2003). Language function and dysfunction in corticobasal degeneration. *Neurology*, *61*(4), 493–499.

Graham, S., Jiang, J., Manning, V., Nejad, A. B., Zhisheng, K., Salleh, S. R., . . . McKenna, P. J. (2010). IQ-related fMRI differences during cognitive set shifting. *Cerebral Cortex*, *20*(3), 641–649. doi: 10.1093/cercor/bhp130

Grant, C. M., Apperly, I., & Oliver, C. (2007). Is theory of mind understanding impaired in males with fragile X syndrome? *Journal of Abnormal Child Psychology*, *35*(1), 17–28. doi: 10.1007/s10802-006-9077-0

Green, C. R., Mihic, A. M., Nikkel, S. M., Stade, B. C., Rasmussen, C., Munoz, D. P., & Reynolds, J. N. (2009). Executive function deficits in children with fetal alcohol spectrum disorders (FASD) measured using the Cambridge Neuropsychological Tests Automated Battery (CANTAB). *Journal of Child Psychology and Psychiatry*, *50*(6), 688–697.

Greer, J., Riby, D. M., Hamiliton, C., & Riby, L. M. (2013). Attentional lapse and inhibition control in adults with Williams syndrome. *Research in Developmental Disabilities*, *34*(11), 4170–4177. doi: 10.1016/j.ridd.2013.08.041

Grigsby, J., Brega, A. G., Engle, K., Leehey, M. A., Hagerman, R. J., Tassone, F., . . . Reynolds, A. (2008). Cognitive profile of fragile X premutation carriers with and without fragile X–associated tremor/ataxia syndrome. *Neuropsychology*, *22*(1), 48–60.

Grigsby, J., Brega, A. G., Jacquemont, S., Loesch, D. Z., Leehey, M. A., Goodrich, G. K., . . . Hagerman, P. J. (2006). Impairment in the cognitive functioning of men with fragile X–associated tremor/ataxia syndrome (FXTAS). *Journal of the Neurological Sciences*, *248*(1–2), 227–233.

Grigsby, J., Kaye, K., Baxter, J., Shetterly, S. M., & Hamman, R. F. (1998). Executive cognitive abilities and functional status among community-dwelling older persons in the San Luis Valley Health and Aging Study. *Journal of the American Geriatrics Society*, *46*(5), 590–596.

Grootens, K. P., Vermeeren, L., Verkes, R. J., Buitelaar, J. K., Sabbe, B. G. C., Van Veelen, N., . . . Hulstijn, W. (2009). Psychomotor planning is deficient in recent-onset schizophrenia. *Schizophrenia Research*, *107*(2–3), 294–302.

Gross, R. G., McMillan, C. T., Chandrasekaran, K., Dreyfuss, M., Ash, S., Avants, B., . . . Grossman, M. (2012). Sentence processing in Lewy body spectrum disorder: The role of working memory. *Brain and Cognition*, *78*(2), 85–93.

Grossberg, S., Bullock, D., & Dranias, M. R. (2008). Neural dynamics underlying impaired autonomic and conditioned responses following amygdala and orbitofrontal lesions. *Behavioral Neuroscience, 122*(5), 1100–1125.

Gschwandtner, U., Aston, J., Renaud, S., & Fuhr, P. (2001). Pathological gambling in patients with Parkinson's disease. *Clinical Neuropharmacology, 24*(3), 170–172.

Gu, B.-M., Park, J.-Y., Kang, D.-H., Lee, S. J., Yoo, S., Jo, H. J., . . . Kwon, J. S. (2008). Neural correlates of cognitive inflexibility during task-switching in obsessive-compulsive disorder. *Brain: A Journal of Neurology, 131*(1), 155–164.

Guilbaud, O., Loas, G., Corcos, M., Speranza, M., Stephan, P., Perez-Diaz, F., . . . Jeammet, P. (2002). L'alexithymie dans les conduites de dépendance et chez le sujet sain: valeur en populatino française et francophone. *Annales Médico-Psychologiques, 160*(1), 77–85.

Guilford, J. P. (1972). Executive functions and a model of behavior. *Journal of General Psychology, 86*(2), 279–287.

Guoping, S., Kan, Z., Danmin, M., & Fuen, H. (2008). Effects of sleep deprivation on executive function. *Psychological Science (China), 31*(1), 32–34.

Gut-Fayand, A., Dervaux, A., Olié, J.-P., Lôo, H., Poirier, M.-F., & Krebs, M.-O. (2001). Substance abuse and suicidality in schizophrenia: A common risk factor linked to impulsivity. *Psychiatry Research, 102*(1), 65–72.

Gvion, Y., & Apter, A. (2011). Aggression, impulsivity, and suicide behavior: A review of the literature. *Archives of Suicide Research, 15*(2), 93–112.

Gvirts, H. Z., Harari, H., Braw, Y., Shefet, D., Shamay-Tsoory, S. G., & Levkovitz, Y. (2012). Executive functioning among patients with borderline personality disorder (BPD) and their relatives. *Journal of Affective Disorders, 143*(1–3), 261–264.

Haaland, K. Y., & Swanda, R. M. (2008). Vascular dementia. In J. E. Morgan & J. H. Ricker (Eds.), *Textbook of clinical neuropsychology* (pp. 384–391). New York, NY: Psychology Press.

Haaland, V. Ø., Esperaas, L., & Landrø, N. I. (2009). Selective deficit in executive functioning among patients with borderline personality disorder. *Psychological Medicine, 39*(10), 1733–1743.

Hagan, C. C., Hoeft, F., Mackey, A., Mobbs, D., & Reiss, A. L. (2008). Aberrant neural function during emotion attribution in female subjects with fragile X syndrome. *Journal of the American Academy of Child and Adolescent Psychiatry, 47*(12), 1443–1454.

Hagenhoff, M., Franzen, N., Koppe, G., Baer, N., Scheibel, N., Sammer, G., . . . Lis, S. (2013). Executive functions in borderline personality disorder. *Psychiatry Research, 210*(1), 224–231.

Hagerman, P. J., & Hagerman, R. J. (2004). Fragile X–associated tremor/ataxia syndrome (FXTAS). *Mental Retardation and Developmental Disabilities Research Reviews, 10*(1), 25–30.

Hagerman, R., Leehey, M., Heinrichs, W., Tassone, F., Wilson, R., Hills, J., . . . Hagerman, P. J. (2001). Intention tremor, parkinsonism, and generalized brain atrophy in male carriers of fragile X. *Neurology, 57*(1), 127–130.

Halstead, W. C. (1947). *Brain and intelligence: A quantitative study of the frontal lobes*. Chicago, IL: University of Chicago Press.

Halstead, W. C. (1950). Frontal lobe functions and intelligence. *Bulletin of the Los Angeles Neurological Society, 15*, 205–212.

Hammar, Å., & Årdal, G. (2009). Cognitive functioning in major depression—A summary. *Frontiers in Human Neuroscience, 3*(26), doi: 10.3389/neuro.09.026.2009.

Hampshire, A., Gruszka, A., Fallon, S. J., & Owen, A. M. (2008). Inefficiency in self-organized attentional switching in the normal aging population is associated with decreased activity in the ventrolateral prefrontal cortex. *Journal of Cognitive Neuroscience, 20*(9), 1670–1686.

Hampton, L. E., Fletcher, J. M., Cirino, P., Blaser, S., Kramer, L. A., & Dennis, M. (2013). Neuropsychological profiles of children with aqueductal stenosis and spina bifida myelomeningocele. *Journal of the International Neuropsychological Society, 19*(2), 127–136.

Hanyu, H., Sato, T., Kume, K., Takada, Y., Onuma, T., & Iwamoto, T. (2009). Differentiation of dementia with Lewy bodies from Alzheimer disease using the Frontal Assessment Battery test. *International Journal of Geriatric Psychiatry, 24*(9), 1034–1035.

Happé, F., Booth, R., Charlton, R., & Hughes, C. (2006). Executive function deficits in autism spectrum disorders and attention-deficit/hyperactivity disorder: Examining profiles across domains and ages. *Brain and Cognition, 61*(1), 25–39. doi: 10.1016/j.bandc.2006.03.004

Hardy, D. J., & Hinkin, C. H. (2002). Reaction time performance in adults with HIV/AIDS. *Journal of Clinical and Experimental Neuropsychology, 24*(7), 912–929.

Harlow, J. M. (1868). Recovery from the passage of an iron bar through the head. *Publications of the Massachusetts Medical Society, 2*, 327–347.

Harms, M. P., Wang, L., Csernansky, J. G., & Barch, D. M. (2013). Structure-function relationship of working memory activity with hippocampal and prefrontal cortex volumes. *Brain Structure and Function, 218*(1), 173–186.

Harrison, J., Rentz, D. M., McLaughlin, T., Niecko, T., Gregg, K. M., Black, R. S., . . . Grundman, M. (2014). Cognition in MCI and Alzheimer's disease: Baseline data from a longitudinal study of the NTB. *Clinical Neuropsychologist, 28*(2), 252–268. doi: 10.1080/13854046.2013.875595

Hart, R. P., & Bean, M. K. (2011). Executive function, intellectual decline and daily living skills. *Aging, Neuropsychology, and Cognition, 18*(1), 64–85. doi: 10.1080/13825585.2010.510637

Hartman, E., Houwen, S., Scherder, E., & Visscher, C. (2010). On the relationship between motor performance and executive functioning in children with intellectual disabilities. *Journal of Intellectual Disability Research, 54*(5), 468–477. doi: 10.1111/j.1365-2788.2010.01284.x

Harvey, P. O., Le Bastard, G., Pochon, J. B., Levy, R., Allilaire, J. F., Dubois, B., & Fossati, P. (2004). Executive functions and updating of the contents of working memory in unipolar depressions. *Journal of Psychiatric Research, 38*(6), 567–576.

Harvey, P. O., Pruessner, J., Czechowska, Y., & Lepage, M. (2007). Individual differences in trait anhedonia: A structural and functional magnetic resonance imaging study in non-clinical subjects. *Molecular Psychiatry, 12*(8), 767–775.

Hastings, M. E., Tangney, J. P., & Stuewig, J. (2008). Psychopathy and identification of facial expressions of emotion. *Personality and Individual Differences, 44*(7), 1474–1483.

Haug, E. T., Havnen, A., Hansen, B., Bless, J., & Kvale, G. (2013). Attention training with dichotic listening in OCD patients using an iPhone/iPod app. *Clinical Neuropsychiatry: Journal of Treatment Evaluation, 10*(3, Suppl. 1), 45–47.

Hazlett, E. A., Lamade, R. V., Graff, F. S., McClure, M. M., Kolaitis, J. C., Goldstein, K. E., . . . Moshier, E. (2014). Visual-spatial working memory performance and temporal gray matter volume predict schizotypal personality disorder group membership. *Schizophrenia Research, 152*(2–3), 350–357.

Healey, D. M., Marks, D. J., & Halperin, J. M. (2011). Examining the interplay among negative emotionality, cognitive functioning, and attention deficit/hyperactivity disorder symptom severity. *Journal of the International Neuropsychological Society, 17*(3), 502–510. doi: 10.1017/s1355617711000294

Heaton, R. K., Chelune, G. J., Talley, J. L., Kay, G. G., & Curtiss, G. (1993). *Wisconsin Card Sorting Test manual: Revised and expanded*. Psychological Assessment Resources, Inc., Odessa, FL.

Heck, E. T., & Bryer, J. B. (1986). Superior sorting and categorizing ability in a case of bilateral frontal atrophy: An exception to the rule. *Journal of Clinical and Experimental Neuropsychology, 8*(3), 313–316.

Heilbronner, R. L., Sweet, J. J., Morgan, J. E., Larrabee, G. J., & Millis, S. R. (2009). American Academy of Clinical Neuropsychology consensus conference statement on the neuropsychological assessment of effort, response bias, and malingering. *Clinical Neuropsychologist, 23*(7), 1093–1129. doi: 10.1080/13854040903155063

Heilman, K. M., Leon, S. A., & Rosenbek, J. C. (2004). Affective aprosodia from a medial frontal stroke. *Brain and Language, 89*(3), 411–416.

Heims, H. C., Critchley, H. D., Dolan, R., Mathias, C. J., & Cipolotti, L. (2004). Social and motivational functioning is not critically dependent on feedback of autonomic responses: Neuropsychological evidence from patients with pure autonomic failure. *Neuropsychologia, 42*(14), 1979–1988.

Heinrichs, R. W. (2005). The primacy of cognition in schizophrenia. *American Psychologist, 60*(3), 229–242.

Henry, J. D., Crawford, J. R., & Phillips, L. H. (2004). Verbal fluency performance in dementia of the Alzheimer's type: A meta-analysis. *Neuropsychologia, 42*(9), 1212–1222.

Henry, J. D., Phillips, L. H., Beatty, W. W., McDonald, S., Longley, W. A., Joscelyne, A., & Rendell, P. G. (2009). Evidence for deficits in facial affect recognition and theory of mind in multiple sclerosis. *Journal of the International Neuropsychological Society, 15*(2), 277–285.

Henry, J. D., Phillips, L. H., Crawford, J. R., Theodorou, G., & Summers, F. (2006). Cognitive and psychosocial correlates of alexithymia following traumatic brain injury. *Neuropsychologia, 44*(1), 62–72.

Henry, J. D., Phillips, L. H., Maylor, E. A., Hosie, J., Milne, A. B., & Meyer, C. (2006). A new conceptualization of alexithymia in the general adult population: Implications for research involving older adults. *Journal of Psychosomatic Research, 60*(5), 535–543.

Hensler, M., Wolfe, K., Lebensburger, J., Nieman, J., Barnes, M., Nolan, W., . . . Madan-Swain, A. (2014). Social skills and executive function among youth with sickle cell disease: A preliminary investigation. *Journal of Pediatric Psychology, 39*(5), 493–500.

Hermann, B. P., Dabbs, K., Becker, T., Jones, J. E., Myers y Gutierrez, A., Wendt, G., . . . Seidenberg, M. (2010). Brain development in children with new onset epilepsy: A prospective controlled cohort investigation. *Epilepsia, 51*(10), 2038–2046.

Hessl, D., Rivera, S., Koldewyn, K., Cordeiro, L., Adams, J., Tassone, F., . . . Hagerman, R. J. (2007). Amygdala dysfunction in men with the fragile X premutation. *Brain: A Journal of Neurology, 130*(2), 404–416.

Hetherington, R., Dennis, M., & Spiegler, B. (2000). Perception and estimation of time in long-term survivors of childhood posterior fossa tumors. *Journal of the International Neuropsychological Society, 6*(6), 682–692.

Heyes, C. (2011). Automatic imitation. *Psychological Bulletin, 137*(3), 463–483.

Hieger, E. D. (2006). Neuropsychological profiles of adults with Asperger's syndrome: Exploring the utility of the D-KEFS executive function system for diagnostic facilitation. 67, ProQuest Information & Learning, US. Retrieved from http://search.ebscohost.com/login.aspx?direct=true&db=psyh&AN=2006-99022-214&site=ehost-live Available from EBSCOhost psyh database.

Hill, E. L., & Bird, C. M. (2006). Executive processes in Asperger syndrome: Patterns of performance in a multiple case series. *Neuropsychologia, 44*(14), 2822–2835. doi: 10.1016/j.neuropsychologia.2006.06.007

Hills, T. T., Mata, R., Wilke, A., & Samanez-Larkin, G. R. (2013). Mechanisms of age-related decline in memory search across the adult life span. *Developmental Psychology, 49*(12), 2396–2404.

Himle, M. B., Hayes, L. P., Suchy, Y., Thorgusen, S. R., Herbert, S., Zelaya, J., . . . Chang, S. (2012, November). *The effects of tic suppression on current and subsequent cognitive functioning: Cognitive mechanisms of tic control.* Paper presented at the Association for Behavioral and Cognitive Therapies, National Harbor, MD.

Hinkelmann, K., Moritz, S., Botzenhardt, J., Riedesel, K., Wiedemann, K., Kellner, M., & Otte, C. (2009). Cognitive impairment in major depression: Association with salivary cortisol. *Biological Psychiatry, 66*(9), 879–885. doi: 10.1016/j.biopsych.2009.06.023

Hippolyte, L., Iglesias, K., Van der Linden, M., & Barisnikov, K. (2010). Social reasoning skills in adults with Down syndrome: The role of language, executive functions and socio-emotional behaviour. *Journal of Intellectual Disability Research, 54*(8), 714–726. doi: 10.1111/j.1365-2788.2010.01299.x

Hirshorn, E. A., & Thompson-Schill, S. L. (2006). Role of the left inferior frontal gyrus in covert word retrieval: Neural correlates of switching during verbal fluency. *Neuropsychologia, 44*(12), 2547–2557.

Hobson, C. W., Scott, S., & Rubia, K. (2011). Investigation of cool and hot executive function in ODD/CD independently of ADHD. *Journal of Child Psychology and Psychiatry, 52*(10), 1035–1043.

Hoelzel, B. K., Ott, U., Gard, T., Hempel, H., Weygandt, M., Morgen, K., & Vaitl, D. (2008). Investigation of mindfulness meditation practitioners with voxel-based morphometry. *Social Cognitive and Affective Neuroscience*, 3(1), 55–61.

Hoffstaedter, F., Grefkes, C., Caspers, S., Roski, C., Palomero-Gallagher, N., Laird, A. R., . . . Eickhoff, S. B. (2014). The role of anterior midcingulate cortex in cognitive motor control: Evidence from functional connectivity analyses. *Human Brain Mapping*, 35(6), 2741–2753.

Hoffstaedter, F., Sarlon, J., Grefkes, C., & Eickhoff, S. B. (2012). Internally vs. externally triggered movements in patients with major depression. *Behavioural Brain Research*, 228(1), 125–132.

Hohler, A. D., Ransom, B. R., Chun, M. R., Troster, A. I., & Samii, A. (2003). The youngest reported case of corticobasal degeneration. *Parkinsonism and Related Disorders*, 10(1), 47–50.

Holdnack, J., Goldstein, G., & Drozdick, L. (2011). Social perception and WAIS-IV performance in adolescents and adults diagnosed with Asperger's syndrome and autism. *Assessment*, 18(2), 192–200.

Holmén, A., Juuhl-Langseth, M., Thormodsen, R., Sundet, K., Melle, I., & Rund, B. R. (2012). Executive function tests in early-onset psychosis: Which one to choose? *Scandinavian Journal of Psychology*, 53(3), 200–205.

Homack, S., & Riccio, C. A. (2004). A meta-analysis of the sensitivity and specificity of the Stroop Color and Word Test with children. *Archives of Clinical Neuropsychology*, 19(6), 725–743. doi: 10.1016/j.acn.2003.09.003

Hooker, C. I., Verosky, S. C., Germine, L. T., Knight, R. T., & D'Esposito, M. (2010). Neural activity during social signal perception correlates with self-reported empathy. *Brain Research*, 1308, 100–113.

Hooper, S. R., Hatton, D., Sideris, J., Sullivan, K., Hammer, J., Schaaf, J., . . . Bailey, D. B., Jr. (2008). Executive functions in young males with fragile X syndrome in comparison to mental age–matched controls: Baseline findings from a longitudinal study. *Neuropsychology*, 22(1), 36–47. doi: 10.1037/0894-4105.22.1.36

Hopkins, R. O. (2008). Does near drowning in ice water prevent anoxic induced brain injury? *Journal of the International Neuropsychological Society*, 14(4), 656–659.

Hopkins, R. O., & Bigler, E. D. (2008). Hypoxic and anoxic conditions of the CNS. In J. E. Morgan & J. H. Ricker (Eds.), *Textbook of clinical neuropsychology* (pp. 521–535). New York, NY: Psychology Press.

Hopkins, R. O., & Woon, F. L. M. (2006). Neuroimaging, cognitive, and neurobehavioral outcomes following carbon monoxide poisoning. *Behavioral and Cognitive Neuroscience Reviews, 5*(3), 141–155.

Hoppitt, T., Pall, H., Calvert, M., Gill, P., Yao, G., Ramsay, J., . . . Sackley, C. (2011). A systematic review of the incidence and prevalence of long-term neurological conditions in the UK. *Neuroepidemiology, 36*(1), 19–28.

Hoptman, M. J., Ardekani, B. A., Butler, P. D., Nierenberg, J., Javitt, D. C., & Lim, K. O. (2004). DTI and impulsivity in schizophrenia: A first voxelwise correlational analysis. *NeuroReport: For Rapid Communication of Neuroscience Research, 15*(16), 2467–2470.

Hoptman, M. J., Volavka, J., Johnson, G., Weiss, E., Bilder, R. M., & Lim, K. O. (2002). Frontal white matter microstructure, aggression, and impulsivity in men with schizophrenia: A preliminary study. *Biological Psychiatry, 52*(1), 9–14.

Hornak, J., Bramham, J., Rolls, E. T., Morris, R. G., O'Doherty, J., Bullock, P. R., & Polkey, C. E. (2003). Changes in emotion after circumscribed surgical lesions of the orbitofrontal and cingulate cortices. *Brain: A Journal of Neurology, 126*(7), 1691–1712.

Hornak, J., O'Doherty, J., Bramham, J., Rolls, E. T., Morris, R. G., Bullock, P. R., & Polkey, C. E. (2004). Reward-related reversal learning after surgical excisions in orbito-frontal or dorsolateral prefrontal cortex in humans. *Journal of Cognitive Neuroscience, 16*(3), 463–478. doi: 10.1162/089892904322926791

Hornberger, M., & Piguet, O. (2012). Episodic memory in frontotemporal dementia: A critical review. *Brain: A Journal of Neurology, 135*(3), 678–692.

Hoshino, O. (2013). Ambient GABA responsible for age-related changes in multistable perception. *Neural Computation, 25*(5), 1164–1190.

Hou, X., Ma, L., Wu, L., Zhang, Y., Ge, H., Li, Z., . . . Gao, C. (2013). Diffusion tensor imaging for predicting the clinical outcome of delayed encephalopathy of acute carbon monoxide poisoning. *European Neurology, 69*(5), 275–280.

Howard, K., Anderson, P. J., & Taylor, H. G. (2008). Executive functioning and attenion in children born preterm. In V. Anderson, R. Jacobs, & B. J. Anderson (Eds.), *Executive functions and the frontal lobes: A lifespan perspective* (pp. 219–242). New York, NY: Taylor and Francis.

Hubbard, K., & Trauner, D. A. (2007). Intonation and emotion in autistic spectrum disorders. *Journal of Psycholinguistic Research, 36*(2), 159–173.

Huebner, T., Vloet, T. D., Marx, I., Konrad, K., Fink, G. R., Herpertz, S. C., & Herpertz-Dahlmann, B. (2008). Morphometric brain abnormalities in boys with conduct disorder. *Journal of the American Academy of Child and Adolescent Psychiatry, 47*(5), 540–547.

Hughes, G., Velmans, M., & De Fockert, J. (2009). Unconscious priming of a no-go response. *Psychophysiology, 46*(6), 1258–1269.

Hughes, S. K., Nilsson, D. E., Boyer, R. S., Bolte, R. G., Hoffman, R. O., Lewine, J. D., & Bigler, E. D. (2002). Neurodevelopmental outcome for extended cold water drowning: A longitudinal case study. *Journal of the International Neuropsychological Society, 8*(4), 588–595.

Humphrey, A., Golan, O., Wilson, B. A., & Sopena, S. (2011). Measuring executive function in children with high-functioning autism spectrum disorders: What is ecologically valid? In I. Roth & P. Rezaie (Eds.), *Researching the autism spectrum: Contemporary perspectives* (pp. 347–363). New York, NY: Cambridge University Press.

Humphreys, K., Minshew, N., Leonard, G. L., & Behrmanna, M. (2007). A fine-grained analysis of facial expression processing in high-functioning adults with autism. *Neuropsychologia, 45*(4), 685–695.

Hurlemann, R., Wagner, M., Hawellek, B., Reich, H., Pieperhoff, P., Amunts, K., . . . Dolan, R. J. (2007). Amygdala control of emotion-induced forgetting and remembering: Evidence from Urbach-Wiethe disease. *Neuropsychologia, 45*(5), 877–884.

Hyman, S. E. (2007). Obsessed with grooming. *Nature, 448*(7156), 871–872.

Iampietro, M., Giovannetti, T., Drabick, D. A. G., & Kessler, R. K. (2012). Empirically defined patterns of executive function deficits in schizophrenia and their relation to everyday functioning: A person-centered approach. *Clinical Neuropsychologist, 26*(7), 1166–1185.

Iancu, I., Bodner, E., Roitman, S., Piccone Sapir, A., Poreh, A., & Kotler, M. (2010). Impulsivity, aggression and suicide risk among male schizophrenia patients. *Psychopathology, 43*(4), 223–229.

Ibáñez, A., Petroni, A., Urquina, H., Torrente, F., Torralva, T., Hurtado, E., . . . Manes, F. (2011). Cortical deficits of emotional face processing in adults with ADHD: Its relation to social cognition and executive function. *Social Neuroscience, 6*(5–6), 464–481.

Iddon, J. L., Morgan, D. J. R., Loveday, C., Sahakian, B. J., & Pickard, J. D. (2004). Neuropsychological profile of young adults with spina bifida with or without hydrocephalus. *Journal of Neurology, Neurosurgery and Psychiatry, 75*(8), 1112–1118.

Ilonen, T., Taiminen, T., Lauerma, H., Karlsson, H., Helenius, H. Y. M., Tuimala, P., . . . Salokangas, R. K. R. (2000). Impaired Wisconsin Card Sorting

Test performance in first-episode schizophrenia: Resource or motivation deficit? *Comprehensive Psychiatry*, 41(5), 385–391.

Imamizu, H., Kuroda, T., Yoshioka, T., & Kawato, M. (2004). Functional magnetic resonance imaging examination of two modular architectures for switching multiple internal models. *Journal of Neuroscience*, 24(5), 1173–1181.

Irwin, D., Lippa, C. F., & Swearer, J. M. (2007). Cognition and amyotrophic lateral sclerosis (ALS). *American Journal of Alzheimer's Disease and Other Dementias*, 22(4), 300–312.

Iwasaki, Y., Mimuro, M., Yoshida, M., Kitamoto, T., & Hashizume, Y. (2011). Survival to akinetic mutism state in Japanese cases of MM1-type sporadic Creutzfeldt–Jakob disease is similar to Caucasians. *European Journal of Neurology*, 18(7), 999–1002.

Jacobs, R., Harvey, A. S., & Anderson, V. (2007). Executive function following focal frontal lobe lesions: Impact of timing of lesion on outcome. *Cortex: A Journal Devoted to the Study of the Nervous System and Behavior*, 43(6), 792–805.

Jacobson, L. A., Murphy-Bowman, S. C., Pritchard, A. E., Tart-Zelvin, A., Zabel, T. A., & Mahone, E. M. (2012). Factor structure of a sluggish cognitive tempo scale in clinically-referred children. *Journal of Abnormal Child Psychology*, 40(8), 1327–1337.

Jain, N., Brouwers, P., Okcu, M. F., Cirino, P. T., & Krull, K. R. (2009). Sex-specific attention problems in long-term survivors of pediatric acute lymphoblastic leukemia. *Cancer*, 115(18), 4238–4245.

Jameson, K. G., Nasrallah, H. A., Northern, T. G., & Welge, J. A. (2011). Executive function impairment in first-degree relatives of persons with schizophrenia: A meta-analysis of controlled studies. *Asian Journal of Psychiatry*, 4(2), 96–99.

Janelsins, M. C., Kesler, S. R., Ahles, T. A., & Morrow, G. R. (2014). Prevalence, mechanisms, and management of cancer-related cognitive impairment. *International Review of Psychiatry*, 26(1), 102–113.

Jansari, A. S., Devlin, A., Agnew, R., Akesson, K., Murphy, L., & Leadbetter, T. (2014). Ecological assessment of executive functions: A new virtual reality paradigm. *Brain Impairment*, 15(2), 71–85. doi: 10.1017/BrImp.2014.14

Janvin, C. C., Aarsland, D., & Larsen, J. P. (2005). Cognitive predictors of dementia in Parkinson's disease: A community-based, 4-year longitudinal study. *Journal of Geriatric Psychiatry and Neurology*, 18(3), 149–154.

Jauregi, J., Arias, C., Vegas, O., Alén, F., Martinez, S., Copet, P., & Thuilleaux, D. (2007). A neuropsychological assessment of frontal cognitive functions in Prader-Willi syndrome. *Journal of Intellectual Disability Research, 51*(5), 350–365. doi: 10.1111/j.1365-2788.2006.00883.x

Jefferson, A. L., Cahn-Weiner, D., Boyle, P., Paul, R. H., Moser, D. J., Gordon, N., & Cohen, R. A. (2006). Cognitive predictors of functional decline in vascular dementia. *International Journal of Geriatric Psychiatry, 21*(8), 752–754.

Jellinger, K. A. (2008). Morphologic diagnosis of "vascular dementia"—A critical update. *Journal of the Neurological Sciences, 270*(1–2), 1–12.

Jha, M. (2012). Theory of mind deficit in schizophrenia and associated cognitive functions. *Psychological Studies, 57*(3), 283–291.

Jimura, K., & Braver, T. S. (2010). Age-related shifts in brain activity dynamics during task switching. *Cerebral Cortex, 20*(6), 1420–1431.

Jin, Y., Mai, C., & Ding, K. (2001). A study of alexithymia of hemodialysis patients. *Chinese Journal of Clinical Psychology, 9*(3), 226–227.

Johns, E. K., Phillips, N. A., Belleville, S., Goupil, D., Babins, L., Kelner, N., . . . Chertkow, H. (2009). Executive functions in frontotemporal dementia and Lewy body dementia. *Neuropsychology, 23*(6), 765–777.

Johnson, M. R., & Johnson, M. K. (2014). Decoding individual natural scene representations during perception and imagery. *Frontiers in Human Neuroscience, 8*(59), doi: 10.3389/fnhum.2014.00059.

Johnson, S. L., Carver, C. S., Mulé, S., & Joormann, J. (2013). Impulsivity and risk for mania: Towards greater specificity. *Psychology and Psychotherapy: Theory, Research and Practice, 86*(4), 401–412.

Jonas, K. G., & Markon, K. E. (2014). A meta-analytic evaluation of the endophenotype hypothesis: Effects of measurement paradigm in the psychiatric genetics of impulsivity. *Journal of Abnormal Psychology, 123*(3), 660–675. doi: 10.1037/a0037094.supp (Supplemental)

Jongbloed-Pereboom, M., Janssen, A. J. W. M., Steenbergen, B., & Nijhuis-van der Sanden, M. W. G. (2012). Motor learning and working memory in children born preterm: A systematic review. *Neuroscience and Biobehavioral Reviews, 36*(4), 1314–1330.

Jongsma, M. L. A., Postma, S. A. E., Souren, P., Arns, M., Gordon, E., Vissers, K., . . . van Goor, H. (2011). Neurodegenerative properties of chronic pain: Cognitive decline in patients with chronic pancreatitis. *PLoS ONE, 6*(8).

Jost, J. T., Glaser, J., Kruglanski, A. W., & Sulloway, F. J. (2003). Political conservatism as motivated social cognition. *Psychological Bulletin, 129*(3), 339–375.

Jovanovski, D., Zakzanis, K., Campbell, Z., Erb, S., & Nussbaum, D. (2012). Development of a novel, ecologically oriented virtual reality measure of executive function: The Multitasking in the City Test. *Applied Neuropsychology: Adult*, 19(3), 171–182. doi: 10.1080/09084282.2011.643955

Jovanovski, D., Zakzanis, K., Ruttan, L., Campbell, Z., Erb, S., & Nussbaum, D. (2012). Ecologically valid assessment of executive dysfunction using a novel virtual reality task in patients with acquired brain injury. *Applied Neuropsychology: Adult*, 19(3), 207–220. doi: 10.1080/09084282.2011.643956

Julian, L. J., & Arnett, P. A. (2009). Relationships among anxiety, depression, and executive functioning in multiple sclerosis. *Clinical Neuropsychologist*, 23(5), 794–804.

Jungwirth, S., Zehetmayer, S., Hinterberger, M., Kudrnovsky-Moser, S., Weissgram, S., Tragi, K. H., & Fischer, P. (2011). The influence of depression on processing speed and executive function in nondemented subjects aged 75. *Journal of the International Neuropsychological Society*, 17(5), 822–831.

Justus, T. C., & Ivry, R. B. (2001). The cognitive neuropsychology of the cerebellum. *International Review of Psychiatry*, 13(4), 276–282.

Kaetsyri, J., Saalasti, S., Tiippana, K., von Wendt, L., & Sams, M. (2008). Impaired recognition of facial emotions from low-spatial frequencies in Asperger syndrome. *Neuropsychologia*, 46(7), 1888–1897.

Kaladjian, A., Jeanningros, R., Azorin, J. M., Anton, J. L., & Mazzola-Pomietto, P. (2011). Impulsivity and neural correlates of response inhibition in schizophrenia. *Psychological Medicine*, 41(2), 291–299.

Kalanthroff, E., Cohen, N., & Henik, A. (2013). Stop feeling: Inhibition of emotional interference following stop-signal trials. *Frontiers in Human Neuroscience*, 7(78), doi: 10.3389/fnhum.2013.00078.

Kalisch, R., Wiech, K., Herrmann, K., & Dolan, R. J. (2006). Neural correlates of self-distraction from anxiety and a process model of cognitive emotion regulation. *Journal of Cognitive Neuroscience*, 18(8), 1266–1276.

Kamphuis, J., Dijk, D.-J., Spreen, M., & Lancel, M. (2014). The relation between poor sleep, impulsivity and aggression in forensic psychiatric patients. *Physiology and Behavior*, 123, 168–173.

Kanakogi, Y., & Itakura, S. (2010). The link between perception and action in early infancy: From the viewpoint of the direct-matching hypothesis. *Japanese Psychological Research*, 52(2), 121–131.

Kao, A. W., Racine, C. A., Quitania, L. C., Kramer, J. H., Christine, C. W., & Miller, B. L. (2009). Cognitive and neuropsychiatric profile of the synucleinopathies: Parkinson disease, dementia with Lewy bodies, and multiple system atrophy. *Alzheimer Disease and Associated Disorders*, 23(4), 365–370.

Karlsson, H., Naaanen, P., & Stenman, H. (2008). Cortical activation in alexithymia as a response to emotional stimuli. *British Journal of Psychiatry*, *192*(1), 32–38.

Karow, C. M., Marquardt, T. P., & Marshall, R. C. (2001). Affective processing in left and right hemisphere brain-damaged subjects with and without subcortical involvement. *Aphasiology*, *15*(8), 715–729.

Karp, J. F., Reynolds, C. F., III, Butters, M. A., Dew, M. A., Mazumdar, S., Begley, A. E., . . . Weiner, D. K. (2006). The relationship between pain and mental flexibility in older adult pain clinic patients. *Pain Medicine*, *7*(5), 444–452.

Karr, J. E., Areshenkoff, C. N., & Garcia-Barrera, M. A. (2014). The neuropsychological outcomes of concussion: A systematic review of meta-analyses on the cognitive sequelae of mild traumatic brain injury. *Neuropsychology*, *28*(3), 321–336. doi: 10.1037/neu0000037.supp (Supplemental)

Karukivi, M., Vahlberg, T., Pölönen, T., Filppu, T., & Saarijärvi, S. (2014). Does alexithymia expose to mental disorder symptoms in late adolescence? A 4-year follow-up study. *General Hospital Psychiatry*, *36*(6), 748–752.

Kasari, C., Freeman, S. F. N., & Hughes, M. A. (2001). Emotion recognition by children with Down syndrome. *American Journal on Mental Retardation*, *106*(1), 59–72.

Kawai, Y., Miura, R., Tsujimoto, M., Sakurai, T., Yamaoka, A., Takeda, A., . . . Toba, K. (2013). Neuropsychological differentiation between Alzheimer's disease and dementia with Lewy bodies in a memory clinic. *Psychogeriatrics*, *13*(3), 157–163.

Kenemans, J. L., Bekker, E. M., Lijffijt, M., Overtoom, C. C. E., Jonkman, L. M., & Verbaten, M. N. (2005). Attention deficit and impulsivity: Selecting, shifting, and stopping. *International Journal of Psychophysiology*, *58*(1), 59–70. doi: 10.1016/j.ijpsycho.2005.03.009

Kennedy, M. R. T., Coelho, C., Turkstra, L., Ylvisaker, M., Sohlberg, M. M., Yorkston, K., . . . Kan, P.-F. (2008). Intervention for executive functions after traumatic brain injury: A systematic review, meta-analysis and clinical recommendations. *Neuropsychological Rehabilitation*, *18*(3), 257–299.

Kenner, N. M., Mumford, J. A., Hommer, R. E., Skup, M., Leibenluft, E., & Poldrack, R. A. (2010). Inhibitory motor control in response stopping and response switching. *Journal of Neuroscience*, *30*(25), 8512–8518.

Kerns, K. A., Don, A., Mateer, C. A., & Streissguth, A. P. (1997). Cognitive deficits in nonretarded adults with fetal alcohol syndrome. *Journal of Learning Disabilities*, *30*(6), 685–693.

Kerns, K. A., & Price, K. J. (2001). An investigation of prospective memory in children with ADHD. *Child Neuropsychology*, *7*(3), 162–171.

Kesler, S. R., Kent, J. S., & O'Hara, R. (2011). Prefrontal cortex and executive function impairments in primary breast cancer. *Archives of Neurology*, 68(11), 1447–1453.

Killgore, W. D. S., Grugle, N. L., Reichardt, R. M., Killgore, D. B., & Balkin, T. J. (2009). Executive functions and the ability to sustain vigilance during sleep loss. *Aviation, Space, and Environmental Medicine*, 80(2), 81–87. doi: 10.3357/asem.2396.2009

Kim, C., Johnson, N. F., & Gold, B. T. (2012). Common and distinct neural mechanisms of attentional switching and response conflict. *Brain Research*, 1469, 92–102.

Kim, E.-J., Sidhu, M., Gaus, S. E., Huang, E. J., Hof, P. R., Miller, B. L., . . . Seeley, W. W. (2012). Selective frontoinsular von Economo neuron and fork cell loss in early behavioral variant frontotemporal dementia. *Cerebral Cortex*, 22(2), 251–259.

Kimhi, Y., Shoam-Kugelmas, D., Agam Ben-Artzi, G., Ben-Moshe, I., & Bauminger-Zviely, N. (2014). Theory of mind and executive function in preschoolers with typical development versus intellectually able preschoolers with autism spectrum disorder. *Journal of Autism and Developmental Disorders*, 44(9), 2341–2454.

Kipman, M., Weber, M., Schwab, Z. J., DelDonno, S. R., & Killgore, W. D. S. (2012). A funny thing happened on the way to the scanner: Humor detection correlates with gray matter volume. *NeuroReport: For Rapid Communication of Neuroscience Research*, 23(18), 1059–1064.

Kipps, C. M., Nestor, P. J., Acosta-Cabronero, J., Arnold, R., & Hodges, J. R. (2009). Understanding social dysfunction in the behavioural variant of frontotemporal dementia: The role of emotion and sarcasm processing. *Brain: A Journal of Neurology*, 132(3), 592–603.

Kircher, T., Pohl, A., Krach, S., Thimm, M., Schulte-Rüther, M., Anders, S., & Mathiak, K. (2013). Affect-specific activation of shared networks for perception and execution of facial expressions. *Social Cognitive and Affective Neuroscience*, 8(4), 370–377.

Kirsch, L. G., & Becker, J. V. (2007). Emotional deficits in psychopathy and sexual sadism: Implications for violent and sadistic behavior. *Clinical Psychology Review*, 27(8), 904–922.

Kleeberg, J., Bruggimann, L., Annoni, J.-M., van Melle, G., Bogousslavsky, J., & Schluep, M. (2004). Altered decision-making in multiple sclerosis: A sign of impaired emotional reactivity? *Annals of Neurology*, 56(6), 787–795.

Kleinhans, N., Akshoomoff, N., & Delis, D. C. (2005). Executive functions in autism and Asperger's disorder: Flexibility, fluency, and inhibition. *Developmental Neuropsychology, 27*(3), 379–401. doi: 10.1207/s15326942dn2703_5

Kliegel, M., Altgassen, M., Hering, A., & Rose, N. S. (2011). A process-model based approach to prospective memory impairment in Parkinson's disease. *Neuropsychologia, 49*(8), 2166–2177.

Klimkeit, E. I., Mattingley, J. B., Sheppard, D. M., Lee, P., & Bradshaw, J. L. (2005). Motor preparation, motor execution, attention, and executive functions in attention deficit/hyperactivity disorder (ADHD). *Child Neuropsychology, 11*(2), 153–173.

Klimkeit, E. I., Tonge, B., Bradshaw, J. L., Melvin, G. A., & Gould, K. (2011). Neuropsychological deficits in adolescent unipolar depression. *Archives of Clinical Neuropsychology, 26*(7), 662–676.

Klinger, E., Cao, X., Douguet, A.-S., & Fuchs, P. (2009). Designing an ecological and adaptable virtual task in the context of executive functions. *Annual Review of CyberTherapy and Telemedicine, 7*, 248–252.

Knobl, P., Kielstra, L., & Almeida, Q. (2012). The relationship between motor planning and freezing of gait in Parkinson's disease. *Journal of Neurology, Neurosurgery and Psychiatry, 83*(1), 98–101.

Knutson, K. M., Monte, O. D., Raymont, V., Wassermann, E. M., Krueger, F., & Grafman, J. (2014). Neural correlates of apathy revealed by lesion mapping in participants with traumatic brain injuries. *Human Brain Mapping, 35*(3), 943–953.

Koechlin, E., Basso, G., Pietrini, P., Panzer, S., & Grafman, J. (1999). The role of the anterior prefrontal cortex in human cognition. *Nature, 399*(6732), 148–151.

Koechlin, E., Ody, C., & Kounelher, F. d. r. (2003). The architecture of cognitive control in the human prefrontal cortex. *Science, 302*(5648), 1181–1185.

Koehler, M., Kliegel, M., Wiese, B., Bickel, H., Kaduszkiewicz, H., van den Bussche, H., . . . Pentzek, M. (2011). Malperformance in verbal fluency and delayed recall as cognitive risk factors for impairment in instrumental activities of daily living. *Dementia and Geriatric Cognitive Disorders, 31*(1), 81–88.

Koenigs, M., Barbey, A. K., Postle, B. R., & Grafman, J. (2009). Superior parietal cortex is critical for the manipulation of information in working memory. *Journal of Neuroscience, 29*(47), 14980–14986.

Kofler, M. J., Alderson, R. M., Raiker, J. S., Bolden, J., Sarver, D. E., & Rapport, M. D. (2014). Working memory and intraindividual variability as neurocognitive indicators in ADHD: Examining competing model predictions. *Neuropsychology, 28*(3), 459–471.

Kogan, C. S., Boutet, I., Cornish, K., Graham, G. E., Berry-Kravis, E., Drouin, A., & Milgram, N. W. (2009). A comparative neuropsychological test battery differentiates cognitive signatures of fragile X and Down syndrome. *Journal of Intellectual Disability Research*, 53(2), 125–142. doi: 10.1111/j.1365-2788.20 08.01135.x

Kojima, M. (2012). Alexithymia as a prognostic risk factor for health problems: A brief review of epidemiological studies. *BioPsychoSocial Medicine*, 6(1), doi: 10.1186/1751-0759-6-21.

Kopald, B. E., Mirra, K. M., Egan, M. F., Weinberger, D. R., & Goldberg, T. E. (2012). Magnitude of impact of executive functioning and IQ on episodic memory in schizophrenia. *Biological Psychiatry*, 71(6), 545–551.

Koponen, S., Taiminen, T., Honkalampi, K., Joukamaa, M., Viinamaki, H., Kurki, T., . . . Tenovuo, O. (2005). Alexithymia after traumatic brain injury: Its relation to magnetic resonance imaging findings and psychiatric disorders. *Psychosomatic Medicine*, 67(5), 807–812.

Korkman, M., Kettunen, S., & Autti-Rämö, I. (2003). Neurocognitive impairment in early adolescence following prenatal alcohol exposure of varying duration. *Child Neuropsychology*, 9(2), 117–128.

Kornreich, C., Blairy, S., Philippot, P., Dan, B., Foisy, M.-L., Hess, U., . . . Verbanck, P. (2001). Impaired emotional facial expression recognition in alcoholism compared with obsessive-compulsive disorder and normal controls. *Psychiatry Research*, 102(3), 235–248.

Koso, M., & Hansen, S. (2006). Executive function and memory in posttraumatic stress disorder: A study of Bosnian war veterans. *European Psychiatry*, 21(3), 167–173.

Kosson, D. S., Suchy, Y., Mayer, A. R., & Libby, J. (2002). Facial affect recognition in criminal psychopaths. *Emotion*, 2(4), 398–411.

Koster, E. H. W., De Lissnyder, E., & De Raedt, R. (2013). Rumination is characterized by valence-specific impairments in switching of attention. *Acta Psychologica*, 144(3), 563–570.

Kostopoulos, P., & Petrides, M. (2008). Left mid-ventrolateral prefrontal cortex: Underlying principles of function. *European Journal of Neuroscience*, 27(4), 1037–1049.

Kovarsky, D., Schiemer, C., & Murray, A. (2011). Humor, rapport, and uncomfortable moments in interactions with adults with traumatic brain injury. *Topics in Language Disorders*, 31(4), 325–335.

Kowalczyk, E., Szewczyk, P., Budrewicz, S., Koszewicz, M., Gruszka, E., Slotwinski, K., & Podemski, R. (2013). Dynamics of magnetic resonance image changes in a patient with Creutzfeldt-Jakob disease. *European Neurology*, 70(3–4), 139–140.

Kramer, J. H., Jurik, J., Sha, S. J., Rankin, K. P., Rosen, H. J., Johnson, J. K., & Miller, B. L. (2003). Distinctive neuropsychological patterns in frontotemporal dementia, semantic dementia, and alzheimer disease. *Cognitive and Behavioral Neurology*, 16(4), 211–218.

Kraybill, M. L., Larson, E. B., Tsuang, D. W., Teri, L., McCormick, W. C., Bowen, J. D., . . . Cherrier, M. M. (2005). Cognitive differences in dementia patients with autopsy-verified AD, Lewy body pathology, or both. *Neurology*, 64(12), 2069–2073.

Kraybill, M. L., & Suchy, Y. (2008). Evaluating the role of motor regulation in figural fluency: Partialing variance in the Ruff Figural Fluency Test. *Journal of Clinical and Experimental Neuropsychology*, 30(8), 903–912.

Kraybill, M. L., & Suchy, Y. (2011). Executive functioning, motor programming, and functional independence: Accounting for variance, people, and time. *Clinical Neuropsychologist*, 25, 210–223.

Kraybill, M. L., Thorgusen, S. R., & Suchy, Y. (2013). The Push-Turn-Taptap task outperforms measures of executive functioning in predicting declines in functionality: Evidence-based approach to test validation. *Clinical Neuropsychologist*, 27(2), 238–255.

Kringelbach, M. L., & Rolls, E. T. (2004). The functional neuroanatomy of the human orbitofrontal cortex: Evidence from neuroimaging and neuropsychological studies. *Progress in Neurobiology*, 72(5), 341–372.

Ku, H.-L., Yang, K.-C., Lee, Y.-C., Lee, M.-B., & Chou, Y.-H. (2010). Predictors of carbon monoxide poisoning–induced delayed neuropsychological sequelae. *General Hospital Psychiatry*, 32(3), 310–314.

Kudlicka, A., Clare, L., & Hindle, J. V. (2013). Awareness of executive deficits in people with Parkinson's disease. *Journal of the International Neuropsychological Society*, 19(5), 559–570.

Kuha, A., Tuulio-Henriksson, A., Eerola, M., Perälä, J., Suvisaari, J., Partonen, T., & Lönnqvist, J. (2007). Impaired executive performance in healthy siblings of schizophrenia patients in a population-based study. *Schizophrenia Research*, 92(1–3), 142–150.

Kumbhani, S. (2008). Alcoholism and familial vulnerability to neuropsychological deficits: A discordant twin study. 69, ProQuest Information & Learning, US. Retrieved from http://search.ebscohost.com/login.aspx?direct=true&db=psyh&AN=2008-99140-240&site=ehost-live Available from EBSCOhost psyh database.

Kuntsi, J., Pinto, R., Price, T. S., van der Meere, J. J., Frazier-Wood, A. C., & Asherson, P. (2014). The separation of ADHD inattention and hyperactivity-impulsivity symptoms: Pathways from genetic effects to cognitive impairments and symptoms. *Journal of Abnormal Child Psychology, 42*(1), 127–136.

Kuroiwa, T., & Okeda, R. (1994). Neuropathology of cerebral ischemia and hypoxia: Recent advances in experimental studies on its pathogenesis. *Pathology International, 44*(3), 171–181.

Kwok, F. Y., Lee, T. M. C., Leung, C. H. S., & Poon, W. S. (2008). Changes of cognitive functioning following mild traumatic brain injury over a 3-month period. *Brain Injury, 22*(10), 740–751. doi: 10.1080/02699050802336989

Laloyaux, J., Van der Linden, M., Levaux, M.-N., Mourad, H., Pirri, A., Bertrand, H., . . . Larøi, F. (2014). Multitasking capacities in persons diagnosed with schizophrenia: A preliminary examination of their neurocognitive underpinnings and ability to predict real world functioning. *Psychiatry Research, 217*(3), 163–170.

Lamar, M., Podell, K., Carew, T. G., Cloud, B. S., Resh, R., Kennedy, C., . . . Libon, D. J. (1997). Perseverative behavior in Alzheimer's disease and subcortical ischemic vascular dementia. *Neuropsychology, 11*(4), 523–534. doi: 10.1037/0894-4105.11.4.523

Lamar, M., Swenson, R., Kaplan, E., & Libon, D. J. (2004). Characterizing alterations in executive functioning across distinct subtypes of cortical and subcortical dementia. *Clinical Neuropsychologist, 18*(1), 22–31.

LaMarre, A. K., & Kramer, J. H. (2013). Accurate assessment of behavioral variant frontotemporal dementia. In L. D. Ravdin & H. L. Katzen (Eds.), *Handbook on the neuropsychology of aging and dementia* (pp. 313–332). New York, NY: Springer Science + Business Media.

LaMarre, A. K., Rascovsky, K., Bostrom, A., Toofanian, P., Wilkins, S., Sha, S. J., . . . Kramer, J. H. (2013). Interrater reliability of the new criteria for behavioral variant frontotemporal dementia. *Neurology, 80*(21), 1973–1977.

Landa, A., Bossis, A. P., Boylan, L. S., & Wang, P. S. (2012). Beyond the unexplainable pain: Relational world of patients with somatization syndromes. *Journal of Nervous and Mental Disease, 200*(5), 413–422.

Landa, R. J., & Goldberg, M. C. (2005). Language, social, and executive functions in high functioning autism: A continuum of performance. *Journal of Autism and Developmental Disorders, 35*(5), 557–573. doi: 10.1007/s10803-005-0001-1

Lanfranchi, S., Jerman, O., Dal Pont, E., Alberti, A., & Vianello, R. (2010). Executive function in adolescents with Down syndrome. *Journal of Intellectual Disability Research, 54*(4), 308–319. doi: 10.1111/j.1365-2788.2010.01262.x

Langa, K. M., Foster, N. L., & Larson, E. B. (2004). Mixed dementia: Emerging concepts and therapeutic implications. *Journal of the American Medical Association, 292*(23), 2901–2908.

Langner, R., & Eickhoff, S. B. (2013). Sustaining attention to simple tasks: A meta-analytic review of the neural mechanisms of vigilant attention. *Psychological Bulletin, 139*(4), 870–900. doi: 10.1037/a0030694.supp (Supplemental)

Lansbergen, M. M., Kenemans, J. L., & van Engeland, H. (2007). Stroop interference and attention-deficit/hyperactivity disorder: A review and meta-analysis. *Neuropsychology, 21*(2), 251–262. doi: 10.1037/0894-4105.21.2.251 10.1037/0894-4105.21.2.251.supp (Supplemental)

Larsen, J. K., Brand, N., Bermond, B., & Hijman, R. (2003). Cognitive and emotional characteristics of alexithymia: A review of neurobiological studies. *Journal of Psychosomatic Research, 54*(6), 533–541.

Larson, M. J., Kelly, K. G., Stigge-Kaufman, D. A., Schmalfuss, I. M., & Perlstein, W. M. (2007). Reward context sensitivity impairment following severe TBI: An event-related potential investigation. *Journal of the International Neuropsychological Society, 13*(4), 615–625.

Lau, E. Y. Y., Eskes, G. A., Morrison, D. L., Rajda, M., & Spurr, K. F. (2010). Executive function in patients with obstructive sleep apnea treated with continuous positive airway pressure. *Journal of the International Neuropsychological Society, 16*(6), 1077–1088.

Lavenu, I., & Pasquier, F. (2004). Perception of emotion on faces in fronto-temporal dementia and Alzheimer's disease: A longitudinal study. *Dementia and Geriatric Cognitive Disorders, 19*(1), 37–41.

Laws, K. R., Patel, D. D., & Tyson, P. J. (2008). Awareness of everyday executive difficulties precede overt executive dysfunction in schizotypal subjects. *Psychiatry Research, 160*(1), 8–14.

Lazar, R. M., Festa, J. R., Geller, A. E., Romano, G. M., & Marshall, R. S. (2007). Multitasking disorder from right temporoparietal stroke. *Cognitive and Behavioral Neurology, 20*(3), 157–162.

Lazzaretti, M., Morandotti, N., Sala, M., Isola, M., Frangou, S., De Vidovich, G., . . . Brambilla, P. (2012). Impaired working memory and normal sustained attention in borderline personality disorder. *Acta Neuropsychiatrica, 24*(6), 349–355.

Lebert, F., Pasquier, F., & Petit, H. (1995). Personality traits and frontal lobe dementia. *International Journal of Geriatric Psychiatry, 10*(12), 1047–1049.

LeDoux, J. E., Berntson, G. G., Sarter, M., Cacioppo, J. T., Lang, P. J., Bradley, M. M., . . . Carter, C. S. (2002). Basic processes. In J. T. Cacioppo,

G. G. Berntson, R. Adolphs, C. S. Carter, R. J. Davidson, M. K. McClintock, B. S. McEwen, M. J. Meaney, D. L. Schacter, E. M. Sternberg, S. S. Suomi, & S. E. Taylor (Eds.), *Foundations in social neuroscience* (pp. 389–490). Cambridge, MA: MIT Press.

Lee, G. P., & Clason, C. L. (2008). Classification of seizure disorders and syndromes, and neuropsychological impairment in adults with epilepsy. In J. E. Morgan & J. H. Ricker (Eds.), *Textbook of clinical neuropsychology* (pp. 437–465). New York, NY: Psychology Press.

Lee, S., Burns, G. L., Snell, J., & McBurnett, K. (2014). Validity of the sluggish cognitive tempo symptom dimension in children: Sluggish cognitive tempo and ADHD-inattention as distinct symptom dimensions. *Journal of Abnormal Child Psychology*, 42(1), 7–19.

Lee, T.-W., Josephs, O., Dolan, R. J., & Critchley, H. D. (2006). Imitating expressions: Emotion-specific neural substrates in facial mimicry. *Social Cognitive and Affective Neuroscience*, 1(2), 122–135.

Leeson, V. C., Barnes, T. R. E., Harrison, M., Matheson, E., Harrison, I., Mutsatsa, S. H., . . . Joyce, E. M. (2010). The relationship between IQ, memory, executive function, and processing speed in recent-onset psychosis: 1-year stability and clinical outcome. *Schizophrenia Bulletin*, 36(2), 400–409.

Leeson, V. C., Robbins, T. W., Franklin, C., Harrison, M., Harrison, I., Ron, M. A., . . . Joyce, E. M. (2009). Dissociation of long-term verbal memory and fronto-executive impairment in first-episode psychosis. *Psychological Medicine*, 39(11), 1799–1808.

Lehto, J. (1996). Are executive function tests dependent on working memory capacity? *Quarterly Journal of Experimental Psychology A: Human Experimental Psychology*, 49A(1), 29–50.

Lemay, M., Lê, T.-T., & Lamarre, C. (2012). Deficits in two versions of a sustained attention test in adolescents with cerebral palsy. *Developmental NeuroRehabilitation*, 15(4), 253–258.

Lerner, M. D., & Lonigan, C. J. (2014). Executive function among preschool children: Unitary versus distinct abilities. *Journal of Psychopathology and Behavioral Assessment*, 36(4), 626–639.

Leterme, A., Brun, L., Dittmar, A., & Robin, O. (2008). Autonomic nervous system responses to sweet taste: Evidence for habituation rather than pleasure. *Physiology and Behavior*, 93(4), 994–999.

Levine, B., Dawson, D., Boutet, I., Schwartz, M. L., & Stuss, D. T. (2000). Assessment of strategic self-regulation in traumatic brain injury: Its relationship to injury severity and psychosocial outcome. *Neuropsychology*, 14(4), 491–500.

Levine, D. A., & Langa, K. M. (2011). Vascular cognitive impairment: Disease mechanisms and therapeutic implications. *Neurotherapeutics, 8*(3), 361–373.

Levy, J. A., & Chelune, G. J. (2007). Cognitive-behavioral profiles of neurodegenerative dementias: Beyond Alzheimer's disease. *Journal of Geriatric Psychiatry and Neurology, 20*(4), 227–238.

Lewin, A. B., Larson, M. J., Park, J. M., McGuire, J. F., Murphy, T. K., & Storch, E. A. (2014). Neuropsychological functioning in youth with obsessive compulsive disorder: An examination of executive function and memory impairment. *Psychiatry Research, 216*(1), 108–115.

Lezak, M. D. (1982). The problem of assessing executive functions. *International Journal of Psychology, 17*(2–3), 281–297.

Lezak, M. D. (1983). *Neuropsychological assessment*. New York, NY: Oxford University Press.

Lezak, M. D., Howieson, D. B., Bigler, E. D., & Tranel, D. (2013). *Neuropsychological assessment* (5th ed.). New York, NY: Oxford University Press.

Lezak, M. D., Howieson, D. B., & Loring, D. W. (Eds.). (2004). *Neuropsychological assessment* (4th ed.). New York, NY: Oxford University Press.

Li, Y.-M., Zou, X.-B., & Li, J.-Y. (2005). A study of executive function in children with high functioning autism and Asperger syndrome. *Chinese Mental Health Journal, 19*(3), 168–170.

Libon, D. J., McMillan, C., Avants, B., Boller, A., Morgan, B., Burkholder, L., . . . Grossman, M. (2012). Deficits in concept formation in amyotrophic lateral sclerosis. *Neuropsychology, 26*(4), 422–429.

Libon, D. J., Xie, S. X., Moore, P., Farmer, J., Antani, S., McCawley, G., . . . Grossman, M. (2007). Patterns of neuropsychological impairment in frontotemporal dementia. *Neurology, 68*(5), 369–375.

Lichter, D. G., & Cummings, J. L. (2001). *Frontal-subcortical circuits in psychiatric and neurological disorders*. New York, NY: Guilford Press.

Liebermann, D., Giesbrecht, G. F., & Maller, U. (2007). Cognitive and emotional aspects of self-regulation in preschoolers. *Cognitive Development, 22*(4), 511–529.

Lim, C., Alexander, M. P., LaFleche, G., Schnyer, D. M., & Verfaellie, M. (2004). The neurological and cognitive sequelae of cardiac arrest. *Neurology, 63*(10), 1774–1778.

Lim, D. C., & Pack, A. I. (2014). Obstructive sleep apnea and cognitive impairment: Addressing the blood-brain barrier. *Sleep Medicine Reviews, 18*(1), 35–48.

Lindsay, A. R. (1997). Nonverbal learning disabilities and adults with spina bifida: Differentiating subgroups based on higher order cognitive skills and family environment. 57, ProQuest Information & Learning, US. Retrieved from http://search.ebscohost.com/login.aspx?direct=true&db=psyh&AN=1997-95006-389&site=ehost-live Available from EBSCOhost psyh database.

Lippé, S., Bulteau, C., Dorfmuller, G., Audren, F., Delalande, O., & Jambaqué, I. (2010). Cognitive outcome of parietooccipital resection in children with epilepsy. *Epilepsia, 51*(10), 2047–2057.

Lippert-Grüner, M., Kuchta, J., Hellmich, M., & Klug, N. (2006). Neurobehavioural deficits after severe traumatic brain injury (TBI). *Brain Injury, 20*(6), 569–574.

Liu, K. C. M., Chan, R. C. K., Chan, K. K. S., Tang, J. Y. M., Chiu, C. P. Y., Lam, M. M. L., . . . Chen, E. Y. H. (2011). Executive function in first-episode schizophrenia: A three-year longitudinal study of an ecologically valid test. *Schizophrenia Research, 126*(1–3), 87–92.

Loesel, F., & Schmucker, M. (2004). Psychopathy, risk taking, and attention: A differentiated test of the somatic marker hypothesis. *Journal of Abnormal Psychology, 113*(4), 522–529.

Logan, G. D., & Irwin, D. E. (2000). Don't look! Don't touch! Inhibitory control of eye and hand movements. *Psychonomic Bulletin and Review, 7*(1), 107–112.

Logie, R. H., Law, A., Trawley, S., & Nissan, J. (2010). Multitasking, working memory and remembering intentions. *Psychologica Belgica, 50*(3–4), 309–326.

Longo, C. A., Kerr, E. N., & Smith, M. L. (2013). Executive functioning in children with intractable frontal lobe or temporal lobe epilepsy. *Epilepsy and Behavior, 26*(1), 102–108.

Loring, D. W. (1999). *INS dictionary of neuropsychology*. New York, NY: Oxford University Press.

Lough, S., Kipps, C. M., Treise, C., Watson, P., Blair, J. R., & Hodges, J. R. (2006). Social reasoning, emotion and empathy in frontotemporal dementia. *Neuropsychologia, 44*(6), 950–958.

Lovejoy, T. I., & Suhr, J. A. (2009). The relationship between neuropsychological functioning and HAART adherence in HIV-positive adults: A systematic review. *Journal of Behavioral Medicine, 32*(5), 389–405.

Lunazzi de Jubany, H. (2000). Investigación de variables en el constructo Alexitimia en 550 casos. *Revista Iberoamericana de Diagnóstico y Evaluación Psicológica, 10*(2), 101–119.

Luria, A. R. (1973). The frontal lobes and the regulation of behavior *Psychophysiology of the frontal lobes*. Oxford, England: Academic Press.

Luton, L. M., Burns, T. G., & Defilippis, N. (2010). Frontal lobe epilepsy in children and adolescents: A preliminary neuropsychological assessment of executive function. *Archives of Clinical Neuropsychology, 25*(8), 762–770.

Lyons, V., & Fitzgerald, M. (2004). Humor in autism and Asperger syndrome. *Journal of Autism and Developmental Disorders, 34*(5), 521–531. doi: 10.1007/s10803-004-2547-8

MacKillop, J., Miller, J. D., Fortune, E., Maples, J., Lance, C. E., Campbell, W. K., & Goodie, A. S. (2014). Multidimensional examination of impulsivity in relation to disordered gambling. *Experimental and Clinical Psychopharmacology, 22*(2), 176–185.

Mackinlay, R., Charman, T., & Karmiloff-Smith, A. (2006). High functioning children with autism spectrum disorder: A novel test of multitasking. *Brain and Cognition, 61*(1), 14–24.

Macmillan, M. (2000). *An odd kind of fame: Stories of Phineas Gage*. Cambridge, MA: MIT Press.

MacPherson, S. E., Phillips, L. H., Della Sala, S., & Cantagallo, A. (2008). Iowa Gambling Task impairment is not specific to ventromedial prefrontal lesions. *Clinical Neuropsychologist, 23*(3), 510–522.

Madore, K. P., & Schacter, D. L. (2014). An episodic specificity induction enhances means-end problem solving in young and older adults. *Psychology and Aging, 29*(4), 913–924.

Maeda, K., Kasai, K., Watanabe, A., Henomatsu, K., Rogers, M. A., & Kato, N. (2006). Effect of subjective reasoning and neurocognition on medication adherence for persons with schizophrenia. *Psychiatric Services, 57*(8), 1203–1205. doi: 10.1176/appi.ps.57.8.1203

Magai, C., Cohen, C. I., Culver, C., Gomberg, D., & Malatesta, C. (1997). Relation between premorbid personality and patterns of emotion expression in mid- to late-stage dementia. *International Journal of Geriatric Psychiatry, 12*(11), 1092–1099.

Mahone, E. M., & Slomine, B. S. (2008). Neurodevelopmental disorders. In J. E. Morgan & J. H. Ricker (Eds.), *Textbook of clinical neuropsychology* (pp. 105–127). New York, NY: Psychology Press.

Mahurin, R. K., Velligan, D. I., Hazleton, B., Davis, J. M., Eckert, S., & Miller, A. L. (2006). Trail making test errors and executive function in schizophrenia and depression. *Clinical Neuropsychologist, 20*(2), 271–288.

Maier, M. E., Di Pellegrino, G., & Steinhauser, M. (2012). Enhanced error-related negativity on flanker errors: Error expectancy or error significance? *Psychophysiology, 49*(7), 899–908.

Makin, S. D. J., Turpin, S., Dennis, M. S., & Wardlaw, J. M. (2013). Cognitive impairment after lacunar stroke: Systematic review and meta-analysis of incidence, prevalence and comparison with other stroke subtypes. *Journal of Neurology, Neurosurgery and Psychiatry, 84*(8), 893–900.

Mangelli, L., Semprini, F., Sirri, L., Fava, G., & Sonino, N. (2006). Use of the Diagnostic Criteria for Psychosomatic Research (DCPR) in a community sample. *Psychosomatics: Journal of Consultation Liaison Psychiatry, 47*(2), 143–146.

Manji, H., Jager, H. R., & Winston, A. (2013). HIV, dementia and antiretroviral drugs: 30 years of an epidemic. *Journal of Neurology, Neurosurgery and Psychiatry, 84*(10), 1126–1136.

Manly, J. J. (2005). Advantages and disadvantages of separate norms for African Americans. *Clinical Neuropsychologist, 19*(2), 270–275. doi: 10.1080/13854040590945346

Manning, L., Pierot, L., & Dufour, A. (2005). Anterior and non-anterior ruptured aneurysms: Memory and frontal lobe function performance following coiling. *European Journal of Neurology, 12*(6), 466–474. doi: 10.1111/j.1468-1331.2005.01012.x

Mansfield, E. L., Karayanidis, F., Jamadar, S., Heathcote, A., & Forstmann, B. U. (2011). Adjustments of response threshold during task switching: A model-based functional magnetic resonance imaging study. *Journal of Neuroscience, 31*(41), 14688–14692.

Mantani, T., Okamoto, Y., Shirao, N., Okada, G., & Yamawaki, S. (2005). Reduced activation of posterior cingulate cortex during imagery in subjects with high degrees of alexithymia: A functional magnetic resonance imaging study. *Biological Psychiatry, 57*(9), 982–990.

Marin, R. S., & Wilkosz, P. A. (2005). Disorders of diminished motivation. *Journal of Head Trauma Rehabilitation, 20*(4), 377–388.

Marini, A. (2012). Characteristics of narrative discourse processing after damage to the right hemisphere. *Seminars in Speech and Language, 33*(1), 68–78. doi: 10.1055/s-0031-1301164

Marini, A., Carlomagno, S., Caltagirone, C., & Nocentini, U. (2005). The role played by the right hemisphere in the organization of complex textual structures. *Brain and Language, 93*(1), 46–54. doi: 10.1016/j.bandl.2004.08.002

Marklund, P., & Persson, J. (2012). Context-dependent switching between proactive and reactive working memory control mechanisms in the right inferior frontal gyrus. *Neuroimage, 63*(3), 1552–1560.

Marsh, A. A., Finger, E. C., Mitchell, D. G. V., Reid, M. E., Sims, C., Kosson, D. S., . . . Blair, R. J. R. (2008). Reduced amygdala response to fearful expressions in children and adolescents with callous-unemotional traits and disruptive behavior disorders. *American Journal of Psychiatry, 165*(6), 712–720.

Marshall, G. A., Hendrickson, R., Kaufer, D. I., Ivanco, L. S., & Bohnen, N. I. (2006). Cognitive correlates of brain MRI subcortical signal hyperintensities in non-demented elderly. *International Journal of Geriatric Psychiatry, 21*(1), 32–35. doi: 10.1002/gps.1419

Martel, M. M., Nikolas, M., & Nigg, J. T. (2007). Executive function in adolescents with ADHD. *Journal of the American Academy of Child and Adolescent Psychiatry, 46*(11), 1437–1444. doi: 10.1097/chi.0b013e31814cf953

Martel, M. M. (2009). Research review: A new perspective on attention-deficit hyperactivity disorder: Emotion dysregulation and trait models. *Journal of Child Psychology and Psychiatry, 50*(9), 1042–1051.

Martin, I., & McDonald, S. (2006). That can't be right! What causes pragmatic language impairment following right hemisphere damage? *Brain Impairment, 7*(3), 202–211. doi: 10.1375/brim.7.3.202

Martin, R. C., Griffith, H. R., Faught, E., Gilliam, F., Mackey, M., & Vogtle, L. (2005). Cognitive functioning in community dwelling older adults with chronic partial epilepsy. *Epilepsia, 46*(2), 298–303.

Martinaud, O., Perin, B., Gérardin, E., Proust, F., Bioux, S., Le Gars, D., . . . Godefroy, O. (2009). Anatomy of executive deficit following ruptured anterior communicating artery aneurysm. *European Journal of Neurology, 16*(5), 595–601.

Martinez-Aran, A., Scott, J., Colom, F., Torrent, C., Tabares-Seisdedos, R., Daban, C., . . . Vieta, E. (2009). Treatment nonadherence and neurocognitive impairment in bipolar disorder. *Journal of Clinical Psychiatry, 70*(7), 1017–1023. doi: 10.4088/JCP.08m04408

Martins, I. P., Maruta, C., Freitas, V., & Mares, I. (2013). Executive performance in older Portuguese adults with low education. *Clinical Neuropsychologist, 27*(3), 410–425. doi: 10.1080/13854046.2012.748094

Martyr, A., & Clare, L. (2012). Executive function and activities of daily living in Alzheimer's disease: A correlational meta-analysis. *Dementia and Geriatric Cognitive Disorders, 33*(2–3), 189–203. doi: 10.1159/000338233

Mathalon, D. H., Whitfield, S. L., & Ford, J. M. (2003). Anatomy of an error: ERP and fMRI. *Biological Psychology, 64*(1–2), 119–141.

Mathews, C. A., Perez, V. B., Delucchi, K. L., & Mathalon, D. H. (2012). Error-related negativity in individuals with obsessive-compulsive symptoms: Toward an understanding of hoarding behaviors. *Biological Psychology*, *89*(2), 487–494.

Matsui, M., Sumiyoshi, T., Kato, K., Yoneyama, E., & Kurachi, M. (2004). Neuropsychological profile in patients with schizotypal personality disorder or schizophrenia. *Psychological Reports*, *94*(2), 387–397.

Matthews, G., Warm, J. S., Reinerman-Jones, L. E., Langheim, L. K., Washburn, D. A., & Tripp, L. (2010). Task engagement, cerebral blood flow velocity, and diagnostic monitoring for sustained attention. *Journal of Experimental Psychology: Applied*, *16*(2), 187–203.

Matthys, W., Vanderschuren, L. J. M. J., & Schutter, D. J. L. G. (2013). The neurobiology of oppositional defiant disorder and conduct disorder: Altered functioning in three mental domains. *Development and Psychopathology*, *25*(1), 193–207.

Mattson, S. N., Roesch, S. C., Fagerlund, Å., Autti-Rämö, I., Jones, K. L., May, P. A., . . . Riley, E. P. (2010). Toward a neurobehavioral profile of fetal alcohol spectrum disorders. *Alcoholism: Clinical and Experimental Research*, *34*(9), 1640–1650.

Mattson, S. N., Schoenfeld, A. M., & Riley, E. P. (2001). Teratogenic effects of alcohol on brain and behavior. *Alcohol Research and Health*, *25*(3), 185–191.

Mazzola, F., Seigal, A., MacAskill, A., Corden, B., Lawrence, K., & Skuse, D. H. (2006). Eye tracking and fear recognition deficits in Turner syndrome. *Social Neuroscience*, *1*(3), 259–269.

McAlister, C., & Schmitter-Edgecombe, M. (2013). Naturalistic assessment of executive function and everyday multitasking in healthy older adults. *Aging, Neuropsychology, and Cognition*, *20*(6), 735–756.

McCabe, D. P., Roediger, H. L., III, McDaniel, M. A., Balota, D. A., & Hambrick, D. Z. (2010). The relationship between working memory capacity and executive functioning: Evidence for a common executive attention construct. *Neuropsychology*, *24*(2), 222–243.

McClure, M. M., Romero, M. J., Bowie, C. R., Reichenberg, A., Harvey, P. D., & Siever, L. J. (2007). Visual-spatial learning and memory in schizotypal personality disorder: Continued evidence for the importance of working memory in the schizophrenia spectrum. *Archives of Clinical Neuropsychology*, *22*(1), 109–116.

McCown, W., Johnson, J., & Austin, S. (1986). Inability of delinquents to recognize facial affects. *Journal of Social Behavior and Personality*, *1*(4), 489–496.

McCown, W. G., Johnson, J. L., & Austin, S. H. (1988). Patterns of facial affect recognition errors in delinquent adolescent males. *Journal of Social Behavior and Personality*, *3*(3), 215–224.

McCusker, C. G., Kennedy, P. J., Anderson, J., Hicks, E. M., & Hanrahan, D. (2002). Adjustment in children with intractable epilepsy: Importance of seizure duration and family factors. *Developmental Medicine and Child Neurology*, *44*(10), 681–687.

McDonald, B. C., Conroy, S. K., Smith, D. J., West, J. D., & Saykin, A. J. (2013). Frontal gray matter reduction after breast cancer chemotherapy and association with executive symptoms: A replication and extension study. *Brain, Behavior, and Immunity*, *30*(Suppl.), S117–S125.

McDonald, C. R., Delis, D. C., Norman, M. A., Tecoma, E. S., & Iragui-Madoz, V. J. (2005). Is impairment in set-shifting specific to frontal-lobe dysfunction? Evidence from patients with frontal-lobe or temporal-lobe epilepsy. *Journal of the International Neuropsychological Society*, *11*(4), 477–481.

McDonald, S. (2013). Impairments in social cognition following severe traumatic brain injury. *Journal of the International Neuropsychological Society*, *19*(3), 231–246.

McDonald, S., Flanagan, S., & Rollins, J. (2002). *The Awareness of Social Interference Test (TASIT)*. San Antonio, TX: Pearson.

McGee, C. L., Schonfeld, A. M., Roebuck-Spencer, T. M., Riley, E. P., & Mattson, S. N. (2008). Children with heavy prenatal alcohol exposure demonstrate deficits on multiple measures of concept formation. *Alcoholism: Clinical and Experimental Research*, *32*(8), 1388–1397.

McGuire, L. C., Ford, E. S., & Ajani, U. A. (2006). Cognitive functioning as a predictor of functional disability in later life. *American Journal of Geriatric Psychiatry*, *14*(1), 36–42. doi: 10.1097/01.JGP.0000192502.10692.d6

McIntosh, R. D., Pritchard, C. L., Dijkerman, H. C., Milner, A. D., & Roberts, R. C. (2001). Prehension and perception of size in left visual neglect. *Behavioural Neurology*, *13*(1–2), 3–15.

McKeith, I. G. (2002). Dementia with Lewy bodies. *British Journal of Psychiatry*, *180*(2), 144–147.

McLaughlin, N. C. R., Chang, A. C., & Malloy, P. (2012). Verbal and nonverbal learning and recall in dementia with Lewy bodies and Alzheimer's disease. *Applied Neuropsychology: Adult*, *19*(2), 86–89.

McRae, K., Jacobs, S. E., Ray, R. D., John, O. P., & Gross, J. J. (2012). Individual differences in reappraisal ability: Links to reappraisal frequency, well-being, and cognitive control. *Journal of Research in Personality*, *46*(1), 2–7.

Meager, M. R., Kramer, M., Frim, D. M., & Lacy, M. A. (2010). An introduction to hydrocephalus: Congenital and late-life onset. In C. L. Armstrong & L. Morrow (Eds.), *Handbook of medical neuropsychology: Applications of cognitive neuroscience* (pp. 223–236). New York, NY: Springer Science + Business Media.

Medeiros-Ward, N., Watson, J. M., & Strayer, D. L. (2014). On supertaskers and the neural basis of efficient multitasking. *Psychonomic Bulletin and Review*, 22(3), 876–883.

Mega, M. S., & Cohenour, R. C. (1997). Akinetic mutism: Disconnection of frontal-subcortical circuits. *Neuropsychiatry, Neuropsychology, and Behavioral Neurology*, 10(4), 254–259.

Meiran, N., & Marciano, H. (2002). Limitations in advance task preparation: Switching the relevant stimulus dimension in speeded same-different comparisons. *Memory and Cognition*, 30(4), 540–550.

Meiron, O., Hermesh, H., Katz, N., & Weizman, A. (2013). Executive attention deficits in schizophrenia: Putative mandatory and differential cognitive pathology domains in medicated schizophrenia patients. *Psychiatry Research*, 209(1), 1–8.

Melnick, S. M., & Hinshaw, S. P. (2000). Emotion regulation and parenting in AD/HD and comparison boys: Linkages with social behaviors and peer preference. *Journal of Abnormal Child Psychology*, 28(1), 73–86.

Menon, V., & Uddin, L. Q. (2010). Saliency, switching, attention and control: A network model of insula function. *Brain Structure and Function*, 214(5–6), 655–667.

Messina, A., Beadle, J. N., & Paradiso, S. (2014). Towards a classification of alexithymia: Primary secondary and organic. *Journal of Wslashes? use just eng? Psychopathology / Giornale di Psicopatologia*, 20(1), 38–49.

Metzler, C., & Parkin, A. J. (2000). Reversed negative priming following frontal lobe lesions. *Neuropsychologia*, 38(4), 363–379. doi: 10.1016/s0028-3932(99)00097-4

Middelkamp, W., Moulaert, V. R. M. P., Verbunt, J. A., van Heugten, C. M., Bakx, W. G., & Wade, D. T. (2007). Life after survival: Long-term daily life functioning and quality of life of patients with hypoxic brain injury as a result of a cardiac arrest. *Clinical Rehabilitation*, 21(5), 425–431.

Miele, D. B., Wager, T. D., Mitchell, J. P., & Metcalfe, J. (2011). Dissociating neural correlates of action monitoring and metacognition of agency. *Journal of Cognitive Neuroscience*, 23(11), 3620–3636.

Milan, G., Iavarone, A., Lorè, E., Vitaliano, S., Lamenza, F., Sorrentino, P., & Postiglione, A. (2007). When behavioral assessment detects frontotemporal dementia and cognitive testing does not: Data from the Frontal Behavioral Inventory. *International Journal of Geriatric Psychiatry*, 22(3), 266–267.

Miller, E. K., & Cohen, J. D. (2001). An integrative theory of prefrontal cortex function. *Annual Review of Neuroscience*, 24, 167–202.

Miller, G. (2010). New clues about what makes the human brain special. *Science*, 330(6008), 1167.

Miller, M. R., Giesbrecht, G. F., Müller, U., McInerney, R. J., & Kerns, K. A. (2012). A latent variable approach to determining the structure of executive function in preschool children. *Journal of Cognition and Development*, 13(3), 395–423.

Millis, S. R., Rosenthal, M., Novack, T. A., Sherer, M., Nick, T. G., Kreutzer, J. S., . . . Ricker, J. H. (2001). Long-term neuropsychological outcome after traumatic brain injury. *Journal of Head Trauma Rehabilitation*, 16(4), 343–355.

Milner, A. D., Dijkerman, H. C., Pisella, L., McIntosh, R. D., Tilikete, C., Vighetto, A., & Rossetti, Y. (2001). Grasping the past: Delay can improve visuomotor performance. *Current Biology*, 11(23), 1896–1901.

Minzenberg, M. J., Laird, A. R., Thelen, S., Carter, C. S., & Glahn, D. C. (2009). Meta-analysis of 41 functional neuroimaging studies of executive function in schizophrenia. *Archives of General Psychiatry*, 66(8), 811–822.

Miraghaie, A. M., Moradi, A. R., Hasani, J., Rahimi, V., & Mirzaie, J. (2013). A comparative study on the performance of PTSD and OCD in executive functions. *Journal of Psychology*, 17(1), 83–103.

Miralbell, J., Soriano, J. J., Spulber, G., López-Cancio, E., Arenillas, J. F., Bargalló, N., . . . Mataró, M. (2012). Structural brain changes and cognition in relation to markers of vascular dysfunction. *Neurobiology of Aging*, 33(5), e9–e17.

Mitchell, M., & Miller, L. S. (2008). Prediction of functional status in older adults: The ecological validity of four Delis-Kaplan Executive Function System tests. *Journal of Clinical and Experimental Neuropsychology*, 30(6), 683–690. doi: 10.1080/13803390701679893

Mitchell, R. L. C., & Ross, E. D. (2013). Attitudinal prosody: What we know and directions for future study. *Neuroscience and Biobehavioral Reviews*, 37(3), 471–479.

Mitropoulou, V., Harvey, P. D., Zegarelli, G., New, A. S., Silverman, J. M., & Siever, L. J. (2005). Neuropsychological performance in schizotypal personality disorder: Importance of working memory. *American Journal of Psychiatry*, 162(10), 1896–1903.

Mittenberg, W., & Roberts, D. M. (2008). Mild traumatic brain injury and postconcussion syndrome. In J. E. Morgan & J. H. Ricker (Eds.), *Textbook of clinical neuropsychology* (pp. 430–436). New York, NY: Psychology Press.

Miyake, A., Friedman, N. P., Emerson, M. J., Witzki, A. H., & Howerter, A. (2000). The unity and diversity of executive functions and their contributions to complex "frontal lobe" tasks: A latent variable analysis. *Cognitive Psychology*, 41(1), 49–100.

Molano, J., Boeve, B., Ferman, T., Smith, G., Parisi, J., Dickson, D., . . . Petersen, R. (2010). Mild cognitive impairment associated with limbic and neocortical Lewy body disease: A clinicopathological study. *Brain: A Journal of Neurology*, 133(2), 540–556.

Monnot, M., Lovallo, W. R., Nixon, S. J., & Ross, E. (2002). Neurological basis of deficits in affective prosody comprehension among alcoholics and fetal alcohol–exposed adults. *Journal of Neuropsychiatry and Clinical Neuroscience*, 14(3), 321–328.

Monnot, M., Nixon, S., Lovallo, W., & Ross, E. (2001). Altered emotional perception in alcoholics: Deficits in affective prosody comprehension. *Alcoholism: Clinical and Experimental Research*, 25(3), 362–369.

Montgomery, J. M., Stoesz, B. M., & McCrimmon, A. W. (2013). Emotional intelligence, theory of mind, and executive functions as predictors of social outcomes in young adults with Asperger syndrome. *Focus on Autism and Other Developmental Disabilities*, 28(1), 4–13.

Moore, A. B., Li, Z., Tyner, C. E., Hu, X., & Crosson, B. (2013). Bilateral basal ganglia activity in verbal working memory. *Brain and Language*, 125(3), 316–323.

Morice, R. (1986). Beyond language: Speculations on the prefrontal cortex and schizophrenia. *Australian and New Zealand Journal of Psychiatry*, 20(1), 7–10.

Moriguchi, Y., Decety, J., Ohnishi, T., Maeda, M., Mori, T., Nemoto, K., . . . Komaki, G. (2007). Empathy and judging other's pain: An fMRI study of alexithymia. *Cerebral Cortex*, 17(9), 2223–2234.

Morris, J. S., de Gelder, B., Weiskrantz, L., & Dolan, R. J. (2001). Differential extrageniculostriate and amygdala responses to presentation of emotional faces in a cortically blind field. *Brain: A Journal of Neurology*, 124(6), 1241–1252.

Morrow, L. A., Robards, M., Saxton, J. A., & Metheny, K. (2008). Toxins in the CNS: Alcohol, illicit drugs, heavy metals, solvents, and related exposure. In J. E. Morgan & J. H. Ricker (Eds.), *Textbook of clinical neuropsychology* (pp. 588–598). New York, NY: Psychology Press.

Moscovitch, M., & Winocur, G. (2002). The frontal cortex and working with memory. In D. T. Stuss & R. T. Knight (Eds.), *Principles of frontal lobe function* (pp. 188–209). New York, NY: Oxford University Press.

Moser, J. S., Moran, T. P., Schroder, H. S., Donnellan, M. B., & Yeung, N. (2013). On the relationship between anxiety and error monitoring: A meta-analysis and conceptual framework. *Frontiers in Human Neuroscience*, 7(466), doi: 10.3389/fnhum.2013.00466.

Moss, J., & Howlin, P. (2009). Autism spectrum disorders in genetic syndromes: Implications for diagnosis, intervention and understanding the wider autism spectrum disorder population. *Journal of Intellectual Disability Research*, 53(10), 852–873. doi: 10.1111/j.1365-2788.2009.01197.x

Mula, M., & Trimble, M. R. (2009). Antiepileptic drug–induced cognitive adverse effects: Potential mechanisms and contributing factors. *CNS Drugs*, 23(2), 121–137.

Mulder, H., Pitchford, N. J., Hagger, M. S., & Marlow, N. (2009). Development of executive function and attention in preterm children: A systematic review. *Developmental Neuropsychology*, 34(4), 393–421.

Muraven, M., Tice, D. M., & Baumeister, R. F. (1998). Self-control as a limited resource: Regulatory depletion patterns. *Journal of Personality and Social Psychology*, 74(3), 774–789.

Murdock, K. W., Oddi, K. B., & Bridgett, D. J. (2013). Cognitive correlates of personality: Links between executive functioning and the big five personality traits. *Journal of Individual Differences*, 34(2), 97–104.

Murphy, M. M., & Mazzocco, M. M. M. (2009). The trajectory of mathematics skills and working memory thresholds in girls with fragile X syndrome. *Cognitive Development*, 24(4), 430–449. doi: 10.1016/j.cogdev.2009.09.004

Murrough, J. W., Iacoviello, B., Neumeister, A., Charney, D. S., & Iosifescu, D. V. (2011). Cognitive dysfunction in depression: Neurocircuitry and new therapeutic strategies. *Neurobiology of Learning and Memory*, 96(4), 553–563.

Muslimović, D., Post, B., Speelman, J. D., & Schmand, B. (2005). Cognitive profile of patients with newly diagnosed Parkinson disease. *Neurology*, 65(8), 1239–1245.

Mutschler, I., Reinbold, C., Wankerl, J., Seifritz, E., & Ball, T. (2013). Structural basis of empathy and the domain general region in the anterior insular cortex. *Frontiers in Human Neuroscience*, 7(177). doi: 10.3389/fnhum.2013.00177.

Mutter, B., Alcorn, M. B., & Welsh, M. (2006). Theory of mind and executive function: Working-memory capacity and inhibitory control as predictors of false-belief task performance. *Perceptual and Motor Skills*, 102(3), 819–835.

Nacher, V., Ojeda, S., Cadarso-Suarez, C., Roca-Pardinas, J., & Acuna, C. (2006). Neural correlates of memory retrieval in the prefrontal cortex. *European Journal of Neuroscience*, 24(3), 925–936.

Nagel, B. J., Herting, M. M., Maxwell, E. C., Bruno, R., & Fair, D. (2013). Hemispheric lateralization of verbal and spatial working memory during adolescence. *Brain and Cognition*, 82(1), 58–68.

Naghavi, H. R., & Nyberg, L. (2005). Common fronto-parietal activity in attention, memory, and consciousness: Shared demands on integration? *Consciousness and Cognition: An International Journal*, 14(2), 390–425.

Naismith, S., Winter, V., Gotsopoulos, H., Hickie, I., & Cistulli, P. (2004). Neurobehavioral functioning in obstructive sleep apnea: Differential effects of sleep quality, hypoxemia and subjective sleepiness. *Journal of Clinical and Experimental Neuropsychology*, 26(1), 43–54.

Nakaaki, S., Murata, Y., Sato, J., Shinagawa, Y., Hongo, J., Tatsumi, H., . . . Furukawa, T. A. (2008). Association between apathy/depression and executive function in patients with Alzheimer's disease. *International Psychogeriatrics*, 20(5), 964–975.

Neill, E., & Rossell, S. L. (2013). Executive functioning in schizophrenia: The result of impairments in lower order cognitive skills? *Schizophrenia Research*, 150(1), 76–80.

Nelson, B. D., McGowan, S. K., Sarapas, C., Robison-Andrew, E. J., Altman, S. E., Campbell, M. L., . . . Shankman, S. A. (2013). Biomarkers of threat and reward sensitivity demonstrate unique associations with risk for psychopathology. *Journal of Abnormal Psychology*, 122(3), 662–671.

Nelson, W. L., & Suls, J. (2013). New approaches to understand cognitive changes associated with chemotherapy for non–central nervous system tumors. *Journal of Pain and Symptom Management*, 46(5), 707–721.

Nes, L. S., Roach, A. R., & Segerstrom, S. C. (2009). Executive functions, self-regulation, and chronic pain: A review. *Annals of Behavioral Medicine*, 37(2), 173–183.

Newcombe, V. F. J., Outtrim, J. G., Chatfield, D. A., Manktelow, A., Hutchinson, P. J., Coles, J. P., . . . Menon, D. K. (2011). Parcellating the neuroanatomical basis of impaired decision-making in traumatic brain injury. *Brain: A Journal of Neurology*, 134(3), 759–768.

Niccols, A. (2007). Fetal alcohol syndrome and the developing socio-emotional brain. *Brain and Cognition*, 65(1), 135–142.

Nicolai, J., van Putten, M. J. A. M., & Tavy, D. L. J. (2001). BIPLEDs in akinetic mutism caused by bilateral anterior cerebral artery infarction. *Clinical Neurophysiology*, 112(9), 1726–1728.

Niedenthal, P. M. (2007). Embodying emotion. *Science*, 316(5827), 1002–1005.

Niedenthal, P. M., Winkielman, P., Mondillon, L., & Vermeulen, N. (2009). Embodiment of emotion concepts. *Journal of Personality and Social Psychology*, 96(6), 1120–1136.

Niewoehner, P. M., Henderson, R. R., Dalchow, J., Beardsley, T. L., Stern, R. A., & Carr, D. B. (2012). Predicting road test performance in adults with cognitive or visual impairment referred to a Veterans Affairs medical center driving clinic. *Journal of the American Geriatrics Society*, 60(11), 2070–2074.

Norman, D. A., & Shallice, T. (1986). Attention to action: Willed and automatic control of behavior. In D. L. Shapiro & G. Schwartz (Eds.), *Consciousness and self-regulation in research: Advances in research*. New York, NY: Plenum Press.

Nuñez, S. C., Roussotte, F., & Sowell, E. R. (2011). Focus on: Structural and functional brain abnormalities in fetal alcohol spectrum disorders. *Alcohol Research and Health*, 34(1), 121–131.

O'Brien, J. W., Dowell, L. R., Mostofsky, S. H., Denckla, M. B., & Mahone, E. M. (2010). Neuropsychological profile of executive function in girls with attention-deficit/hyperactivity disorder. *Archives of Clinical Neuropsychology*, 25(7), 656–670.

O'Connell, R. G., Bellgrove, M. A., Dockree, P. M., Lau, A., Hester, R., Garavan, H., . . . Robertson, I. H. (2009). The neural correlates of deficient error awareness in attention-deficit hyperactivity disorder (ADHD). *Neuropsychologia*, 47(4), 1149–1159.

O'Connell, R. G., Dockree, P. M., Bellgrove, M. A., Kelly, S. P., Hester, R., Garavan, H., . . . Foxe, J. J. (2007). The role of cingulate cortex in the detection of errors with and without awareness: A high-density electrical mapping study. *European Journal of Neuroscience*, 25(8), 2571–2579.

Ochsner, K. N., Bunge, S. A., Gross, J. J., & Gabrieli, J. D. E. (2002). Rethinking feelings: An fMRI study of the cognitive regulation of emotion. *Journal of Cognitive Neuroscience*, 14(8), 1215–1229.

Ochsner, K. N., & Gross, J. J. (2007). The neural architecture of emotion regulation. In J. Gross (Ed.), *Handbook of emotion regulation* (pp. 87–109). New York, NY: Guilford Press.

Ochsner, K. N., & Gross, J. J. (2008). Cognitive emotion regulation: Insights from social cognitive and affective neuroscience. *Current Directions in Psychological Science*, 17(2), 153–158.

O'Driscoll, G. A., Dépatie, L., Holahan, A.-L. V., Savion-Lemieux, T., Barr, R. G., Jolicoeur, C., & Douglas, V. I. (2005). Executive functions and methylphenidate response in subtypes of attention-deficit/hyperactivity disorder. *Biological Psychiatry*, 57(11), 1452–1460.

Ogawa, A., & Koyasu, M. (2008). The relation between components of executive function and theory of mind in young children. *Japanese Journal of Developmental Psychology, 19*(2), 171–182.

Ogilvie, J. M., Stewart, A. L., Chan, R. C. K., & Shum, D. H. K. (2011). Neuropsychological measures of executive function and antisocial behavior: A meta-analysis. *Criminology: An Interdisciplinary Journal, 49*(4), 1063–1107.

Oh, S., Park, A., Kim, H.-J., Oh, K.-W., Choi, H., Kwon, M.-J., . . . Kim, S. H. (2014). Spectrum of cognitive impairment in Korean ALS patients without known genetic mutations. *PLoS ONE, 9*(2).

Ohman, A. (2002). Automaticity and the amygdala: Nonconscious responses to emotional faces. *Current Directions in Psychological Science, 11*(2), 62–66.

Ohman, A. (2005). The role of the amygdala in human fear: Automatic detection of threat. *Psychoneuroendocrinology, 30*(10), 953–958.

Ohman, A., & Mineka, S. (2001). Fears, phobias, and preparedness: Toward an evolved module of fear and fear learning. *Psychological Review, 108*, 483–522.

Ohsugi, H., Ohgi, S., Shigemori, K., & Schneider, E. B. (2013). Differences in dual-task performance and prefrontal cortex activation between younger and older adults. *BMC Neuroscience, 14*(10), doi: 10.1186/1471-2202-14-10

Olff, M., Polak, A. R., Witteveen, A. B., & Denys, D. (2014). Executive function in posttraumatic stress disorder (PTSD) and the influence of comorbid depression. *Neurobiology of Learning and Memory, 112*, 114–121. doi: 10.1016/j.nlm.2014.01.003.

Olley, A., Malhi, G., & Sachdev, P. (2007). Memory and executive functioning in obsessive-compulsive disorder: A selective review. *Journal of Affective Disorders, 104*(1–3), 15–23.

Olver, J. H., Ponsford, J. L., & Curran, C. A. (1996). Outcome following traumatic brain injury: A comparison between 2 and 5 years after injury. *Brain Injury, 10*(11), 841–848.

Oosterman, J. M., Derksen, L. C., van Wijck, A. J. M., Kessels, R. P. C., & Veldhuijzen, D. S. (2012). Executive and attentional functions in chronic pain: Does performance decrease with increasing task load? *Pain Research and Management, 17*(3), 159–165.

Oosterman, J. M., Oosterveld, S., Olde Rikkert, M. C., Claassen, J. A., & Kessels, R. P. C. (2012). Medial temporal lobe atrophy relates to executive dysfunction in Alzheimer's disease. *International Psychogeriatrics, 24*(9), 1474–1482.

Oram, J., Geffen, G. M., Geffen, L. B., Kavanagh, D. J., & McGrath, J. J. (2005). Executive control of working memory in schizophrenia. *Psychiatry Research, 135*(2), 81–90.

Ordemann, G. J., Opper, J., & Davalos, D. (2014). Prospective memory in schizophrenia: A review. *Schizophrenia Research, 155*(1–3), 77–89.

Orfei, M. D., Robinson, R. G., Bria, P., Caltagirone, C., & Spalleta, G. (2008). Unawareness of illness in neuropsychiatric disorders: Phenomenological certainty versus etiopathogenic vagueness. *Neuroscientist, 14*(2), 203–222.

Orr, C., & Hester, R. (2012). Error-related anterior cingulate cortex activity and the prediction of conscious error awareness. *Frontiers in Human Neuroscience, 6*(177), doi: 10.3389/fnhum.2012.00177.

Ortega, R. O., Chapelo, l. B., & Santoncini, C. U. (2012). Disordered eating behaviors and binge drinking in female high-school students: The role of impulsivity. =*Salud Mental, 35*(2), 83–89.

Østby, Y., Tamnes, C. K., Fjell, A. M., & Walhovd, K. B. (2011). Morphometry and connectivity of the fronto-parietal verbal working memory network in development. *Neuropsychologia, 49*(14), 3854–3862.

Ouzir, M. (2013). Impulsivity in schizophrenia: A comprehensive update. *Aggression and Violent Behavior, 18*(2), 247–254.

Ownsworth, T., & McKenna, K. (2004). Investigation of factors related to employment outcome following traumatic brain injury: A critical review and conceptual model. *Disability and Rehabilitation: An International, Multidisciplinary Journal, 26*(13), 765–784.

Ozonoff, S., Cook, I., Coon, H., Dawson, G., Joseph, R. M., Klin, A., . . . Wrathall, D. (2004). Performance on Cambridge Neuropsychological Test Automated Battery subtests sensitive to frontal lobe function in people with autistic disorder: Evidence from the Collaborative Programs of Excellence in Autism Network. *Journal of Autism and Developmental Disorders, 34*(2), 139–150.

Ozonoff, S., South, M., & Provencal, S. (2007). Executive functions in autism: Theory and practice. In J. M. Pérez, P. M. González, M. Llorente Comí, & C. Nieto (Eds.), *New developments in autism: The future is today* (pp. 185–213). London, England: Jessica Kingsley.

Paelecke-Habermann, Y., Pohl, J., & Leplow, B. (2005). Attention and executive functions in remitted major depression patients. *Journal of Affective Disorders, 89*(1–3), 125–135.

Palmer, H. M., & McDonald, S. (2000). The role of frontal and temporal lobe processes in prospective remembering. *Brain and Cognition, 44*(1), 103–107.

Papagno, C., Rizzo, S., Ligori, L., Lima, J., & Riggio, A. (2003). Memory and executive functions in aneurysms of the anterior communicating artery. *Journal of Clinical and Experimental Neuropsychology, 25*(1), 24–35.

Paquier, P. F., & Mariën, P. (2005). A synthesis of the role of the cerebellum in cognition. *Aphasiology, 19*(1), 3–19.

Pardini, M., Gialloreti, L. E., Mascolo, M., Benassi, F., Abate, L., Guida, S., . . . Cocito, L. (2013). Isolated theory of mind deficits and risk for frontotemporal dementia: A longitudinal pilot study. *Journal of Neurology, Neurosurgery and Psychiatry, 84*(7), 818–821.

Parikh, M., Hynan, L. S., Weiner, M. F., Lacritz, L., Ringe, W., & Cullum, C. M. (2014). Single neuropsychological test scores associated with rate of cognitive decline in early Alzheimer disease. *Clinical Neuropsychologist, 28*(6), 926–940. doi: 10.1080/13854046.2014.944937

Park, S., Kim, B.-N., Choi, N.-H., Ryu, J., McDermott, B., Cobham, V., . . . Cho, S.-C. (2014). The effect of persistent posttraumatic stress disorder symptoms on executive functions in preadolescent children witnessing a single incident of death. *Anxiety, Stress and Coping: An International Journal, 27*(3), 241–252.

Parkin, A. J. (1998). The central executive does not exist. *Journal of the International Neuropsychological Society, 4*(5), 518–522.

Parmenter, B. A., Zivadinov, R., Kerenyi, L., Gavett, R., Weinstock-Guttman, B., Dwyer, M. G., . . . Benedict, R. H. B. (2007). Validity of the Wisconsin Card Sorting and Delis-Kaplan Executive Function System (DKEFS) Sorting Tests in multiple sclerosis. *Journal of Clinical and Experimental Neuropsychology, 29*(2), 215–223.

Pas, P., Custers, R., Bijleveld, E., & Vink, M. (2014). Effort responses to suboptimal reward cues are related to striatal dopaminergic functioning. *Motivation and Emotion, 38*(6), 759–770.

Paternoster, R., & Pogarsky, G. (2009). Rational choice, agency and thoughtfully reflective decision making: The short and long-term consequences of making good choices. *Journal of Quantitative Criminology, 25*(2), 103–127.

Paternoster, R., Pogarsky, G., & Zimmerman, G. (2011). Thoughtfully reflective decision making and the accumulation of capital: Bringing choice back in. *Journal of Quantitative Criminology, 27*(1), 1–26.

Paul, L. K., Lautzenhiser, A., Brown, W. S., Hart, A., Neumann, D., Spezio, M., & Adolphs, R. (2006). Emotional arousal in agenesis of the corpus callosum. *International Journal of Psychophysiology, 61*(1), 47–56.

Paul, R., Cohen, R., Navia, B., & Tashima, K. (2002). Relationships between cognition and structural neuroimaging findings in adults with human immunodeficiency virus type-1. *Neuroscience and Biobehavioral Reviews*, 26(3), 353–359.

Pauli-Pott, U., & Becker, K. (2011). Neuropsychological basic deficits in preschoolers at risk for ADHD: A meta-analysis. *Clinical Psychology Review*, 31(4), 626–637. doi: 10.1016/j.cpr.2011.02.005

Pearson. (2009). *Advanced clinical solutions for the WAIS-IV/WMS-IV*. San Antonio, TX: Pearson.

Peavy, G. M., Salmon, D. P., Edland, S. D., Tam, S., Hansen, L. A., Masliah, E., . . . Hamilton, J. M. (2013). Neuropsychiatric features of frontal lobe dysfunction in autopsy-confirmed patients with Lewy bodies and "pure" Alzheimer disease. *American Journal of Geriatric Psychiatry*, 21(6), 509–519.

Pennington, C., Hodges, J. R., & Hornberger, M. (2011). Neural correlates of episodic memory in behavioral variant frontotemporal dementia. *Journal of Alzheimer's Disease*, 24(2), 261–268.

Perera, S., Crewther, D., Croft, R., Keage, H., Hermens, D., & Clark, C. R. (2012). Comorbid externalising behaviour in AD/HD: Evidence for a distinct pathological entity in adolescence. *PLoS ONE*, 7(9).

Perfetti, B., Saggino, A., Ferretti, A., Caulo, M., Romani, G. L., & Onofrj, M. (2009). Differential patterns of cortical activation as a function of fluid reasoning complexity. *Human Brain Mapping*, 30(2), 497–510. doi: 10.1002/hbm.20519

Perna, R., Loughan, A. R., & Talka, K. (2012). Executive functioning and adaptive living skills after acquired brain injury. *Applied Neuropsychology: Adult*, 19(4), 263–271. doi: 10.1080/09084282.2012.670147

Peskine, A., Rosso, C., Picq, C., Caron, E., & Pradat-Diehl, P. (2010). Neurological sequelae after cerebral anoxia. *Brain Injury*, 24(5), 755–761.

Pessoa, L. (2009). How do emotion and motivation direct executive control? *Trends in Cognitive Sciences*, 13(4), 160–166.

Pettit, L. D., Bastin, M. E., Smith, C., Bak, T. H., Gillingwater, T. H., & Abrahams, S. (2013). Executive deficits, not processing speed relates to abnormalities in distinct prefrontal tracts in amyotrophic lateral sclerosis. *Brain: A Journal of Neurology*, 136(11), 3290–3304.

Pettit, L. D., McCarthy, M., Davenport, R., & Abrahams, S. (2013). Heterogeneity of letter fluency impairment and executive dysfunction in Parkinson's disease. *Journal of the International Neuropsychological Society*, 19(9), 986–994.

Pfeifer, J. H., & Dapretto, M. (2009). "Mirror, mirror, in my mind": Empathy, interpersonal competence, and the mirror neuron system. In J. Decety & W.

Ickes (Eds.), *The social neuroscience of empathy* (pp. 183–197). Cambridge, MA: MIT Press.

Phelps, E. A. (2004). Human emotion and memory: Interactions of the amygdala and hippocampal complex. *Current Opinion in Neurobiology, 14*(2), 198–202.

Phelps, E. A., Fiske, S. T., Kazdin, A. E., & Schacter, D. L. (2006). Emotion and cognition: Insights from studies of the human amygdala. *Annual review of psychology, 57,* 27–53.

Philipp, A. M., Weidner, R., Koch, I., & Fink, G. R. (2013). Differential roles of inferior frontal and inferior parietal cortex in task switching: Evidence from stimulus-categorization switching and response-modality switching. *Human Brain Mapping, 34*(8), 1910–1920.

Philippot, P., Kornreich, C., Blairy, S., Den Dulk, A., Le Bon, O., Streel, E., . . . Verbanck, P. (1999). Alcoholics' deficits in the decoding of emotional facial expression. *Alcoholism: Clinical and Experimental Research, 23*(6), 1031–1038.

Phillips, K. M., Jim, H. S., Small, B. J., Laronga, C., Andrykowski, M. A., & Jacobsen, P. B. (2012). Cognitive functioning after cancer treatment: A 3-year longitudinal comparison of breast cancer survivors treated with chemotherapy or radiation and noncancer controls. *Cancer, 118*(7), 1925–1932.

Pickup, G. J. (2008). Relationship between theory of mind and executive function in schizophrenia: A systematic review. *Psychopathology, 41*(4), 206–213.

Picton, T. W., Stuss, D. T., Shallice, T., Alexander, M. P., & Gillingham, S. (2006). Keeping time: Effects of focal frontal lesions. *Neuropsychologia, 44*(7), 1195–1209.

Pietrzak, R. H., Snyder, P. J., Jackson, C. E., Olver, J., Norman, T., Piskulic, D., & Maruff, P. (2009). Stability of cognitive impairment in chronic schizophrenia over brief and intermediate re-test intervals. *Human Psychopharmacology: Clinical and Experimental, 24*(2), 113–121.

Pihlajamäki, M., Tanila, H., Hänninen, T., Könönen, M., Laakso, M., Partanen, K., . . . Aronen, H. J. (2000). Verbal fluency activates the left medial temporal lobe: A functional magnetic resonance imaging study. *Annals of Neurology, 47*(4), 470–476.

Pineda, J. A., Moore, A. R., Elfenbeinand, H., & Cox, R. (2009). Hierarchically organized mirroring processes in social cognition: The functional neuroanatomy of empathy. In J. A. Pineda (Ed.), *Mirror neuron systems: The role of mirroring processes in social cognition* (pp. 135–160). Totowa, NJ: Humana Press.

Piovesana, A. M., Ross, S., Whittingham, K., Ware, R. S., & Boyd, R. N. (2015). Stability of executive functioning measures in 8–17-year-old children with unilateral cerebral palsy. *Clinical Neuropsychologist, 29*(1), 133–149. doi: 10.1080/13854046.2014.999125

Planche, V., Gibelin, M., Cregut, D., Pereira, B., & Clavelou, P. (2015). Cognitive impairment in a population-based study of patients with multiple sclerosis: Differences between late relapsing-remitting, secondary progressive and primary progressive multiple sclerosis. *European Journal of Neurology.* doi: 10.1111/ene.12715

Plessow, F., Kiesel, A., Petzold, A., & Kirschbaum, C. (2011). Chronic sleep curtailment impairs the flexible implementation of task goals in new parents. *Journal of Sleep Research, 20*(2), 279–287.

Pocheptsova, A., Amir, O., Dhar, R., & Baumeister, R. F. (2009). Deciding without resources: Resource depletion and choice in context. *Journal of Marketing Research, 46*(3), 344–355.

Polak, A. R., Witteveen, A. B., Reitsma, J. B., & Olff, M. (2012). The role of executive function in posttraumatic stress disorder: A systematic review. *Journal of Affective Disorders, 141*(1), 11–21.

Pollatos, O., Gramann, K., & Schandry, R. (2007). Neural systems connecting interoceptive awareness and feelings. *Human Brain Mapping, 28*(1), 9–18.

Pollatos, O., Kirsch, W., & Schandry, R. (2005). On the relationship between interoceptive awareness, emotional experience, and brain processes. *Cognitive Brain Research, 25*(3), 948–962.

Polyakova, M., Sonnabend, N., Sander, C., Mergl, R., Schroeter, M. L., Schroeder, J., & Schönknecht, P. (2014). Prevalence of minor depression in elderly persons with and without mild cognitive impairment: A systematic review. *Journal of Affective Disorders, 152–154,* 28–38.

Porcelli, P., Guidi, J., Sirri, L., Grandi, S., Grassi, L., Ottolini, F., . . . Fava, G. A. (2013). Alexithymia in the medically ill: Analysis of 1190 patients in gastroenterology, cardiology, oncology and dermatology. *General Hospital Psychiatry, 35*(5), 521–527.

Porter, S. S., Hopkins, R. O., Weaver, L. K., Bigler, E. D., & Blatter, D. D. (2002). Corpus callosum atrophy and neuropsychological outcome following carbon monoxide poisoning. *Archives of Clinical Neuropsychology, 17*(2), 195–204.

Porto, C. S., Caramelli, P., & Nitrini, R. (2007). The Dementia Rating Scale (DRS) in the diagnosis of vascular dementia. *Dementia and Neuropsychologia, 1*(3), 282–287.

Power, B. D., Dragović, M., & Rock, D. (2013). Clusters according to patient need in a long-stay inpatient population with schizophrenia: Does executive dysfunction underpin needs-directed care? *Social Psychiatry and Psychiatric Epidemiology*, 48(4), 621–630.

Prehn, K., Schulze, L., Rossmann, S., Berger, C., Vohs, K., Fleischer, M., . . . Herpertz, S. C. (2013). Effects of emotional stimuli on working memory processes in male criminal offenders with borderline and antisocial personality disorder. *World Journal of Biological Psychiatry*, 14(1), 71–78.

Premack, D., & Woodruff, G. (1978). Does the chimpanzee have a theory of mind? *Behavioral and Brain Sciences*, 1(4), 515–526.

Premkumar, P., Fannon, D., Kuipers, E., Simmons, A., Frangou, S., & Kumari, V. (2008). Emotional decision-making and its dissociable components in schizophrenia and schizoaffective disorder: A behavioural and MRI investigation. *Neuropsychologia*, 46(7), 2002–2012.

Preobrazhenskaya, I. S., Mkhitaryan, É. A., & Yakhno, N. N. (2006). Comparative analysis of cognitive impairments in Lewy body dementia and Alzheimer's disease. *Neuroscience and Behavioral Physiology*, 36(1), 1–6.

Pribram, K. H. (1973). The primate frontal cortex: Executive of the brain. In K. H. Pribram & A. R. Luria (Eds.), *Psychophysiology of the frontal lobes*. Oxford, England: Academic Press.

Prigatano, G. P. (2005). Disturbances of self-awareness and rehabilitation of patients with traumatic brain injury: A 20-year perspective. *Journal of Head Trauma Rehabilitation*, 20(1), 19–29.

Prohl, J., Bodenburg, S., & Rustenbach, S. J. (2009). Early prediction of long-term cognitive impairment after cardiac arrest. *Journal of the International Neuropsychological Society*, 15(3), 344–353.

Puente, A. N., Lindbergh, C. A., & Miller, L. S. (2015). The relationship between cognitive reserve and functional ability is mediated by executive functioning in older adults. *Clinical Neuropsychologist*, 29(1), 67–81.

Pulsipher, D. T., Stricker, N. H., Sadek, J. R., & Haaland, K. Y. (2013). Clinical utility of the Neuropsychological Assessment Battery (NAB) after unilateral stroke. *Clinical Neuropsychologist*, 27(6), 924–945. doi: 10.1080/13854046.2013.799714

Quattrocchi, G., & Bestmann, S. (2014). Possible role of the basal ganglia in poor reward sensitivity and apathy after stroke. *Neurology*, 82(20), e171–e173.

Quinn, C., Elman, L., McCluskey, L., Hoskins, K., Karam, C., Woo, J. H., . . . Grossman, M. (2012). Frontal lobe abnormalities on MRS correlate with poor letter fluency in ALS. *Neurology*, 79(6), 583–588.

Radice-Neumann, D., Zupan, B., Babbage, D. R., & Willer, B. (2007). Overview of impaired facial affect recognition in persons with traumatic brain injury. *Brain Injury, 21*(8), 807–816.

Raffard, S., & Bayard, S. (2012). Understanding the executive functioning heterogeneity in schizophrenia. *Brain and Cognition, 79*(1), 60–69.

Rahmani, M., Bennani, M., Benabdeljlil, M., Aidi, S., Jiddane, M., Chkili, T., & Faris, M. E. A. (2006). Troubles cognitifs dus à l'intoxication oxycarbonée: Étude neuropsychologique et IRM de 5 cas [Neuropsychological and magnetic resonance imaging findings in five patients after carbon monoxide poisoning]. *Revue Neurologique, 162*(12), 1240–1247.

Rajendran, G., Law, A. S., Logie, R. H., van der Meulen, M., Fraser, D., & Corley, M. (2011). Investigating multitasking in high-functioning adolescents with autism spectrum disorders using the Virtual Errands Task. *Journal of Autism and Developmental Disorders, 41*(11), 1445–1454.

Rajeswaran, J., & Nalini, A. (2013). Neuropsychological deficits in amyotrophic lateral sclerosis (ALS): A South India experience. *Neuropsychological Trends, 13*, 47–58.

Rajji, T. K., & Mulsant, B. H. (2008). Nature and course of cognitive function in late-life schizophrenia: A systematic review. *Schizophrenia Research, 102*(1–3), 122–140.

Randolph, J. J., Arnett, P. A., & Freske, P. (2004). Metamemory in multiple sclerosis: Exploring affective and executive contributors. *Archives of Clinical Neuropsychology, 19*(2), 259–279.

Rankin, K. P., Baldwin, E., Pace-Savitsky, C., Kramer, J. H., & Miller, B. L. (2005). Self awareness and personality change in dementia. *Journal of Neurology, Neurosurgery and Psychiatry, 76*(5), 632–639.

Rankin, K. P., Kramer, J. H., & Miller, B. L. (2005). Patterns of cognitive and emotional empathy in frontotemporal lobar degeneration. *Cognitive and Behavioral Neurology, 18*(1), 28–36.

Rankin, K. P., Santos-Modesitt, W., Kramer, J. H., Pavlic, D., Beckman, V., & Miller, B. L. (2008). Spontaneous social behaviors discriminate behavioral dementias from psychiatric disorders and other dementias. *Journal of Clinical Psychiatry, 69*(1), 60–73.

Rapp, M. A., Beeri, M. S., Schmeidler, J., Sano, M., Silverman, J. M., & Haroutunian, V. (2005). Relationship of neuropsychological performance to functional status in nursing home residents and community-dwelling older adults. *American Journal of Geriatric Psychiatry, 13*(6), 450–459.

Rascovsky, K., Salmon, D. P., Hansen, L. A., Thal, L. J., & Galasko, D. (2007). Disparate letter and semantic category fluency deficits in autopsy-confirmed frontotemporal dementia and Alzheimer's disease. *Neuropsychology, 21*(1), 20–30.

Reader, S. M., & Laland, K. N. (2002). Social intelligence, innovation, and enhanced brain size in primates. *Proceedings of the National Academy of Sciences, 99*(7), 4436–4441.

Reed, B. R., Eberling, J. L., Mungas, D., Weiner, M., Kramer, J. H., & Jagust, W. J. (2004). Effects of white matter lesions and lacunes on cortical function. *Archives of Neurology, 61*(10), 1545–1550.

Reed, R. A., Harrow, M., Herbener, E. S., & Martin, E. M. (2002). Executive function in schizophrenia: Is it linked to psychosis and poor life functioning? *Journal of Nervous and Mental Disease, 190*(11), 725–732.

Renison, B., Ponsford, J., Testa, R., Richardson, B., & Brownfield, K. (2012). The ecological and construct validity of a newly developed measure of executive function: The Virtual Library Task. *Journal of the International Neuropsychological Society, 18*(3), 440–450. doi: 10.1017/s1355617711001883

Rhodes, S. M., Riby, D. M., Park, J., Fraser, E., & Campbell, L. E. (2010). Executive neuropsychological functioning in individuals with Williams syndrome. *Neuropsychologia, 48*(5), 1216–1226. doi: 10.1016/j.neuropsychologia.2009.12.021

Ridderinkhof, K. R., van den Wildenberg, W. P. M., Segalowitz, S. J., & Carter, C. S. (2004). Neurocognitive mechanisms of cognitive control: The role of prefrontal cortex in action selection, response inhibition, performance monitoring, and reward-based learning. *Brain and Cognition, 56*(2), 129–140. doi: 10.1016/j.bandc.2004.09.016

Ridler, K., Veijola, J. M., Tanskanen, P., Miettunen, J., Chitnis, X., Suckling, J., . . . Bullmore, E. T. (2006). Fronto-cerebellar systems are associated with infant motor and adult executive functions in healthy adults but not in schizophrenia. *Proceedings of the National Academy of Sciences of the United States of America, 103*(42), 15651–15656.

Riesel, A., Endrass, T., Kaufmann, C., & Kathmann, N. (2011). Overactive error-related brain activity as a candidate endophenotype for obsessive-compulsive disorder: Evidence from unaffected first-degree relatives. *American Journal of Psychiatry, 168*(3), 317–324.

Rinehart, N. J., Cornish, K. M., & Tonge, B. J. (2011). Gender differences in neurodevelopmental disorders: Autism and fragile X syndrome. In J. C. Neill & J. Kulkarni (Eds.), *Biological basis of sex differences in psychopharmacology* (Vol. 8, pp. 209–229). New York, NY: Springer-Verlag.

Ringholz, G. M., Appel, S. H., Bradshaw, M., Cooke, N. A., Mosnik, D. M., & Schulz, P. E. (2005). Prevalence and patterns of cognitive impairment in sporadic ALS. *Neurology, 65*(4), 586–590.

Rippon, G. A., Scarmeas, N., Gordon, P. H., Murphy, P. L., Albert, S. M., Mitsumoto, H., . . . Stern, Y. (2006). An observational study of cognitive impairment in amyotrophic lateral sclerosis. *Archives of Neurology, 63*(3), 345–352.

Risse, G. L. (2006). Cognitive outcomes in patients with frontal lobe epilepsy. *Epilepsia, 47*(Suppl. 2), 87–89.

Rissman, B. (2011). Nonverbal learning disability explained: The link to shunted hydrocephalus. *British Journal of Learning Disabilities, 39*(3), 209–215.

Ritchie, K., & Lovestone, S. (2002). The dementias. *Lancet, 360*(9347), 1767–1769.

Rizzolatti, G., & Craighero, L. (2004). The mirror-neuron system. *Annual Review of Neuroscience, 27*, 169–192.

Rizzolatti, G., Craighero, L., & Fadiga, L. (2002). The mirror system in humans. In M. I. Stamenov & V. Gallese (Eds.), *Mirror neurons and the evolution of brain and language* (pp. 37–59). Amsterdam, Netherlands: John Benjamins.

Robinson, G., Shallice, T., Bozzali, M., & Cipolotti, L. (2012). The differing roles of the frontal cortex in fluency tests. *Brain: A Journal of Neurology, 135*(7), 2202–2214.

Robinson, S., Goddard, L., Dritschel, B., Wisley, M., & Howlin, P. (2009). Executive functions in children with autism spectrum disorders. *Brain and Cognition, 71*(3), 362–368. doi: 10.1016/j.bandc.2009.06.007

Robinson, T. E., & Berridge, K. C. (2000). The psychology and neurobiology of addiction: An incentive-sensitization view. *Addiction, 95*, S91–S117.

Roca, M., Manes, F., Gleichgerrcht, E., Watson, P., Ibáñez, A., Thompson, R., . . . Duncan, J. (2013). Intelligence and executive functions in frontotemporal dementia. *Neuropsychologia, 51*(4), 725–730.

Roca, M., Torralva, T., Gleichgerrcht, E., Woolgar, A., Thompson, R., Duncan, J., & Manes, F. (2011). The role of Area 10 (BA10) in human multitasking and in social cognition: A lesion study. *Neuropsychologia, 49*(13), 3525–3531.

Rochat, L., Beni, C., Annoni, J.-M., Vuadens, P., & Van der Linden, M. (2013). How inhibition relates to impulsivity after moderate to severe traumatic brain injury. *Journal of the International Neuropsychological Society, 19*(8), 890–898.

Rochat, L., Beni, C., Billieux, J., Annoni, J.-M., & Van der Linden, M. (2011). How impulsivity relates to compulsive buying and the burden perceived by caregivers after moderate-to-severe traumatic brain injury. *Psychopathology*, 44(3), 158–164.

Rochat, L., Van der Linden, M., Renaud, O., Epiney, J.-B., Michel, P., Sztajzel, R., . . . Annoni, J.-M. (2013). Poor reward sensitivity and apathy after stroke: Implication of basal ganglia. *Neurology*, 81(19), 1674–1680.

Roebuck-Spencer, T., & Sherer, M. (2008). Moderate and severe traumatic brain injury. In J. E. Morgan & J. H. Ricker (Eds.), *Textbook of clinical neuropsychology* (pp. 411–429). New York, NY: Psychology Press.

Roehrs, T., Merrion, M., Pedrosi, B., & Stepanski, E. (1995). Neuropsychological function in obstructive sleep apnea (OSAS) compared to chronic obstructive pulmonary disease (COPD). *Sleep: Journal of Sleep Research and Sleep Medicine*, 18(5), 382–388.

Roessner, V., Albrecht, B., Dechent, P., Baudewig, J., & Roethenberger, A. (2008). A normal response inhibition in boys with Tourette syndrome. *Behavioral and Brain Functions*, 4, 1–4.

Rog, L. A., Park, L. Q., Harvey, D. J., Huang, C.-J., Mackin, S., & Farias, S. T. (2014). The independent contributions of cognitive impairment and neuropsychiatric symptoms to everyday function in older adults. *Clinical Neuropsychologist*, 28(2), 215–236. doi: 10.1080/13854046.2013.876101

Roger, C., Núñez Castellar, E., Pourtois, G., & Fias, W. (2014). Changing your mind before it is too late: The electrophysiological correlates of online error correction during response selection. *Psychophysiology*, 51(8), 746–760.

Rolls, E. T. (2004). The functions of the orbitofrontal cortex. *Brain and Cognition*, 55(1), 11–29.

Romine, C. B., Lee, D., Wolfe, M. E., Homack, S., George, C., & Riccio, C. A. (2004). Wisconsin Card Sorting Test with children: A meta-analytic study of sensitivity and specificity. *Archives of Clinical Neuropsychology*, 19(8), 1027–1041. doi: 10.1016/j.acn.2003.12.009

Roodenrys, S. (2006). Working memory function in attention deficit hyperactivity disorder. In T. P. Alloway & S. E. Gathercole (Eds.), *Working memory and neurodevelopmental disorders* (pp. 187–211). New York, NY: Psychology Press.

Rosen, H. J., Alcantar, O., Zakrzewski, J., Shimamura, A. P., Neuhaus, J., & Miller, B. L. (2014). Metacognition in the behavioral variant of frontotemporal dementia and Alzheimer's disease. *Neuropsychology*, 28(3), 436–447.

Rosenthal, M., Wallace, G. L., Lawson, R., Wills, M. C., Dixon, E., Yerys, B. E., & Kenworthy, L. (2013). Impairments in real-world executive function increase from childhood to adolescence in autism spectrum disorders. *Neuropsychology*, 27(1), 13–18. doi: 10.1037/a0031299

Ross, E. D., & Mesulam, M. M. (2000). Affective prosody and the aprosodias. In M. M. Mesulam (Ed.), *Principles of behavioral and cognitive neurology* (2nd ed., pp. 316–331). New York, NY: Oxford University Press.

Rossetti, Y., & Pisella, L. (2003). Mediate responses as direct evidence for intention: Neuropsychology of not-to, not-now, and not-there tasks. In S. H. Johnson-Frey (Ed.), *Taking action: Cognitive neuroscience perspectives on intentional acts* (pp. 67–105). Cambridge, MA: MIT Press.

Rossetti, Y., Revol, P., McIntosh, R., Pisella, L., Rode, G., Danckert, J., . . . Milner, A. D. (2005). Visually guided reaching: Bilateral posterior parietal lesions cause a switch from fast visuomotor to slow cognitive control. *Neuropsychologia, 43*(2), 162–177.

Roszyk, A., Izdebska, A., & Peichert, K. (2013). Planning and inhibitory abilities in criminals with antisocial personality disorder. *Acta Neuropsychologica, 11*(2), 193–205.

Roth, R. M., Baribeau, J., Milovan, D. L., & O'Connor, K. (2004). Speed and accuracy on tests of executive function in obsessive-compulsive disorder. *Brain and Cognition, 54*(3), 263–265.

Rottschy, C., Langner, R., Dogan, I., Reetz, K., Laird, A. R., Schulz, J. B., . . . Eickhoff, S. B. (2012). Modelling neural correlates of working memory: A coordinate-based meta-analysis. *Neuroimage, 60*(1), 830–846.

Royall, D. R., & Mahurin, R. K. (1996). Neuroanatomy, measurement, and clinical significance of the executive cognitive functions. *American Psychiatric Press Review of Psychiatry, 15,* 175–204.

Royer, A., Schneider, F. C. G., Grosselin, A., Pellet, J., Barral, F.-G., Laurent, B., . . . Lang, F. (2009). Brain activation during executive processes in schizophrenia. *Psychiatry Research: Neuroimaging, 173*(3), 170–176.

Rozen, T. D. (2012). Rapid resolution of akinetic mutism in delayed posthypoxic leukoencephalopathy with intravenous magnesium sulfate. *NeuroRehabilitation, 30*(4), 329–332.

Ruchsow, M., Grön, G., Reuter, K., Spitzer, M., Hermle, L., & Kiefer, M. (2005). Error-related brain activity in patients with obsessive-compulsive disorder and in healthy controls. *Journal of Psychophysiology, 19*(4), 298–304.

Ruet, A., Deloire, M., Charré-Morin, J., Hamel, D., & Brochet, B. (2013). Cognitive impairment differs between primary progressive and relapsing-remitting MS. *Neurology, 80*(16), 1501–1508.

Ruff, R. (2005). Two decades of advances in understanding of mild traumatic brain injury. *Journal of Head Trauma Rehabilitation, 20*(1), 5–18.

Ruffin, H. (1939). Stirnhirnsymptomatologie und Stirnhirnsyndrome [Frontal lobe symptomatology and frontal lobe syndrome]. *Fortschritte der Neurologie und Psychiatrie*, *11*, 34–52.

Ruitenberg, M. F. L., Verwey, W. B., Schutter, D. J. L. G., & Abrahamse, E. L. (2014). Cognitive and neural foundations of discrete sequence skill: A TMS study. *Neuropsychologia*, *56*, 229–238.

Rüsch, N., Spoletini, I., Wilke, M., Bria, P., Di Paola, M., Di Iulio, F., . . . Spalletta, G. (2007). Prefrontal-thalamic-cerebellar gray matter networks and executive functioning in schizophrenia. *Schizophrenia Research*, *93*(1–3), 79–89.

Rüsch, N., van Elst, L. T., Valerius, G., Büchert, M., Thiel, T., Ebert, D., . . . Olbrich, H.-M. (2008). Neurochemical and structural correlates of executive dysfunction in schizophrenia. *Schizophrenia Research*, *99*(1–3), 155–163.

Rushworth, M. F. S., Passingham, R. E., & Nobre, A. C. (2005). Components of attentional set-switching. *Experimental Psychology*, *52*(2), 83–98.

Russell, W. R. (1948). Functions of the frontal lobes. *Lancet*, *251*, 356–360.

Sachse, M., Schlitt, S., Hainz, D., Ciaramidaro, A., Schirman, S., Walter, H., . . . Freitag, C. M. (2013). Executive and visuo-motor function in adolescents and adults with autism spectrum disorder. *Journal of Autism and Developmental Disorders*, *43*(5), 1222–1235. doi: 10.1007/s10803-012-1668-8

Saddichha, S., & Schuetz, C. (2014). Is impulsivity in remitted bipolar disorder a stable trait? A meta-analytic review. *Comprehensive Psychiatry*, *55*(7), 1479–1484.

Salamone, J. D., Correa, M., Farrar, A., & Mingote, S. M. (2007). Effort-related functions of nucleus accumbens dopamine and associated forebrain circuits. *Psychopharmacology*, *191*(3), 461–482.

Salamone, J. D., Cousins, M. S., & Snyder, B. J. (1997). Behavioral functions of nucleus accumbens dopamine: Empirical and conceptual problems with the anhedonia hypothesis. *Neuroscience and Biobehavioral Reviews*, *21*(3), 341–359.

Samson, A. C., Hempelmann, C. F., Huber, O., & Zysset, S. (2009). Neural substrates of incongruity-resolution and nonsense humor. *Neuropsychologia*, *47*(4), 1023–1033.

Samuelson, H., Nekludov, M., & Levander, M. (2008). Neuropsychological outcome following near-drowning in ice water: Two adult case studies. *Journal of the International Neuropsychological Society*, *14*(4), 660–666.

Sánchez-Torres, A. M., Basterra, V., Moreno-Izco, L., Rosa, A., Fañanás, L., Zarzuela, A., . . . Cuesta, M. J. (2013). Executive functioning in schizophrenia spectrum disorder patients and their unaffected siblings: A ten-year follow-up study. *Schizophrenia Research, 143*(2–3), 291–296.

Sandson, J., & Albert, M. L. (1984). Varieties of perseveration. *Neuropsychologia, 22*(6), 715–732.

Santangelo, V., & Macaluso, E. (2013). The contribution of working memory to divided attention. *Human Brain Mapping, 34*(1), 158–175.

Santos, M., Uppal, N., Butti, C., Wicinski, B., Schmeidler, J., Giannakopoulos, P., . . . Hof, P. R. (2011). Von Economo neurons in autism: A stereologic study of the frontoinsular cortex in children. *Brain Research, 1380*, 206–217.

Sanz, J. C., Gómez, V., Vargas, M. L., & Marín, J. J. (2012). Dimensions of attention impairment and negative symptoms in schizophrenia: A multidimensional approach using the Conners Continuous Performance Test in a Spanish population. *Cognitive and Behavioral Neurology, 25*(2), 63–71.

Satoh, K., Shirabe, S., Eguchi, H., Tsujino, A., Motomura, M., Satoh, A., . . . Eguchi, K. (2007). Chronological changes in MRI and CSF biochemical markers in Creutzfeldt-Jakob disease patients. *Dementia and Geriatric Cognitive Disorders, 23*(6), 372–381.

Saunamäki, T., & Jehkonen, M. (2007). A review of executive functions in obstructive sleep apnea syndrome. *Acta Neurologica Scandinavica, 115*(1), 1–11.

Savla, G. N., Twamley, E. W., Thompson, W. K., Delis, D. C., Jeste, D. V., & Palmer, B. W. (2011). Evaluation of specific executive functioning skills and the processes underlying executive control in schizophrenia. *Journal of the International Neuropsychological Society, 17*(1), 14–23.

Schacter, D. L. (2012). Adaptive constructive processes and the future of memory. *American Psychologist, 67*(8), 603–613.

Schacter, D. L., Benoit, R. G., De Brigard, F., & Szpunar, K. K. (2013). Episodic future thinking and episodic counterfactual thinking: Intersections between memory and decisions. *Neurobiology of Learning and Memory, 117*, 14–21.

Schenker, R., Coster, W. J., & Parush, S. (2005). Neuroimpairments, activity performance, and participation in children with cerebral palsy mainstreamed in elementary schools. *Developmental Medicine and Child Neurology, 47*(12), 808–814.

Scherder, E. J. A., Eggermont, L., Plooij, B., Oudshoorn, J., Vuijk, P. J., Pickering, G., . . . Oosterman, J. (2008). Relationship between chronic pain and cognition in cognitively intact older persons and in patients with Alzheimer's disease: The need to control for mood. *Gerontology, 54*(1), 50–58.

Schlund, M. W., Magee, S., & Hudgins, C. D. (2012). Dynamic brain mapping of behavior change: Tracking response initiation and inhibition to changes in reinforcement rate. *Behavioural Brain Research*, 234(2), 205–211.

Schmeichel, B. J., Vohs, K. D., & Baumeister, R. F. (2003). Intellectual performance and ego depletion: Role of the self in logical reasoning and other information processing. *Journal of Personality and Social Psychology*, 85(1), 33–46.

Schmeichel, B. J., Volokhov, R. N., & Demaree, H. A. (2008). Working memory capacity and the self-regulation of emotional expression and experience. *Journal of Personality and Social Psychology*, 95(6), 1526–1540.

Schmeichel, B. J., & Zell, A. (2007). Trait self-control predicts performance on behavioral tests of self-control. *Journal of Personality*, 75(4), 743–755.

Schmitter-Edgecombe, M., McAlister, C., & Weakley, A. (2012). Naturalistic assessment of everyday functioning in individuals with mild cognitive impairment: The day-out task. *Neuropsychology*, 26(5), 631–641. doi: 10.1037/a0029352.supp (Supplemental)

Schoemaker, K., Mulder, H., Deković, M., & Matthys, W. (2013). Executive functions in preschool children with externalizing behavior problems: A meta-analysis. *Journal of Abnormal Child Psychology*, 41(3), 457–471.

Schretlen, D. J., & Shapiro, A. M. (2003). A quantitative review of the effects of traumatic brain injury on cognitive functioning. *International Review of Psychiatry*, 15(4), 341–349.

Schurr, A. (2002). Energy metabolism, stress hormones and neural recovery from cerebral ischemia/hypoxia. *Neurochemistry International*, 41(1), 1–8.

Scott, J. C., Woods, S. P., Vigil, O., Heaton, R. K., Schweinsburg, B. C., Ellis, R. J., . . . Marcotte, T. D. (2011). A neuropsychological investigation of multitasking in HIV infection: Implications for everyday functioning. *Neuropsychology*, 25(4), 511–519.

Scott, T. F., Lang, D., Girgis, R. M., & Price, T. (1995). Prolonged akinetic mutism due to multiple sclerosis. *Journal of Neuropsychiatry and Clinical Neurosciences*, 7(1), 90–92.

Seeley, W. W., Allman, J. M., Carlin, D. A., Crawford, R. K., Macedo, M. N., Greicius, M. D., . . . Miller, B. L. (2007). Divergent social functioning in behavioral variant frontotemporal dementia and Alzheimer disease: Reciprocal networks and neuronal evolution. *Alzheimer Disease and Associated Disorders*, 21(4), S50–S57.

Seeley, W. W., Carlin, D. A., Allman, J. M., Macedo, M. N., Bush, C., Miller, B. L., & DeArmond, S. J. (2006). Early frontotemporal dementia targets neurons unique to apes and humans. *Annals of Neurology*, 60(6), 660–667.

Seeley, W. W., Merkle, F. T., Gaus, S. E., Craig, A. D., Allman, J. M., & Hof, P. R. (2012). Distinctive neurons of the anterior cingulate and frontoinsular cortex: A historical perspective. *Cerebral Cortex, 22*(2), 245–250.

Segarra, N., Bernardo, M., Valdes, M., Caldu, X., Falcón, C., Rami, L., . . . Junque, C. (2008). Cerebellar deficits in schizophrenia are associated with executive dysfunction. *NeuroReport: For Rapid Communication of Neuroscience Research, 19*(15), 1513–1517.

Semkovska, M., & McLoughlin, D. M. (2010). Objective cognitive performance associated with electroconvulsive therapy for depression: A systematic review and meta-analysis. *Biological Psychiatry, 68*(6), 568–577.

Semrud-Clikeman, M., Fine, J. G., & Bledsoe, J. (2014). Comparison among children with children with autism spectrum disorder, nonverbal learning disorder and typically developing children on measures of executive functioning. *Journal of Autism and Developmental Disorders, 44*(2), 331–342. doi: 10.1007/s10803-013-1871-2

Semrud-Clikeman, M., Walkowiak, J., Wilkinson, A., & Butcher, B. (2010). Executive functioning in children with Asperger syndrome, ADHD-combined type, ADHD-predominately inattentive type, and controls. *Journal of Autism and Developmental Disorders, 40*(8), 1017–1027. doi: 10.1007/s10803-010-0951-9

Seo, S. W., Jung, K., You, H., Lee, B. H., Kim, G.-M., Chung, C.-S., . . . Na, D. L. (2009). Motor-intentional disorders in right hemisphere stroke. *Cognitive and Behavioral Neurology, 22*(4), 242–248.

Serrien, D. J., & Sovijärvi-Spapé, M. M. (2013). Cognitive control of response inhibition and switching: Hemispheric lateralization and hand preference. *Brain and Cognition, 82*(3), 283–290.

Sgaramella, T. M., Carrieri, L., & Barone, C. (2012). A screening battery for the assessment of executive functioning in young and adult individuals with intellectual disability. *International Journal on Disability and Human Development, 11*(1), 31–37. doi: 10.1515/ijdhd.2012.013

Shah, K., Qureshi, S. U., Johnson, M., Parikh, N., Schulz, P. E., & Kunik, M. E. (2009). Does use of antihypertensive drugs affect the incidence or progression of dementia? A systematic review. *American Journal of Geriatric Pharmacotherapy, 7*(5), 250–261.

Shallice, T. (1990). *From neuropsychology to mental structure*. New York, NY: Oxford University Press.

Shallice, T., & Burgess, P. W. (1991a). Deficits in strategy application following fronal lobe damage in man. *Brain, 114*, 727–741.

Shallice, T., & Burgess, P. W. (1991b). Higher-order cognitive impairments and frontal lobe lesions in man. In H. S. Levin, H. M. Eisenberg, & A. L. Benton (Eds.), *Frontal lobe function and dysfunction* (pp. 125–138). New York, NY: Oxford University Press.

Shamay-Tsoory, S. G., Aharon-Peretz, J., & Perry, D. (2009). Two systems for empathy: A double dissociation between emotional and cognitive empathy in inferior frontal gyrus versus ventromedial prefrontal lesions. *Brain: A Journal of Neurology, 132*(3), 617–627.

Shamay-Tsoory, S. G., Shur, S., Harari, H., & Levkovitz, Y. (2007). Neurocognitive basis of impaired empathy in schizophrenia. *Neuropsychology, 21*(4), 431–438.

Shamay-Tsoory, S. G., Tomer, R., Berger, B. D., & Aharon-Peretz, J. (2003). Characterization of empathy deficits following prefrontal brain damage: The role of the right ventromedial prefrontal cortex. *Journal of Cognitive Neuroscience, 15*(3), 324–337.

Shamay-Tsoory, S. G., Tomer, R., Goldsher, D., Berger, B. D., & Aharon-Peretz, J. (2004). Impairment in cognitive and affective empathy in patients with brain lesions: Anatomical and cognitive correlates. *Journal of Clinical and Experimental Neuropsychology, 26*(8), 1113–1127.

Shamay-Tsoory, S. G., Tomer, R., Yaniv, S., & Aharon-Peretz, J. (2002). Empathy deficits in Asperger syndrome: A cognitive profile. *Neurocase, 8*(3), 245–252.

Shankman, S. A., Nelson, B. D., Sarapas, C., Robison-Andrew, E. J., Campbell, M. L., Altman, S. E., . . . Gorka, S. M. (2013). A psychophysiological investigation of threat and reward sensitivity in individuals with panic disorder and/or major depressive disorder. *Journal of Abnormal Psychology, 122*(2), 322–338.

Sherer, M., Nick, T. G., Millis, S. R., & Novack, T. A. (2003). Use of the WCST and the WCST-64 in the assessment of traumatic brain injury. *Journal of Clinical and Experimental Neuropsychology, 25*(4), 512–520.

Shimamura, A. P. (2002). Memory retrieval and executive control processes. In D. T. Stuss & R. T. Knight (Eds.), *Principles of frontal lobe function* (pp. 210–220). New York, NY: Oxford University Press.

Shimamura, A. P. (2011). Episodic retrieval and the cortical binding of relational activity. *Cognitive, Affective and Behavioral Neuroscience, 11*(3), 277–291.

Shimamura, A. P., Stuss, D. T., & Knight, R. T. (2002). Memory retrieval and executive control processes. In D. T. Stuss & R. T. Knight (Eds.), *Principles of frontal lobe function* (pp. 210–220). New York, NY: Oxford University Press.

Shprecher, D., & Mehta, L. (2010). The syndrome of delayed post-hypoxic leukoencephalopathy. *NeuroRehabilitation, 26*(1), 65–72.

Shum, D., Levin, H., & Chan, R. C. K. (2011). Prospective memory in patients with closed head injury: A review. *Neuropsychologia, 49*(8), 2156–2165.

Siebert, M., Markowitsch, H. J., & Bartel, P. (2003). Amygdala, affect and cognition: Evidence from 10 patients with Urbach-Wiethe disease. *Brain: A Journal of Neurology, 126*(12), 2627–2637.

Sierra-Hidalgo, F., Martínez-Salio, A., Moreno-García, S., de Pablo-Fernández, E., Correas-Callero, E., & Ruiz-Morales, J. (2009). Akinetic mutism induced by tacrolimus. *Clinical Neuropharmacology, 32*(5), 293–294.

Siklos, S., & Kerns, K. A. (2004). Assessing multitasking in children with ADHD using a modified Six Elements Test. *Archives of Clinical Neuropsychology, 19*(3), 347–361.

Silva Neto, Â. R., Brandão Câmara, R. L., & Valença, M. M. (2012). Carotid siphon geometry and variants of the circle of Willis in the origin of carotid aneurysms. *Arquivos de Neuro-Psiquiatria, 70*(12), 917–921.

Silver, H., & Goodman, C. (2007). Impairment in error monitoring predicts poor executive function in schizophrenia patients. *Schizophrenia Research, 94*(1–3), 156–163.

Silvestrini, N., & Rainville, P. (2013). After-effects of cognitive control on pain. *European Journal of Pain, 17*(8), 1225–1233.

Silvia, P. J., Kelly, C. S., Zibaie, A., Nardello, J. L., & Moore, L. C. (2013). Trait self-focused attention increases sensitivity to nonconscious primes: Evidence from effort-related cardiovascular reactivity. *International Journal of Psychophysiology, 88*(2), 143–148.

Silvia, P. J., Nusbaum, E. C., Eddington, K. M., Beaty, R. E., & Kwapil, T. R. (2014). Effort deficits and depression: The influence of anhedonic depressive symptoms on cardiac autonomic activity during a mental challenge. *Motivation and Emotion, 38*(6), 779–789.

Simard, S., Rouleau, I., Brosseau, J., Laframboise, M., & Bojanowsky, M. (2003). Impact of executive dysfunctions on episodic memory abilities in patients with ruptured aneurysm of the anterior communicating artery. *Brain and Cognition, 53*(2), 354–358.

Simó, M., Rifà-Ros, X., Rodriguez-Fornells, A., & Bruna, J. (2013). Chemobrain: A systematic review of structural and functional neuroimaging studies. *Neuroscience and Biobehavioral Reviews, 37*(8), 1311–1321.

Simpson, G. K., Sabaz, M., & Daher, M. (2013). Prevalence, clinical features, and correlates of inappropriate sexual behavior after traumatic brain injury: A multicenter study. *Journal of Head Trauma Rehabilitation, 28*(3), 202–210.

Siri, C., Duerr, S., Canesi, M., Delazer, M., Esselink, R., Bloem, B. R., . . . Antonini, A. (2013). A cross-sectional multicenter study of cognitive and behavioural features in multiple system atrophy patients of the parkinsonian and cerebellar type. *Journal of Neural Transmission, 120*(4), 613–618.

Skuse, D. H., Morris, J. S., & Dolan, R. J. (2005). Functional dissociation of amygdala-modulated arousal and cognitive appraisal, in Turner syndrome. *Brain: A Journal of Neurology, 128*(9), 2084–2096.

Slawik, H., Salmond, C. H., Taylor-Tavares, J. V., Williams, G. B., Sahakian, B. J., & Tasker, R. C. (2009). Frontal cerebral vulnerability and executive deficits from raised intracranial pressure in child traumatic brain injury. *Journal of Neurotrauma, 26*(11), 1891–1903.

Smith, A. (2006). Cognitive empathy and emotional empathy in human behavior and evolution. *Psychological Record, 56*(1), 3–21.

Smith, A. B., Taylor, E., Brammer, M., Halari, R., & Rubia, K. (2008). Reduced activation in right lateral prefrontal cortex and anterior cingulate gyrus in medication-naïve adolescents with attention deficit hyperactivity disorder during time discrimination. *Journal of Child Psychology and Psychiatry, 49*(9), 977–985.

Smith, A. B., Taylor, E., Brammer, M., & Rubia, K. (2004). Neural correlates of switching set as measured in fast, event-related functional magnetic resonance imaging. *Human Brain Mapping, 21*(4), 247–256.

Smith, G. E., & Bondi, M. W. (2008). Normal aging, mild cognitive impairment, and Alzheimer's disease. In J. E. Morgan & J. H. Ricker (Eds.), *Textbook of clinical neuropsychology* (pp. 762–780). New York, NY: Psychology Press.

Smith, G. E., & Bondi, M. W. (2013). *Mild cognitive impairment and dementia*. New York, NY: Oxford University Press.

Smith, M. M., & Arnett, P. A. (2010). Awareness of executive functioning deficits in multiple sclerosis: Self versus informant ratings of impairment. *Journal of Clinical and Experimental Neuropsychology, 32*(7), 780–787.

Snowden, J. S. (2013). Neuropsychology of frontotemporal lobar degeneration: Frontotemporal dementia, semantic dementia and progressive non-fluent aphasia. In L. H. Goldstein & J. E. McNeil (Eds.), *Clinical neuropsychology: A practical guide to assessment and management for clinicians* (2nd ed., pp. 375–396). Hoboken, NJ: Wiley-Blackwell.

Snowden, J. S., Austin, N. A., Sembi, S., Thompson, J. C., Craufurd, D., & Neary, D. (2008). Emotion recognition in Huntington's disease and frontotemporal dementia. *Neuropsychologia, 46*(11), 2638–2649.

Soliveri, P., Monza, D., & Paridi, D. (1999). Cognitive and magnetic resonance imaging aspects of corticobasal degeneration and progressive supranuclear palsy. *Neurology, 53*(3), 502–507.

Soliveri, P., Monza, D., Paridi, D., Carella, F., Genitrini, S., Testa, D., & Girotti, F. (2000). Neuropsychological follow up in patients with Parkinson's disease, striatonigral degeneration-type multisystem atrophy, and progressive supranuclear palsy. *Journal of Neurology, Neurosurgery and Psychiatry, 69*(3), 313–318.

South, M. D., Ozonoff, S., Suchy, Y., Kesner, R. P., McMahon, W. M., & Lainhart, J. E. (2008). Intact emotion facilitation for non-social stimuli in autism: Is amygdala impairment in autism specific for social information? *Journal of the International Neuropsychological Society, 14*(1), 42–54.

Sowell, E. R., Mattson, S. N., Kan, E., Thompson, P. M., Riley, E. P., & Toga, A. W. (2008). Abnormal cortical thickness and brain-behavior correlation patterns in individuals with heavy prenatal alcohol exposure. *Cerebral Cortex, 18*(1), 136–144. doi: 10.1093/cercor/bhm039

Sparto, P. J., Aizenstein, H. J., VanSwearingen, J. M., Rosano, C., Perera, S., Studenski, S. A., . . . Redfern, M. S. (2008). Delays in auditory-cued step initiation are related to increased volume of white matter hyperintensities in older adults. *Experimental Brain Research, 188*(4), 633–640.

Spíndola, L., & Dozzi Brucki, S. M. (2011). Prospective memory in Alzheimer's disease and mild cognitive impairment. *Dementia and Neuropsychologia, 5*(2), 64–68.

Stablum, F., Umiltà, C., Mogentale, C., Carlan, M., & Guerrini, C. (2000). Rehabilitation of executive deficits in closed head injury and anterior communicating artery aneurysm patients. *Psychological Research, 63*(3–4), 265–278.

Staios, M., Fisher, F., Lindell, A. K., Ong, B., Howe, J., & Reardon, K. (2013). Exploring sarcasm detection in amyotrophic lateral sclerosis using ecologically valid measures. *Frontiers in Human Neuroscience, 7*(178) doi: 10.3389/fnhum.2013.00178.

Starr, J. M., & Lonie, J. (2008). Estimated pre-morbid IQ effects on cognitive and functional outcomes in Alzheimer disease: A longitudinal study in a treated cohort. *BMC Psychiatry, 8*(27), doi: 10.1186/1471-244x-8-27

Stautz, K., & Cooper, A. (2014). Brief report: Personality correlates of susceptibility to peer influence in adolescence. *Journal of Adolescence, 37*(4), 401–405. doi: 10.1016/j.adolescence.2014.03.006

Stavitsky, K., Neargarder, S., Bogdanova, Y., McNamara, P., & Cronin-Golomb, A. (2012). The impact of sleep quality on cognitive functioning in Parkinson's disease. *Journal of the International Neuropsychological Society, 18*(1), 108–117.

Stelmach, G. E., Teasdale, N., & Phillips, J. (1992). Response initiation delays in Parkinson's disease patients. *Human Movement Science*, *11*(1–2), 37–45.

Stelzel, C., Kraft, A., Brandt, S. A., & Schubert, T. (2008). Dissociable neural effects on task order control and task set maintenance during dual-task processing. *Journal of Cognitive Neuroscience*, *20*(4), 613–628.

Stone, L. A., & Nielson, K. A. (2001). Intact physiological responses to arousal with impaired emotional recognition in alexithymia. *Psychotherapy and Psychosomatics*, *70*(2), 92–102.

Stoodley, C. J. (2012). The cerebellum and cognition: Evidence from functional imaging studies. *Cerebellum*, *11*(2), 352–365.

Stordal, K. I., Lundervold, A. J., Egeland, J., Mykletun, A., Asbjørnsen, A., Landrø, N. I., . . . Lund, A. (2004). Impairment across executive functions in recurrent major depression. *Nordic Journal of Psychiatry*, *58*(1), 41–47.

Strauss, E., Sherman, E. M. S., & Spreen, O. (2006). *A compendium of neuropsychological tests*. New York: Oxford University Press.

Strong, M. J., Lomen-Hoerth, C., Caselli, R. J., Bigio, E. H., & Yang, W. (2003). Cognitive impairment, frontotemporal dementia, and the motor neuron diseases. *Annals of Neurology*, *54*(Suppl. 5), S20–S23.

Stucke, T. S., & Baumeister, R. F. (2006). Ego depletion and aggressive behavior: Is the inhibition of aggression a limited resource? *European Journal of Social Psychology*, *36*(1), 1–13.

Štukovnik, V., Zidar, J., Podnar, S., & Repovš, G. (2010). Amyotrophic lateral sclerosis patients show executive impairments on standard neuropsychological measures and an ecologically valid motor-free test of executive functions. *Journal of Clinical and Experimental Neuropsychology*, *32*(10), 1095–1109.

Stuss, D. T. (1992). Biological and psychological development of executive functions. *Brain and Cognition*, *20*(1), 8–23.

Stuss, D. T. (2007). New approaches to prefrontal lobe testing. In B. L. Miller & J. L. Cummings (Eds.), *The human frontal lobes: Functions and disorders.* (2nd ed., pp. 292–305). New York, NY: Guilford Press.

Stuss, D. T. (2011). Functions of the frontal lobes: Relation to executive functions. *Journal of the International Neuropsychological Society*, *17*(5), 759–765.

Stuss, D. T., & Alexander, M. P. (2000). Executive functions and the frontal lobes: A conceptual view. *Psychological Research/Psychologische Forschung*, *63*(3), 289–298.

Stuss, D. T., & Alexander, M. P. (2008). Is there a dysexecutive syndrome? In J. Driver, P. Haggard, & T. Shallice (Eds.), *Mental processes in the human brain* (pp. 225–248). New York, NY: Oxford University Press.

Stuss, D. T., & Benson, D. F. (1987). The frontal lobes and control of cognition and memory. In E. Perecman (Ed.), *The frontal lobes revisited* (pp. 141–158). New York, NY: IRBN Press.

Stuss, D. T., Picton, T. W., & Alexander, M. P. (2001). Consciousness, self-awareness and the frontal lobes. In S. P. Salloway & P. F. Malloy (Eds.), *The frontal lobes and neuropsychiatric illness* (pp. 101–109). Arlington, VA: American Psychiatric Publishing.

Su, C. Y., Chen, C. C., Wuang, Y. P., Lin, Y. H., & Wu, Y. Y. (2008). Neuropsychological predictors of everyday functioning in adults with intellectual disabilities. *Journal of Intellectual Disability Research*, 52(1), 18–28.

Suchy, Y. (2009). Executive functioning: Overview, assessment, and research issues for non-neuropsychologists. *Annals of Behavioral Medicine*, 37(2), 106–116. doi: 10.1007/s12160-009-9097-4

Suchy, Y. (2011). *Clinical neuropsychology of emotion*. New York, NY: Guilford Press.

Suchy, Y., Blint, A., & Osmon, D. S. (1997). Behavioral Dyscontrol Scale: Criterion and predictive validity in an inpatient rehabilitation unit population. *Clinical Neuropsychologist*, 11(3), 258–265.

Suchy, Y., & Kraybill, M. L. (2007). The relationship between motor programming and executive abilities: Constructs measured by the Push-Turn-Taptap task from the BDS-EV. *Journal of Clinical and Experimental Neuropsychology*, 29(6), 648–659.

Suchy, Y., Kraybill, M. L., & Franchow, E. I. (2011). Instrumental activities of daily living among community-dwelling older adults: Discrepancies between self-report and performance are mediated by cognitive reserve. *Journal of Clinical and Experimental Neuropsychology*, 33(1), 92–100. doi: 10.1080/13803395.2010.493148

Suchy, Y., Kraybill, M. L., & Larson, J. G. L. (2010). Understanding design fluency: Motor and executive contributions. *Journal of the International Neuropsychological Society*, 16(1), 26–37.

Suchy, Y., Lee, J. N., & Marchand, W. R. (2013). Aberrant cortico-subcortical functional connectivity among women with poor motor control: Toward uncovering the substrate of hyperkinetic perseveration. *Neuropsychologia*, 51(11), 2130–2141.

Suchy, Y., Whittaker, W. J., Strassberg, D. S., & Eastvold, A. (2009). Neurocognitive differences between pedophilic and nonpedophilic child molesters. *Journal of the International Neuropsychological Society*, 15(2), 248–257.

Suchy, Y., Whittaker, W. J., Strassberg, D., & Eastvold, A. (2008). Facial and prosodic affect recognition among pedophilic and non-pedophilic criminal child molesters. *Sexual Abuse: A Journal of Research and Treatment 21*(1), 93–110.

Suchy, Y., Williams, P. G., Kraybill, M. L., Franchow, E. I., & Butner, J. (2010). Instrumental activities of daily living among community-dwelling older adults: Personality associations with self-report, performance, and awareness of functional difficulties. *The Journals of Gerontology: Series B: Psychological Sciences and Social Sciences*, 65B(5), 542–550. doi: 10.1093/geronb/gbq037

Sudo, F. K., Alves, C. E. O., Alves, G. S., Ericeira-Valente, L., Tiel, C., Moreira, D. M., . . . Engelhardt, E. (2012). Dysexecutive syndrome and cerebrovascular disease in non-amnestic mild cognitive impairment: A systematic review of the literature. *Dementia and Neuropsychologia*, 6(3), 145–151.

Sutter, C., Zöllig, J., Allemand, M., & Martin, M. (2012). Sleep quality and cognitive function in healthy old age: The moderating role of subclinical depression. *Neuropsychology*, 26(6), 768–775.

Suzuki, C., Tsukiura, T., Mochizuki-Kawai, H., Shigemune, Y., & Iijima, T. (2009). Prefrontal and medial temporal contributions to episodic memory-based reasoning. *Neuroscience Research*, 63(3), 177–183.

Swann, A. C., Lijffijt, M., Lane, S. D., Kjome, K. L., Steinberg, J. L., & Moeller, F. G. (2011). Criminal conviction, impulsivity, and course of illness in bipolar disorder. *Bipolar Disorders*, 13(2), 173–181.

Tabibnia, G., & Zaidel, E. (2005). Alexithymia, interhemispheric transfer, and right hemispheric specialization: A critical review. *Psychotherapy and Psychosomatics*, 74(2), 81–92.

Taconnat, L., Baudouin, A., Fay, S., Raz, N., Bouazzaoui, B., El-Hage, W., . . . Ergis, A.-M. (2010). Episodic memory and organizational strategy in free recall in unipolar depression: The role of cognitive support and executive functions. *Journal of Clinical and Experimental Neuropsychology*, 32(7), 719–727.

Tamber-Rosenau, B. J., Esterman, M., Chiu, Y.-C., & Yantis, S. (2011). Cortical mechanisms of cognitive control for shifting attention in vision and working memory. *Journal of Cognitive Neuroscience*, 23(10), 2905–2919.

Tanabe, T., Hara, K., Shimakawa, S., Fukui, M., & Tamai, H. (2011). Hippocampal damage after prolonged febrile seizure: One case in a consecutive prospective series. *Epilepsia*, 52(4), 837–840.

Taner, Y. I., Erdogan Bakar, E., & Oner, O. (2011). Impaired executive functions in paediatric obsessive-compulsive disorder patients. *Acta Neuropsychiatrica*, 23(6), 272–281.

Taylor, W. D., Aizenstein, H. J., & Alexopoulos, G. S. (2013). The vascular depression hypothesis: Mechanisms linking vascular disease with depression. *Molecular Psychiatry*, 18(9), 963–974.

Tengvar, C., Johansson, B., & Sörensen, J. (2004). Frontal lobe and cingulate cortical metabolic dysfunction in acquired akinetic mutism: A PET study of the interval form of carbon monoxide poisoning. *Brain Injury*, 18(6), 615–625.

Terroni, L., Sobreiro, M. F. M., Conforto, A. B., Adda, C. C., Guajardo, V. D., de Lucia, M. C. S., & Fráguas, R. (2012). Association among depression, cognitive impairment and executive dysfunction after stroke. *Dementia and Neuropsychologia*, 6(3), 152–157.

Testa, R., Bennett, P., & Ponsford, J. (2012). Factor analysis of nineteen executive function tests in a healthy adult population. *Archives of Clinical Neuropsychology*, 27(2), 213–224.

Thomas, A. J., Gallagher, P., Robinson, L. J., Porter, R. J., Young, A. H., Ferrier, I. N., & O'Brien, J. T. (2009). A comparison of neurocognitive impairment in younger and older adults with major depression. *Psychological Medicine*, 39(5), 725–733.

Thompson, J. C., Stopford, C. L., Snowden, J. S., & Neary, D. (2005). Qualitative neuropsychological performance characteristics in frontotemporal dementia and Alzheimer's disease. *Journal of Neurology, Neurosurgery and Psychiatry*, 76(7), 920–927.

Tibbetts, P. E. (2001). The anterior cingulate cortex, akinetic mutism, and human volition. *Brain and Mind*, 2(3), 323–341.

Till, C., Ho, C., Dudani, A., Garcia-Lorenzo, D., Collins, D. L., & Banwell, B. L. (2012). Magnetic resonance imaging predictors of executive functioning in patients with pediatric-onset multiple sclerosis. *Archives of Clinical Neuropsychology*, 27(5), 459–509.

Timmann, D., & Daum, I. (2010). How consistent are cognitive impairments in patients with cerebellar disorders? *Behavioural Neurology*, 23(1–2), 81–100.

Ting, Z., Ruiming, W., Hong, L., Zelazo, P. D., Li, Z., Yu, L., & Xiaojing, L. (2006). Predictions on different components of early theory of mind by diverse tasks of executive function. *Acta Psychologica Sinica*, 38(1), 56–62.

Tomer, R., Aharon-Peretz, J., & Tsitrinbaum, Z. (2007). Dopamine asymmetry interacts with medication to affect cognition in Parkinson's disease. *Neuropsychologia*, 45(2), 357–367.

Topçuoğlu, V., Fistikci, N., Ekinci, Ö., Gönentür, A. G., & Agouridas, B. C. (2009). Assessment of executive functions in social phobia patients using the Wisconsin Card Sorting Test. *Türk Psikiyatri Dergisi, 20*(4), 1–9.

Tops, M., & Boksem, M. A. S. (2011). Cortisol involvement in mechanisms of behavioral inhibition. *Psychophysiology, 48*(5), 723–732.

Tranel, D., Bechara, A., & Denburg, N. L. (2002). Asymmetric functional roles of right and left ventromedial prefrontal cortices in social conduct, decision making and emotional processing. *Cortex, 38*(4), 589–612.

Treble, A., Hasan, K. M., Iftikhar, A., Stuebing, K. K., Kramer, L. A., Cox, C. S., Jr., . . . Ewing-Cobbs, L. (2013). Working memory and corpus callosum microstructural integrity after pediatric traumatic brain injury: A diffusion tensor tractography study. *Journal of Neurotrauma, 30*(19), 1609–1619.

Tremblay, P.-L., Bedard, M.-A., Langlois, D., Blanchet, P. J., Lemay, M., & Parent, M. (2010). Movement chunking during sequence learning is a dopamine-dependent process: A study conducted in Parkinson's disease. *Experimental Brain Research, 205*(3), 375–385.

Triarhou, L. C. (2006). The signalling contributions of Constantin von Economo to basic, clinical and evolutionary neuroscience. *Brain Research Bulletin, 69*(3), 223–243.

Tripathi, R., Kumar, K., Bharath, S., Marimuthu, P., & Varghese, M. (2014). Age, education and gender effects on neuropsychological functions in healthy Indian older adults. *Dementia and Neuropsychologia, 8*(2), 148–154.

Trivedi, M. H., & Greer, T. L. (2014). Cognitive dysfunction in unipolar depression: Implications for treatment. *Journal of Affective Disorders, 152–154*, 19–27.

Tröster, A. I. (2008). Neuropsychological characteristics of dementia with Lewy bodies and Parkinson's disease with dementia: Differentiation, early detection, and implications for "mild cognitive impairment" and biomarkers. *Neuropsychology Review, 18*(1), 103–119.

Tröster, A. I., & Fields, J. A. (2008). Parkinson's disease, progressive supranuclear palsy, corticobasal degeneration, and related disorders of the frontostriatal system. In J. E. Morgan & J. H. Ricker (Eds.), *Textbook of clinical neuropsychology* (pp. 536–577). New York, NY: Psychology Press.

Tsai, J. C. G. (2010). Neurological and neurobehavioral sequelae of obstructive sleep apnea. *NeuroRehabilitation, 26*(1), 85–94.

Tsoi, D. T. Y., Lee, K. H., Gee, K. A., Holden, K. L., Parks, R. W., & Woodruff, P. W. R. (2008). Humour experience in schizophrenia: Relationship with executive dysfunction and psychosocial impairment. *Psychological Medicine, 38*(6), 801–810.

Tsuchida, A., Doll, B. B., & Fellows, L. K. (2010). Beyond reversal: A critical role for human orbitofrontal cortex in flexible learning from probabilistic feedback. *Journal of Neuroscience, 30*(50), 16868–16875. doi: 10.1523/jneurosci.1958-10.2010

Tsuchida, A., & Fellows, L. K. (2013). Are core component processes of executive function dissociable within the frontal lobes? Evidence from humans with focal prefrontal damage. *Cortex: A Journal Devoted to the Study of the Nervous System and Behavior, 49*(7), 1790–1800.

Tucker, A. M., Whitney, P., Belenky, G., Hinson, J. M., & Van Dongen, H. P. A. (2010). Effects of sleep deprivation on dissociated components of executive functioning. *Sleep: Journal of Sleep and Sleep Disorders Research, 33*(1), 47–57.

Turner, M. S., Cipolotti, L., & Shallice, T. (2010). Spontaneous confabulation, temporal context confusion and reality monitoring: A study of three patients with anterior communicating artery aneurysms. *Journal of the International Neuropsychological Society, 16*(6), 984–994. doi: 10.1017/s1355617710001104

Turner, S. L., Suchy, Y., Queen, T. L., Duraccio, K., Wiebe, D. J., Butner, J. E., & Berg, C. A. (2015, June). *Assessing executive function in adolescents with type 1 diabetes: Relations to adherence and glycemic control*. Paper presented at the annual meeting of the American Diabetes Association, Boston, MA.

Tuzer, V., Bulut, S. D., Bastug, B., Kayalar, G., Göka, E., & Beştepe, E. (2011). Causal attributions and alexithymia in female patients with fibromyalgia or chronic low back pain. *Nordic Journal of Psychiatry, 65*(2), 138–144.

Uekermann, J., Daum, I., Schlebusch, P., & Trenckmann, U. (2005). Processing of affective stimuli in alcoholism. *Cortex, 41*(2), 189–194.

Ullsperger, M., Harsay, H. A., Wessel, J. R., & Ridderinkhof, K. R. (2010). Conscious perception of errors and its relation to the anterior insula. *Brain Structure and Function, 214*(5–6), 629–643. doi: 10.1007/s00429-010-0261-1

Ursu, S., & Carter, C. S. (2005). Outcome representations, counterfactual comparisons and the human orbitofrontal cortex: Implications for neuroimaging studies of decision-making. *Cognitive Brain Research, 23*(1), 51–60.

Vago, L., Bonetto, S., Nebuloni, M., Duca, P., Carsana, L., Zerbi, P., & D'Arminio-Monforte, A. (2002). Pathological findings in the central nervous system of AIDS patients on assumed antiretroviral therapeutic regimens: Retrospective study of 1597 autopsies. *AIDS, 16*, 1925–1928.

Vandierendonck, A. (2012). Role of working memory in task switching. *Psychologica Belgica, 52*(2–3), 229–253.

Verghese, J., Wang, C., Lipton, R. B., Holtzer, R., & Xue, X. (2007). Quantitative gait dysfunction and risk of cognitive decline and dementia. *Journal of Neurology, Neurosurgery and Psychiatry*, 78(9), 929–935.

Verma, M., & Howard, R. J. (2012). Semantic memory and language dysfunction in early Alzheimer's disease: A review. *International Journal of Geriatric Psychiatry*, 27(12), 1209–1217.

Verte, S., Geurts, H. M., Roeyers, H., Oosterlaan, J., & Sergeant, J. A. (2005). Executive functioning in children with autism and Tourette syndrome. *Development and Psychopathology*, 17(2), 415–445.

Verwey, W. B., Abrahamse, E. L., Ruitenberg, M. F. L., Jiménez, L., & de Kleine, E. (2011). Motor skill learning in the middle-aged: Limited development of motor chunks and explicit sequence knowledge. *Psychological Research*, 75(5), 406–422.

Vinberg, M., Miskowiak, K. W., & Kessing, L. V. (2013). Impairment of executive function and attention predicts onset of affective disorder in healthy high-risk twins. *Journal of Clinical Psychiatry*, 74(8), 747–753.

Viskontas, I. V., Possin, K. L., & Miller, B. L. (2007). Symptoms of frontotemporal dementia provide insights into orbitofrontal cortex function and social behavior. In G. Schoenbaum, J. A. Gottfried, E. A. Murray, & S. J. Ramus (Eds.), *Linking affect to action: Critical contributions of the orbitofrontal cortex* (Vol. 1121, pp. 528–545). Malden, MA: Blackwell.

Vöhringer, P. A., Barroilhet, S. A., Amerio, A., Reale, M. L., Alvear, K., Vergne, D., & Ghaemi, S. N. (2013). Cognitive impairment in bipolar disorder and schizophrenia: A systematic review. *Frontiers in Psychiatry*, 4(87), doi: 10.3389/fpsyt.2013.00087.

Volle, E., de Lacy Costello, A., Coates, L. M., McGuire, C., Towgood, K., Gilbert, S., . . . Burgess, P. W. (2012). Dissociation between verbal response initiation and suppression after prefrontal lesions. *Cerebral Cortex*, 22(10), 2428–2440.

Volle, E., Gonen-Yaacovi, G., de Lacy Costello, A., Gilbert, S. J., & Burgess, P. W. (2011). The role of rostral prefrontal cortex in prospective memory: A voxel-based lesion study. *Neuropsychologia*, 49(8), 2185–2198.

von Rimscha, S., Moergeli, H., Weidt, S., Straumann, D., Hegemann, S., & Rufer, M. (2013). Alexithymia and health-related quality of life in patients with dizziness. *Psychopathology*, 46(6), 377–383.

Vu, M.-A. T., Thermenos, H. W., Terry, D. P., Wolfe, D. J., Voglmaier, M. M., Niznikiewicz, M. A., . . . Dickey, C. C. (2013). Working memory in schizotypal personality disorder: fMRI activation and deactivation differences. *Schizophrenia Research*, 151(1–3), 113–123.

Waechter, R. L., Goel, V., Raymont, V., Kruger, F., & Grafman, J. (2013). Transitive inference reasoning is impaired by focal lesions in parietal cortex rather than rostrolateral prefrontal cortex. *Neuropsychologia, 51*(3), 464–471.

Waldron, E. J., Barrash, J., Swenson, A., & Tranel, D. (2014). Personality disturbances in amyotrophic lateral sclerosis: A case study demonstrating changes in personality without cognitive deficits. *Journal of the International Neuropsychological Society, 20*(7), 764–771.

Walker, M. P., Ayre, G. A., Cummings, J. L., Wesnes, K., McKeith, I. G., O'Brien, J. T., & Ballard, C. G. (2000). Quantifying fluctuation in dementia with Lewy bodies, Alzheimer's disease, and vascular dementia. *Neurology, 54*(8), 1616–1624.

Walley, R. M., & Donaldson, M. D. C. (2005). An investigation of executive function abilities in adults with Prader-Willi syndrome. *Journal of Intellectual Disability Research, 49*(8), 613–625. doi: 10.1111/j.1365-2788.2005.00717.x

Walter, H. (2012). Social cognitive neuroscience of empathy: Concepts, circuits, and genes. *Emotion Review, 4*(1), 9–17.

Walter, K. H., Palmieri, P. A., & Gunstad, J. (2010). More than symptom reduction: Changes in executive function over the course of PTSD treatment. *Journal of Traumatic Stress, 23*(2), 292–295.

Warschausky, S., Kaufman, J. N., & Felix, L. (2013). Cerebral palsy. In I. S. Baron & C. Rey-Casserly (Eds.), *Pediatric neuropsychology: Medical advances and lifespan outcomes* (pp. 80–98). New York, NY: Oxford University Press.

Watabe, Y., Owens, J. S., Evans, S. W., & Brandt, N. E. (2014). The relationship between sluggish cognitive tempo and impairment in children with and without ADHD. *Journal of Abnormal Child Psychology, 42*(1), 105–115.

Waters, F., & Bucks, R. S. (2011). Neuropsychological effects of sleep loss: Implication for neuropsychologists. *Journal of the International Neuropsychological Society, 17*(4), 571–586.

Watkins, L. H., Sahakian, B. J., Robertson, M. M., Veale, D. M., Rogers, R. D., Pickard, K. M., . . . Robbins, T. W. (2005). Executive function in Tourette's syndrome and obsessive-compulsive disorder. *Psychological Medicine, 35*(4), 571–582.

Watson, J. M., & Strayer, D. L. (2010). Supertaskers: Profiles in extraordinary multitasking ability. *Psychonomic Bulletin and Review, 17*(4), 479–485.

Watson, K. K., Matthews, B. J., & Allman, J. M. (2007). Brain activation during sight gags and language-dependent humor. *Cerebral Cortex, 17*(2), 314–324.

Weaver, L. K., Hopkins, R. O., Chan, K. J., Churchill, S., Elliott, C. G., Clemmer, T. P., ... Morris, A. H. (2002). Hyperbaric oxygen for acute carbon monoxide poisoning. *New England Journal of Medicine, 347*(14), 1057–1067.

Weaver, T. E., & Chasens, E. R. (2007). Continuous positive airway pressure treatment for sleep apnea in older adults. *Sleep Medicine Reviews, 11*(2), 99–111.

Wechsler, D. (1997). *WAIS-III administration and scoring manual.* San Antonio, TX: Psychological Corporation.

Wechsler, D. (2008). *Wechsler Adult Intelligence Scale* (4th ed.). San Antonio, TX: Harcourt Assessment.

Wefel, J. S., Saleeba, A. K., Buzdar, A. U., & Meyers, C. A. (2010). Acute and late onset cognitive dysfunction associated with chemotherapy in women with breast cancer. *Cancer, 116*(14), 3348–3356.

Wefel, J. S., Vidrine, D. J., Veramonti, T. L., Meyers, C. A., Marani, S. K., Hoekstra, H. J., ... Gritz, E. R. (2011). Cognitive impairment in men with testicular cancer prior to adjuvant therapy. *Cancer, 117*(1), 190–196.

Weigard, A., Chein, J., Albert, D., Smith, A., & Steinberg, L. (2014). Effects of anonymous peer observation on adolescents' preference for immediate rewards. *Developmental Science, 17*(1), 71–78. doi: 10.1111/desc.12099

Weller, J. A. (2007). *The role of affect in decisions under varying levels of uncertainty: Converging evidence from neurological and temperament perspectives.* 68, ProQuest Information & Learning, US. Retrieved from http://search.ebscohost.com/login.aspx?direct=true&db=psyh&AN=2007-99240-094&site=ehost-live

Wells, A., & Matthews, G. (2006). Cognitive vulnerability to anxiety disorders: An integration. In L. B. Alloy & J. H. Riskind (Eds.), *Cognitive vulnerability to emotional disorders* (pp. 303–325). Mahwah, NJ: Erlbaum.

Welsh, M. C., & Huizinga, M. (2005). Tower of Hanoi disk-transfer task: Influences of strategy knowledge and learning on performance. *Learning and Individual Differences, 15*(4), 283–298.

Welsh, M. C., & Pennington, B. F. (1988). Assessing frontal lobe functioning in children: Views from developmental psychology. *Developmental Neuropsychology, 4*(3), 199–230.

Wendelken, C., Bunge, S. A., & Carter, C. S. (2008). Maintaining structured information: An investigation into functions of parietal and lateral prefrontal cortices. *Neuropsychologia, 46*(2), 665–678.

Weniger, G., Lange, C., Rather, E., & Irle, E. (2004). Differential impairments of facial affect recognition in schizophrenia subtypes and major depression. *Psychiatry Research, 128*(2), 135–146.

Werring, D. J., Frazer, D. W., Coward, L. J., Losseff, N. A., Watt, H., Cipolotti, L., . . . Jäger, H. R. (2004). Cognitive dysfunction in patients with cerebral microbleeds on T2*-weighted gradient-echo MRI. *Brain: A Journal of Neurology, 127*(10), 2265–2275.

West, R., & Travers, S. (2008). Differential effects of aging on processes underlying task switching. *Brain and Cognition, 68*(1), 67–80.

Whalen, P. J., Raila, H., Bennett, R., Mattek, A., Brown, A., Taylor, J., . . . Palmer, A. (2013). Neuroscience and facial expressions of emotion: The role of amygdala-prefrontal interactions. *Emotion Review, 5*(1), 78–83.

Whalley, H. C., Papmeyer, M., Sprooten, E., Lawrie, S. M., Sussmann, J. E., & McIntosh, A. M. (2012). Review of functional magnetic resonance imaging studies comparing bipolar disorder and schizophrenia. *Bipolar Disorders, 14*(4), 411–431.

Whitney, P., Arnett, P. A., Driver, A., & Budd, D. (2001). Measuring central executive functioning: What's in a reading span? *Brain and Cognition, 45*(1), 1–14.

Wickremaratchi, M. M., Ben-Shlomo, Y., & Morris, H. R. (2009). The effect of onset age on the clinical features of Parkinson's disease. *European Journal of Neurology, 16*(4), 450–456.

Wiebe, S. A., Sheffield, T., Nelson, J. M., Clark, C. A. C., Chevalier, N., & Espy, K. A. (2011). The structure of executive function in 3-year-olds. *Journal of Experimental Child Psychology, 108*(3), 436–452.

Wilberg, T., Karterud, S., Pedersen, G., Urnes, Ø., & Costa, P. T. (2009). Nineteen-month stability of Revised NEO Personality Inventory domain and facet scores in patients with personality disorders. *Journal of Nervous and Mental Disease, 197*(3), 187–195.

Wilding, J., Cornish, K., & Munir, F. (2002). Further delineation of the executive deficit in males with fragile-X syndrome. *Neuropsychologia, 40*(8), 1343–1349. doi: 10.1016/s0028-3932(01)00212-3

Wilk, H. A., Ezekiel, F., & Morton, J. B. (2012). Brain regions associated with moment-to-moment adjustments in control and stable task-set maintenance. *Neuroimage, 59*(2), 1960–1967.

Willcutt, E. G., Chhabildas, N., Kinnear, M., DeFries, J. C., Olson, R. K., Leopold, D. R., . . . Pennington, B. F. (2014). The internal and external validity of sluggish cognitive tempo and its relation with DSM-IV ADHD. *Journal of Abnormal Child Psychology, 42*(1), 21–35.

Willcutt, E. G., Doyle, A. E., Nigg, J. T., Faraone, S. V., & Pennington, B. F. (2005). Validity of the executive function theory of attention-deficit/hyperactivity disorder: A meta-analytic review. *Biological Psychiatry, 57*(11), 1336–1346. doi: 10.1016/j.biopsych.2005.02.006

Williams, D., Boucher, J., Lind, S., & Jarrold, C. (2013). Time-based and event-based prospective memory in autism spectrum disorder: The roles of executive function and theory of mind, and time-estimation. *Journal of Autism and Developmental Disorders, 43*(7), 1555–1567. doi: 10.1007/s10803-012-1703-9

Williams, L. M., Hermens, D. F., Palmer, D., Kohn, M., Clarke, S., Keage, H., . . . Gordon, E. (2008). Misinterpreting emotional expressions in attention-deficit/hyperactivity disorder: Evidence for a neural marker and stimulant effects. *Biological Psychiatry, 63*(10), 917–926.

Williams, P. G., Suchy, Y., & Kraybill, M. L. (2010). Five-factor model personality traits and executive functioning among older adults. *Journal of Research in Personality, 44*(4), 485–491.

Williams, P. G., Suchy, Y., & Kraybill, M. L. (2013). Preliminary evidence for low openness to experience as a pre-clinical marker of incipient cognitive decline in older adults. *Journal of Research in Personality, 47*(6), 945–951.

Williams, P. G., Suchy, Y., & Rau, H. (2009). Individual differences in executive functioning: Implications for stress regulation. *Annals of Behavioral Medicine, 37*(2), 126–140.

Wilson, B., Alderman, N., Burgess, P. W., Emslie, H., & Evans, J. J. (1996). *Behavioural Assessment of the Dysexecutive Syndrome (BADS)*. San Antonio, TX: Pearson.

Wilson, F. C., Harpur, J., Watson, T., & Morrow, J. I. (2003). Adult survivors of severe cerebral hypoxia—Case series survey and comparative analysis. *NeuroRehabilitation, 18*(4), 291–298.

Windmann, S., Kirsch, P., Mier, D., Stark, R., Walter, B., Guentuerkuen, O., & Vaitl, D. (2006). On framing effects in decision making: Linking lateral versus medial orbitofrontal cortex activation to choice outcome processing. *Journal of Cognitive Neuroscience, 18*(7), 1198–1211.

Wingbermühle, E., Theunissen, H., Verhoeven, W. M. A., Kessels, R. P. C., & Egger, J. I. M. (2012). The neurocognition of alexithymia: Evidence from neuropsychological and neuroimaging studies. *Acta Neuropsychiatrica, 24*(2), 67–80.

Wishart, J. G., Cebula, K. R., Willis, D. S., & Pitcairn, T. K. (2007). Understanding of facial expressions of emotion by children with intellectual disabilities of differing aetiology. *Journal of Intellectual Disability Research, 51*(7), 551–563.

Wittenborn, J. R., & Mettler, F. A. (1951). Some psychological changes following psychosurgery. *Journal of Abnormal and Social Psychology, 46*(4), 548–556.

Wolff, J. C., & Ollendick, T. H. (2006). The comorbidity of conduct problems and depression in childhood and adolescence. *Clinical Child and Family Psychology Review, 9*(3), 201–220.

Wood, R. L. L., & Williams, C. (2007). Neuropsychological correlates of organic alexithymia. *Journal of the International Neuropsychological Society, 13*(3), 471–479.

Wood, R. L. L., Williams, C., & Kalyani, T. (2009). The impact of alexithymia on somatization after traumatic brain injury. *Brain Injury, 23*(7–8), 649–654.

Woods, S. P., Moore, D. J., Weber, E., & Grant, I. (2009). Cognitive neuropsychology of HIV-associated neurocognitive disorders. *Neuropsychology Review, 19*(2), 152–168.

Wright, S. N., Kochunov, P., Mut, F., Bergamino, M., Brown, K. M., Mazziotta, J. C., . . . Ascoli, G. A. (2013). Digital reconstruction and morphometric analysis of human brain arterial vasculature from magnetic resonance angiography. *Neuroimage, 82*, 170–181.

Wu, T.-C., & Grotta, J. C. (2013). Hypothermia for acute ischaemic stroke. *Lancet Neurology, 12*(3), 275–284.

Wyvell, C. L., & Berridge, K. C. (2000). Intra-accumbens amphetamine increases the conditioned incentive salience of sucrose reward: Enhancement of reward "wanting" without enhanced "liking" or response reinforcement. *Journal of Neuroscience, 20*(21), 8122–8130.

Xiong-Zhao, Z., Xiao-Yan, W., & Ying, H. (2006). A comparative study of Wisconsin Card Sorting Test in individuals with different degrees of alexithymia. *Chinese Journal of Clinical Psychology, 14*(2), 132–133.

Yan, J., Meng, G.-H., & Li, G. (2012). Executive function characteristics in patients with obsessive-compulsive disorder and patients with schizophrenia. *Chinese Mental Health Journal, 26*(1), 10–14.

Yang, J., Pan, P., Song, W., Huang, R., Li, J., Chen, K., . . . Shang, H. (2012). Voxelwise meta-analysis of gray matter anomalies in Alzheimer's disease and mild cognitive impairment using anatomic likelihood estimation. *Journal of the Neurological Sciences, 316*(1–2), 21–29.

Yeates, K. O., Fletcher, J. M., & Dennis, M. (2008). Spina bifida and hydrocephalus. In J. E. Morgan & J. H. Ricker (Eds.), *Textbook of clinical neuropsychology* (pp. 128–148). New York, NY: Psychology Press.

Yeates, K. O., Loss, N., Colvin, A. N., & Enrile, B. G. (2003). Do children with myelomeningocele and hydrocephalus display nonverbal learning disabilities? An empirical approach to classification. *Journal of the International Neuropsychological Society*, 9(4), 653–662.

Yen, C.-F., Cheng, C.-P., Huang, C.-F., Ko, C.-H., Yen, J.-Y., Chang, Y.-P., & Chen, C.-S. (2009). Relationship between psychosocial adjustment and executive function in patients with bipolar disorder and schizophrenia in remission: The mediating and moderating effects of insight. *Bipolar Disorders*, 11(2), 190–197.

Yenari, M. A., & Han, H. S. (2012). Neuroprotective mechanisms of hypothermia in brain ischaemia. *Nature Reviews Neuroscience*, 13(4), 267–278.

Yerkes, R. M., & Dodson, J. D. (1908). The relation of strength of stimulus to rapidity of habit formation. *Journal of Comparative Neurology and Psychology*, 18, 459–482.

Yerys, B. E., Hepburn, S. L., Pennington, B. F., & Rogers, S. J. (2007). Executive function in preschoolers with autism: Evidence consistent with a secondary deficit. *Journal of Autism and Developmental Disorders*, 37(6), 1068–1079. doi: 10.1007/s10803-006-0250-7

Yin Foo, R., Guppy, M., & Johnston, L. M. (2013). Intelligence assessments for children with cerebral palsy: A systematic review. *Developmental Medicine and Child Neurology*, 55(10), 911–918.

Yochim, B. P., Mueller, A. E., & Segal, D. L. (2013). Late life anxiety is associated with decreased memory and executive functioning in community dwelling older adults. *Journal of Anxiety Disorders*, 27(6), 567–575.

Yoon, J. H., Lee, J. E., Yong, S. W., Moon, S. Y., & Lee, P. H. (2014). The mild cognitive impairment stage of dementia with Lewy bodies and Parkinson disease: A comparison of cognitive profiles. *Alzheimer Disease and Associated Disorders*, 28(2), 151–155.

Yücel, M., Lubman, D. I., Solowij, N., & Brewer, W. J. (2007). Understanding drug addiction: A neuropsychological perspective. *Australian and New Zealand Journal of Psychiatry*, 41(12), 957–968.

Yun, D. Y., Hwang, S. S.-H., Kim, Y., Lee, Y. H., Kim, Y.-S., & Jung, H. Y. (2011). Impairments in executive functioning in patients with remitted and non-remitted schizophrenia. *Progress in Neuro-Psychopharmacology and Biological Psychiatry*, 35(4), 1148–1154.

Zabel, T. A., Jacobson, L., & Mahone, E. M. (2013). Spina bifida/hydrocephalus. In I. S. Baron & C. Rey-Casserly (Eds.), *Pediatric neuropsychology: Medical advances and lifespan outcomes* (pp. 279–301). New York, NY: Oxford University Press.

Zalonis, I., Christidi, F., Paraskevas, G., Zabelis, T., Evdokimidis, I., & Kararizou, E. (2012). Can executive cognitive measures differentiate between patients with spinal- and bulbar-onset amyotrophic lateral sclerosis? *Archives of Clinical Neuropsychology, 27*(3), 348–354.

Zelazo, P. D., Chandler, M., & Crone, E. (2010). *Developmental social cognitive neuroscience.* New York, NY: Psychology Press.

Zimmerman, E. K., Eslinger, P. J., Simmons, Z., & Barrett, A. M. (2007). Emotional perception deficits in amyotrophic lateral sclerosis. *Cognitive and Behavioral Neurology, 20*(2), 79–82.

Zinke, K., Altgassen, M., Mackinlay, R. J., Rizzo, P., Drechsler, R., & Kliegel, M. (2010). Time-based prospective memory performance and time-monitoring in children with ADHD. *Child Neuropsychology, 16*(4), 338–349.

Zoccolotti, P., Matano, A., Deloche, G., Cantagallo, A., Passadori, A., Leclercq, M., . . . Zimmermann, P. (2000). Patterns of attentional impairment following closed head injury: A collaborative European study. *Cortex: A Journal Devoted to the Study of the Nervous System and Behavior, 36*(1), 93–107.

Zogg, J. B., Woods, S. P., Sauceda, J. A., Wiebe, J. S., & Simoni, J. M. (2012). The role of prospective memory in medication adherence: A review of an emerging literature. *Journal of Behavioral Medicine, 35*(1), 47–62.

Index

Page numbers followed by "f" and "t" indicate figures and tables.

Abulia, 75
AcoAA. *See* Anterior communicating artery aneurysm
Action planning. *See* Initiation
Active inhibition, 52
Acute anoxic events, 207–208
Addictive disorders, 212–213
ADHD. *See* Attention-deficit hyperactivity disorder
Agreeableness, 46, 152
Akinetic mutism, 75, 79–80
Alexithymia, 84, 91, 96
Alphanumeric sequencing, 140
ALS. *See* Amyotrophic lateral sclerosis
Alzheimer's disease and related disorders
  dementia and, 181–182, 215t
  disorganized syndrome and, 49
  dysexecutive syndrome and, 34
  frontotemporal lobar degeneration and, 179, 182
  initiation and maintenance and, 80
  intellectual disability and, 172
  social awareness and, 97
  subcortical ischemic vascular dementia and, 180–181, 182
Amnesia, 207
Amotivational syndrome, 80. *See also* Apathetic syndrome
Amygdala, 62, 64, 93–94, 96, 98, 168
Amyotrophic lateral sclerosis (ALS), 97, 186–187, 215t
Anoxia, 33, 80, 165, 172, 206–209, 213, 215t
Anterior cingulate cortex, 32, 49, 64–66, 77, 79–80, 93–94, 166, 183–184, 192, 209
Anterior cingulate gyrus. *See* Anterior cingulate cortex
Anterior communicating artery aneurysm (AcoAA), 206
Anterior insula, 62, 64–65, 79, 92–94, 192
Antihypertensive medications, 180
Antisocial personality disorder (ASPD), 98, 200–202
Anxiety disorders, 34, 197–198, 215t
Apathetic syndrome. *See also* Initiation and maintenance
  behavioral observations, pathognomonic signs and, 117–118
  interviewing about, 110t
  overview of, 75–77, 215–219t
  records reflecting, 110t
Arousal, threat sensitivity and, 53
ASPD. *See* Antisocial personality disorder

321

Asperger's syndrome, 49, 169, 215t
Assessment. *See also Specific tests*
  daily functioning, prediction of lapses and, 153–156
  diagnostic decision-making and, 150–152
  of executive cognitive functions, 28, 29t
  overview of, 145–146, 156–162
  trait vs. state and, 146–150
Attention, 30, 32–33, 46, 48, 53–54, 64, 123t, 139–140, 142t, 148, 173–174, 182–183, 188, 192, 206, 208–209. *See also* Maintenance; Vigilance
Attention-deficit hyperactivity disorder (ADHD)
  discrepancy detection and, 66
  disorganized syndrome and, 49
  dysexecutive syndrome and, 34
  initiation and maintenance and, 71, 81
  oppositional defiant disorder and, 200
  overview of, 165–167, 215t
  preterm birth and, 174
  sluggish cognitive tempo and, 74
  social cognition and, 96
Autism spectrum disorders, 49, 96, 167–169, 215t
Automatic processes, effort vs., 9–10
Awareness of Social Inference test (TASIT), 92

Background information
  interviewing patients and collateral sources and, 112–115, 114t, 116t
  records review and, 103–112, 104–105t, 106–107t, 108t, 110t
BADS. *See* Behavioural Assessment of the Dysexecutive Syndrome
Basal ganglia, 30, 33, 80, 93, 185, 206–207, 209
Behavioral activation, 71. *See also* Effort mobilization

Behavioral Assessment of Dysexecutive Syndrome (BADS), 143t
Behavioral observations, 115–1198
Behavioral variant frontotemporal lobar degeneration (bvFTD), 177–179, 217t
Behavioural Assessment of the Dysexecutive Syndrome (BADS), 46
Binswanger's disease, 179
Bipolar disorder, 153, 194–195, 216t
Block Design test, 141
Body dysmorphic disorder, 198
Borderline personality disorder (BPD), 201–202
Branching, 39–40
bvFTD. *See* Behavioral variant frontotemporal lobar degeneration

California Verbal Learning Test (CVLT), 142t
Carbon monoxide poisoning, 80
Category fluency. *See* Semantic fluency
Central executive, 6
Central nervous system infections, 209–210, 217t
Cerebellum, 30–35, 93, 185, 192, 203, 205, 207
Cerebral palsy, 172–173, 216t
Cerebrovascular accidents (CVA), 33, 79, 205–206, 216t
Chemotherapy, 211–212, 218t
Cholinesterase inhibitors, 180
Chronic intermittent hypoxemia, 208–209. *Also see* Anoxia
Chronic obstructive pulmonary disease (COPD), 207, 209
Chronic tic disorders (CTD), 170, 216t
Cingulate gyrus, 31, 64–65, 77, 79, 93, 166
Cingulum. *See* Cingulate gyrus
Clinical practice, 130, 137–138
Cognition, hierarchical structure of, 121–124, 123t
Cognitive control, 6

Cognitive decision-making, 23, 51–52
Cognitive empathy. *See* Empathy
Cognitive flexibility. *See* Mental flexibility.
Cognitive reappraisal, 23–24
Cognitive reserve, 153–154
Color-word interference, 76–77. *See also* Delis-Kaplan Executive Function System (D-KEFS); Stroop tests
Communication, emotional, 84–86, 85t, 88t
Complexity of daily life, 155, 161t
Complicated mild traumatic brain injury, 203, 204
Component processes, 121–122, 123t, 129–130, 141
Composite scores, 127, 130, 132t
Concurrent validity, 139–140
Conscientiousness, 45, 46, 152
Construct validity, 139–140
Contingency updating, 53–54, 56, 57t, 61t, 62–64, 143t
Continuous Performance Test (CPT), 141
Continuous positive airway pressure (CPAP) therapy, 208
ConVExA model. *See* Contextually Valid Executive Assessment model
Cooking Breakfast Task, 46
COPD. *See* Chronic obstructive pulmonary disease
Corpus callosum, 31, 93, 96, 173
Cortextually Valid Executive Assessment (ConVExA) model, 101–102, 158–159
Cortical-basal degeneration, 185, 216t
Cortico-cortical networks, 30–31
Cortisol, 196
Cost-benefit analysis, 54
Coup-counter coup injuries, 33
Course of decline, interviewing about, 114t
CPT. *See* Continuous Performance Test
Creutzfeldt-Jakob disease, 80
Criminal records. *See* Records review

Criterion validity, 137
CTD. *See* Chronic tic disorders
CVA. *See* Cerebrovascular accidents
CVLT. *See* California Verbal Learning Test
Cyclothymic disorders, 194–195

Daily functioning, 153–156
Daily life complexity, 155, 161t
Day-Out Task, 46
Decision-making, 51–52, 150–152. *See also* Cognitive decision-making; Emotional decision-making
Definition of executive functions, 10–11
Delis-Kaplan Executive Function System (D-KEFS)
  D-KEFS Color-Word Interference test, 129
  D-KEFS Trail Making, 129, 130
  D-KEFS Verbal Fluency, 127
Dementias
  Alzheimer's dementia, 181–182
  amyotrophic lateral sclerosis and, 97, 186–187, 215t
  dysexecutive syndrome and, 33
  fragile X-associated tremor and ataxia syndrome, 172, 186, 217t
  frontotemporal lobar degeneration, 96–97, 177–179, 217t
  initiation and maintenance and, 80
  with Lewy bodies, 182–183
  Parkinson's disease and related disorders and, 49, 71, 79, 80–81, 183–186, 218t
  subcortical ischemic vascular dementia, 179–181
  vascular, 33–34, 180
Demographics, 151–152
Depletable resource, executive functioning as, 128, 146. *See also* Executive depletion.
Depressive disorders, 34, 81, 188, 195–197, 216t
Design fluency, 29t, 78t, 123–124t, 125t

Digit Symbol Coding test, 76, 140, 141
Discrepancy detection, 52, 54, 56, 57t, 58–59, 60, 61t, 64–66, 122, 142t, 194, 198, 213
Disengagement of resources, 154
Disinhibited syndrome. *See also* Response selection
   behavioral observations, pathognomonic signs and, 117
   dementia with Lewy bodies and, 183
   interviewing about, 110t
   overview of, 58–62, 215–219t
   records reflecting, 110t
Disorganized syndrome. *See also* Meta-tasking
   autism spectrum disorders and, 168
   behavioral observations, pathognomonic signs and, 117
   interviewing about, 110t
   overview of, 44–48, 215–219t
   records reflecting, 110t
Disruptive mood dysregulation disorder, 195
D-KEFS battery. *See* Delis-Kaplan Executive Function System.
Dopaminergic systems, 80, 151–152, 183, 184–185
Dorsolateral prefrontal cortex (DLPFC), 30, 48, 75, 93, 178, 181, 184, 200, 205, 207
Down syndrome, 96, 171, 172
Dysexecutive syndrome. *See also* Executive cognitive functions
   behavioral observations, pathognomonic signs and, 117
   interviewing about, 110t
   overview of, 26t, 29t, 30–33, 215–219t
   records reflecting, 110t
   typical presentation of, 24–30
Dysthymia, 195

ECF. *See* Executive cognitive functions
Echolalia, 117
Ecological validity, 137–138
ECT. *See* Electroconvulsive therapy
Effort, automatic processes vs., 9–10
Effort mobilization, 71–72, 73t, 78t, 79
Electroconvulsive therapy (ECT), 196
Embodied emotions, 93
Emotional communication, 84–86, 85t, 88t
Emotional decision-making, 64. *See also* Decision making, Cognitive decision making.
Emotional empathy. *See* Empathy
Emotional self-awareness, 84, 90–91, 92–93
Emotional suppression, 148, 149t
Emotion regulation, 23–24, 56–58, 89–90, 148–149, 166
Empathy, 86, 88t, 95–97, 168–169
Energization, 72. *See also* Effort mobilization
Epilepsy, 210–211
Episodic memory, 16, 40, 44, 53, 127, 178, 180–182
Error monitoring system, 65, 148, 194, 198–199
Error positivity, 54
Event-based prospective memory, 38, 39–40, 43t, 47t. *See also* Time-based prospective memory.
Evolution, executive functions and, 3–4
Exaggeration of emotional expressions, 148, 149t
Excoriation, 198
Executive assessment. *See* Assessment
Executive cognitive functions (ECF)
   Alzheimer's disease and related disorders and, 181–182
   amyotrophic lateral sclerosis and, 187
   attention-deficit hyperactivity disorder and, 166
   dementia with Lewy bodies and, 183
   depressive disorders and, 196
   dysexecutive syndrome and, 24–30
   etiology of impairments in, 33–34
   executive functions tests and, 28, 29t

frontotemporal lobar degeneration and, 178
initiation and maintenance vs., 69
intellectual disability and, 172
job-related duties and capacities and, 108t
meta-tasking vs., 37
multiple sclerosis and, 188
needed for test performance, 125t
neuroanatomy of, 30–33
other relevant constructs, 20–24
overview of, 15–20, 19f, 21–22t, 34–35
overview of deficits in patient populations, 215–219t
oxygen deprivation and, 208
Parkinson's disease and related disorders and, 184
personality disorders and, 202
post-traumatic stress disorder and, 200
response selection vs., 51
schizophrenia spectrum disorders and, 193
social phobia and, 197–198
spina bifida and hydrocephalus and, 175–176
subcortical ischemic vascular dementia and, 180–181
traumatic brain injury and, 204
Executive depletion, 148, 149t
Explicit learning, 53
Expressive suppression, 56–58, 148, 149t
Extraversion, 152

Factor analysis, 6
Familial intellectual disability, 171
FAS. *See* Fetal alcohol syndrome
Fear conditioning, 53
Feeling awareness, 84
Fetal alcohol syndrome, 96, 173–174, 217t
Figural fluency. *See* Design Fluency
Flexibility. *See* Mental flexibility
Fork neurons, 64

Fragile X-associated tremor and ataxia syndrome (FXATS), 172, 186, 217t
Fragile X syndrome, 96, 171–172, 217t
Frontal Assessment Battery, 185
Frontal lobes, 1, 5, 62, 66
Frontal lobe syndrome, 1
Frontoparietal network, 31, 166
Frontopolar cortex, 48–49
Frontotemporal lobar degeneration (FTD), 49, 66, 80, 96–97, 146, 177–179, 217t
Function, structure vs., 4–5
FXATS. *See* Fragile X-associated tremor and ataxia syndrome

Gage, Phineas, 1, 4–5
Gambling, 212–213
Goal-directed retrieval, 16–17, 20, 21–22t, 23–24, 28, 29t, 31–32, 34, 122, 125t, 142t, 175, 184–185, 187–188

Halstead Category Test
component processes needed for, 123–124t
disorganized syndrome and, 47t
dysexecutive syndrome and, 29t
elemental processes needed for, 125t
initiation and maintenance and, 78t
response selection and, 61t
Hoarding, 198
Heartbeat, 92
Heritability, 151–152
Heuristic calculations, 55–56
Hippocampus, 31, 207
HIV/AIDS, 49, 209–210, 217t
Hopkins Verbal Learning Test (HVLT), 141
Humor and sarcasm, 87–89
Hydrocephalus, 175–176, 219t
Hyperbaric oxygen, 208
Hyperkinetic perseveration. *See* Motor perseveration
Hypoxia. *See* Anoxia

If-then rules, 39–40
I/M. *See* Initiation and maintenance
Implicit-level learning, 53
Impulsivity, 194. *See also* Inhibitory control
Inappropriate syndrome. *See also* Social cognition
　behavioral observations, pathognomonic signs and, 118
　interviewing about, 110t
　overview of, 90–92, 215–219t
　records reflecting, 110t
Incentive sensitivity, 56
Incongruities, 87
Inferior frontal gyrus, 32, 64–65, 95
Inhibitory control, 6, 7, 16, 52–56, 57t, 58–60, 61t, 65–66, 89, 122, 124, 126t, 138, 142t, 148, 170, 172, 178–179, 183, 195, 206, 213
Initiation, 69–71, 73t, 78t
Initiation and maintenance (I/M)
　Alzheimer's disease and related disorders and, 182
　apathetic syndrome and, 75–77
　attention-deficit hyperactivity disorder and, 166
　cerebral vascular accidents and, 205
　defining, 69–74, 73t
　dementia with Lewy bodies and, 183
　depressive disorders and, 196
　etiology of impairments in, 79–80
　executive cognitive functions vs., 69
　job-related duties and capacities and, 108t
　needed for test performance, 126t
　neuroanatomy of, 77–79
　other relevant constructs, 74–75
　overview of deficits in patient populations, 215–219t
　oxygen deprivation and, 208
　schizophrenia spectrum disorders and, 193
　traumatic brain injuries and, 204
Insight, 45
Instrumental activities of daily living (IADL), 153–156

Insula. *See* Anterior insula
Intellectual disability, 34, 170–172, 217t
Intelligence, 2, 153–155, 171
Intermittent explosive disorder, 200–201
International Behavioural Variant FTD Criteria Consortium, 179
Interoceptive awareness, 84, 91, 92
Interpretation. *See* Assessment
Interviewing patients and collateral sources, 112–115, 114t, 116t
Intraparietal sulcus, 31–32, 79
Intrinsic resources, 153–154
IQ. *See* Intelligence

Job categories, 106–107t

Kleptomania, 200

Language, standardized tests and, 123t
Laziness, 75–77. *See also* Motivation
Legal/criminal records. *See* Records review
Letter fluency, 181-182. *See also* Delis-Kaplan Executive Function System (D-KEFS).
Leukoaraiosis, 179
Leukomalacia, 173
Levels of analysis, 8–9
Lewy bodies, 184
Lewy bodies, dementia with, 182–183, 216t
Lezak, Muriel, 2
Linguistic mode of emotional communication, 84–86, 85t, 88t, 94
Long-term goals, 3
Luria, Alexander, 2

Magnetic apraxia, 117
Maintenance, 71, 73t, 78t, 79. *See also* Initiation and maintenance
Major depressive disorder, 195
Manic/bipolar disorder, 66
Mattis Dementia Rating Scale, 181, 185

Medial prefrontal cortex, 32, 64–65, 77, 79, 95, 193, 198
Medial temporal lobe, 31–32, 192
Medical/psychiatric records. *See* Records review
Memantine, 180
Memory. *See* Goal-directed retrieval; Prospective memory; Working memory; Episodic memory
Mental age, 171
Mental flexibility, 16, 17–20, 19f, 21–22t, 32
Mental organization, 15
Mesencephalic infarctions, 80
Mesolimbic dopaminergic system, 79
Meta-monitoring, 38, 42, 43t, 47t
Meta-tasking (MT)
 addressing gaps in typical batteries used for assessment of, 143t
 autism spectrum disorders and, 168, 169
 cerebral vascular accidents and, 205
 defining, 37–42, 38f
 depressive disorders and, 196
 disorganized syndrome and, 44–48
 etiology of impairments in, 49
 executive cognitive functions vs., 37
 job-related duties and capacities and, 108t
 mental flexibility and, 19
 needed for test performance, 125t
 neuroanatomy of, 48–49
 other relevant constructs, 42–44
 overview of, 50
 overview of deficits in patient populations, 215–219t
 schizophrenia spectrum disorders and, 193
 traumatic brain injury and, 204
Midbrain, 79
Mild cognitive impairment (MCI), 49, 180, 196
Mirror neuron system, 93, 94, 95
Modified Six Elements Test, 143t
Motivation, 74
Motor perseveration, 20, 23, 27

Motor planning/programming. *See* Initiation
MS. *See* Multiple sclerosis
MSA. *See* Multiple-system atrophy
MT. *See* Meta-tasking
Multifaceted vs. unitary conceptualization of executive functions, 5–7
Multiple sclerosis (MS), 33, 187–188, 217t
Multiple-system atrophy (MSA), 185–186, 217t
Multitasking in the City Test, 46

NEO Personality Inventory, 25, 46
Nervous system infections, 209–210, 217t
Networks, 18, 30. *See also Specific networks*
Neuroanatomy
 of attention-deficit hyperactivity disorder, 166
 emotional suppression and, 148, 150
 of executive cognitive functions, 30–33
 of initiation and maintenance, 77–79
 of meta-tasking, 48–49
 overview of, 80
 of response selection, 62–65
 of schizophrenia spectrum disorders, 192–193
 of social cognition, 92–95
Neurodegenerative disorders. *See also* Dementias
 executive cognitive functions and, 33–34
 initiation and maintenance and, 79–80
 meta-tasking and, 49
 multiple sclerosis and, 33, 187–188, 217t
 overview of, 187–188, 215–219t
 response selection and, 66
 social cognition and, 95–98

Neurodevelopmental disorders. *See also* Attention-deficit hyperactivity disorder
  autism spectrum disorders, 49, 96, 167–169, 215t
  chronic tic disorders, 170, 216t
  congenital injuries, 172–174, 215–219t
  executive cognitive functions and, 33–34
  initiation and maintenance and, 79–80
  intellectual disability, 170–172, 217t
  meta-tasking and, 49
  overview of, 165, 176
  overview of deficits associated with, 215–219t
  preterm birth, 174–175, 218t
  response selection and, 66
  social cognition and, 95–98
  spina bifida and hydrocephalus, 175–176, 219t
Neuropsychiatric disorders. *See also* Schizophrenia spectrum disorders
  anxiety, 34, 197–198, 215t
  bipolar disorder, 153, 194–195, 216t
  depression, 34, 81, 188, 195–197, 216t
  disruptive, impulse, and conduct disorders, 200–201, 216t
  executive cognitive functions and, 33–34
  initiation and maintenance and, 79–80
  meta-tasking and, 49
  obsessive-compulsive disorders, 170, 198–199, 218t
  overview of deficits associated with, 215–219t
  personality disorders, 201–202
  response selection and, 66
  social cognition and, 95–98
  trauma- and stressor-related, 199–200, 218t
Neuropsychological Assessment (Lezak et al.), 2, 140

Neuroticism, 152
Nonexecutive tests, 141, 142t

Obsessive-compulsive disorders (OCD), 170, 198–199, 218t
ODD. *See* Oppositional defiant disorder
Olivopontocerebellar atrophy, 185–186
Openness to experience, 25–27, 152, 160
Operculum, 79, 92–93
Oppositional defiant disorder (ODD), 200–201
Orbitofrontal cortex, 62–63, 93–95, 98, 183
Organization, 22t, 26t
Oxygen deprivation, 33, 80, 206–209, 215t. *See also* Anoxia

Pain, impacts of, 150
Paragraph-level speech structure, 25
Paralinguistic mode of emotional communication, 84, 85t, 88t, 91, 93–94
Parietal cortex, 31–33, 49, 79, 95, 192, 203, 205
Parkinson's disease and related disorders, 49, 71, 79, 80–81, 183–186, 218t
Passive release, 52
Pathognomonic signs, 115–118
Perseveration, 20, 23, 27
Persistence, 71, 73t, 78t, 79. *See also* Initiation and maintenance
Persistent depressive disorder, 195
Personality, 25–27, 151–152
Personality disorders, 66, 98, 201–202
PFC. *See* Prefrontal cortex
Phonemic fluency. *See* Letter fluency
Planning, 15, 22t, 26t
pnfaFTD. *See* Progressive nonfluent aphasia frontotemporal lobar degeneration
Pons, 93
Posterior cingulate cortex, 93
Post-traumatic stress disorder (PTSD), 199–200, 218t

Prader-Willi syndrome, 171
Precuneus, 49
Prefrontal cortex (PFC), 32, 48, 77, 79, 93. *See also* Inferior frontal gyrus, Superior frontal gyrus, Frontopolar cortex.
Premenstrual dysphoric disorder, 195
Premorbid level of executive functions, 104–108, 112–113, 114t, 150–152
Pre-supplementary motor area (pre-SMA), 32
Preterm birth, 174–175, 218t
Pribram, Karl, 2
Problem-solving, 15, 21t, 26t
Processing speed, 53, 77, 147
Progressive nonfluent aphasia frontotemporal lobar degeneration (pnfaFTD), 177–178
Progressive supranuclear palsy (PSP), 185, 218t
Prospective memory, 40. *See also* Event-based prospective memory; Time-based prospective memory
PSP. *See* Progressive supranuclear palsy
Psychiatric records. *See* Records review
Psychomotor sensitization, 72. *See also* Effort mobilization
PTSD. *See* Post-traumatic stress disorder
Putamen, 79
Pyromania, 200

Radiation therapy, 211–212, 218t
Raven's Matrices, 141
Reasoning, 15, 21t, 26t
Records review, 103–112, 104–105t, 106–107t, 108t, 110t
Referral
  assessment and, 146–150
  daily functioning, prediction of lapses and, 153–156
  diagnostic decision-making and, 150–152
  overview of, 156–162
Refresh cycles, 71
Reinterpretation/reframing, 23–24

Reliability, standardized tests and, 124–130, 131t, 132–136t
Respiratory rate, 92
Response selection (RS)
  antisocial behavior, criminality, aggression and, 201
  attention-deficit hyperactivity disorder and, 166
  cerebral vascular accidents and, 205
  defining, 51–56, 57t
  disinhibited syndrome and, 58–62
  etiology of impairments in, 66
  executive functioning, executive cognitive functions vs., 51
  intellectual disability and, 172
  job-related duties and capacities and, 108t
  needed for test performance, 126t
  neuroanatomy of, 62–65
  obsessive-compulsive disorders and, 199
  other relevant constructs, 56–58
  overview of, 67
  overview of deficits in patient populations, 215–219t
  oxygen deprivation and, 208
  personality disorders and, 202
  schizophrenia spectrum disorders and, 194
  social phobia and, 197–198
  substance-related and addictive disorders and, 213
  traumatic brain injury and, 204
Reward processing, 72
Rey-O Complex Figure test, 140, 141
Right cerebral hemisphere, 25, 30, 64, 75, 79–80, 93–94, 175, 206, 219t
Rostral prefrontal cortex, 48
RS. *See* Response selection
Rule-breaking, 45, 46, 48

Salience network, 64
Sarcasm and humor, 87–89
SC. *See* Social cognition
Schizoaffective disorder, 192

Schizoid personality disorder (SPD), 201–202
Schizophrenia spectrum disorders
  assessment and, 153
  disorganized syndrome and, 49
  dysexecutive syndrome and, 34
  overview of, 191–194, 219t
  schizoid personality disorder, 201–202
  social awareness and, 97
School records. *See* Records review
sdFTD. *See* Semantic dementia frontemporal lobar degeneration
Self-awareness, 84, 90–91, 92–93
Semantic dementia frontemporal lobar degeneration (sdFTD), 177–178
Semantic fluency, 182. *See also* Delis-Kaplan Executive Function System (D-KEFS).
Severity, 109–112, 115
Sexuality, 178
Shifting, 18–19. *See also* Mental flexibility
Shy-Drager syndrome, 185–186
Situational mode of emotional communication, 84–86, 85t, 88t, 94–95
SIVD. *See* Subcortical ischemic vascular dementia
Six Elements Test, 46
Skin temperature/perspiration, 92
Sleep, lack of, 147, 208–209
Sleep apnea, 207, 208–209, 218t
Sluggish cognitive tempo, 74
Social anxiety disorder, 196
Social awareness, 85t, 86, 94–95. *See also* Situational mode of emotional communication
Social cognition (SC)
  addressing gaps in typical batteries used for assessment of, 143t
  amyotrophic lateral sclerosis and, 187
  antisocial behavior, criminality, aggression and, 201
  autism spectrum disorders and, 168
  defining, 83–87

depressive disorders and, 196
etiology of impairments in, 95–98
job-related duties and capacities and, 108t
multiple sclerosis and, 188
needed for test performance, 126t
neuroanatomy of, 92–95
neuropsychiatric disorders and, 191
other relevant constructs, 87–90
overview of, 98–99
overview of deficits of in patient populations, 215–219t
Parkinson's disease and related disorders and, 184
schizophrenia spectrum disorders and, 192, 194
socially inappropriate syndrome and, 90–92
substance-related and addictive disorders and, 213
traumatic brain injury and, 204
Social Cognition subtests of WAIS-IV Advanced Clinical Solutions, 92
Socially inappropriate syndrome. *See* Inappropriate syndrome
Social norms, 83, 86
Social phobia, 196–197
Somatic marker hypothesis, 63–64, 65
Somatosensory cortex, 95
SPD. *See* Schizoid personality disorder
Speech patterns, 25
Spina bifida, 175–176, 219t
Standardized tests. *See also* *Specific tests*
  hierarchical structure of cognition and, 121–124, 123t
  overview of, 142–143t
  reliability and, 124–130, 131t, 132–136t
  selection of, 140–144, 142–143t
  validity and, 137–140
Startle response, 53
State, trait vs., 146–150
Stimulus response, 3–4
Strategy application disorder, 45
Stressor-related disorders, 199–200
Striatonigral degeneration, 185–186

Stroop tests. *See also* Color-word interference, Delis-Kaplan Executive Function System
  component processes needed for, 123–124t
  disorganized syndrome and, 47t
  dysexecutive syndrome and, 29t
  elemental processes needed for, 125t
  hierarchical structure of cognition and, 121, 122, 124
  initiation and maintenance and, 78t
  reliability and, 127
  response selection and, 59, 61t
Structure, function vs., 4–5
Subcortical ischemic vascular dementia (SIVD), 179–181, 219t
Substance abuse disorders, 97, 212–213, 219t
Substantia nigra, 30, 183
Superior frontal gyrus, 79
Superior longitudinal fasciculus, 31
Superior parietal lobule, 31–32
Supertasking, 44
Supplementary motor area, 77, 79
Suppression. *See* Expressive suppression
Switching condition. *See* Trail-making test
Symbol Search test, 141
Sympathetic activation, 53, 72
Synthetic ability, 1

TASIT. *See* Awareness of Social Inference test
Task complexity, 154–155
Task-rule maintenance, 74–75
Task-switching, 19, 42–43
TBI. *See* Traumatic brain injury
Temperament, 155–156
Temporoparietal cortex, 48–49, 79, 95
Thalamic infarctions, 80
Thalamus, 30, 33, 79, 93, 192, 207
Theory of mind (ToM) networks, 89, 94, 95, 179

Thoughtfully-reflective decision-making (TRDM), 23, 51–52
Threat sensitivity, 52–53, 57t, 61t, 62, 143t
Time-based prospective memory, 38, 40–42, 43t, 47t
Time course, 108–109, 113–1115
Time estimation, 40–42
Token Test, 141
ToM. *See* Theory of mind networks
Tower tests
  component processes needed for, 123–124t
  disorganized syndrome and, 47t
  dysexecutive syndrome and, 29t
  elemental processes needed for, 125t
  initiation and maintenance and, 78t
  response selection and, 61t
Trail-making test. *See also* Delis-Kaplan Executive Function System (D-KEFS)
  component processes needed for, 123–124t
  disorganized syndrome and, 47t
  dysexecutive syndrome and, 29t
  elemental processes needed for, 125t
  hierarchical structure of cognition and, 121
  initiation and maintenance and, 78t
  reliability and, 127, 129
  response selection and, 61t
  test selection and, 140
Trait, state vs., 146–150
Trauma-related disorders, 199–200
Traumatic brain injury (TBI)
  assessment and, 153
  dysexecutive syndrome and, 33
  initiation and maintenance and, 80
  overview of, 203–205, 219t
  response selection and, 66
  social cognition and, 96
TRDM. *See* Thoughtfully-reflective decision-making
Trichotillomania, 198
Turner syndrome, 96
Types of difficulties, 109–112, 115

Uncinated fasciculus, 31
Unitary vs. multifaceted conceptualization of executive functions, 5–7
Urbach-Wiethe disease, 98

Valence hypothesis, 63
Validity, standardized tests and, 137–140
Vascular dementia, 33–34, 180. *See also* Subcortical ischemic vascular dementia
Ventral frontal cortex, 62–63
Ventral striatum, 79
Ventromedial prefrontal cortex, 63–64, 79
Verbal fluency. *See also* Letter fluency, Semantic fluency
   component processes needed for, 123–124t
   disorganized syndrome and, 47t
   dysexecutive syndrome and, 29t
   elemental processes needed for, 125t
   initiation and maintenance and, 77, 78t
   reliability and, 127
   response selection and, 61t
   standardized tests and, 122
   test selection and, 140
Vigilance, 53, 75, 206, 208
Vigilant attention, 71. *See also* Maintenance
Visual perception, 123t
von Economo neurons, 64, 66, 94, 96–97, 178

WAIS-IV Advanced Clinical Solutions Social Cognition Battery, 143t
WAIS-IV Comprehension test, 141
WAIS-IV Matrices, 141
WAIS-IV Similarities test, 141
WAIS subtests, 141
Walking pace, 181
Wanting, 72. *See also* Effort mobilization
Watershed areas, 33, 207
WCST. *See* Wisconsin Card Sorting Test
Will and temperament, 1
Williams syndrome, 171
Wisconsin Card Sorting Test (WCST)
   component processes needed for, 123–124t
   disorganized syndrome and, 46, 47t
   dysexecutive syndrome and, 18, 23, 28, 29t
   elemental processes needed for, 125t
   initiation and maintenance and, 78t
   reliability and, 127
   response selection and, 60, 61t
Working memory, 6–7, 16–17, 20, 21–22t, 23–24, 28, 29t, 30–34, 44, 47t, 48, 65, 75, 89, 122, 125t, 142–143t, 148, 155, 166, 170–172, 175, 181, 183–184, 186–188, 193, 201, 212
Work records. *See* Records review

Yerkes-Dodson law, 152, 198

Zoo Map Test, 46, 143t